Life-Threatening Infections: Part 2

Editor

ANAND KUMAR

CRITICAL CARE CLINICS

www.criticalcare.theclinics.com

Consulting Editor
RICHARD W. CARLSON

October 2013 • Volume 29 • Number 4

ELSEVIER

1600 John F. Kennedy Boulevard • Suite 1800 • Philadelphia, Pennsylvania, 19103-2899

http://www.theclinics.com

CRITICAL CARE CLINICS Volume 29, Number 4
October 2013 ISSN 0749-0704, ISBN-13: 978-0-323-22714-8

Editor: Patrick Manley
Developmental Editor: Donald Mumford

Critical Care Clinics (ISSN: 0749-0704) is published quarterly by Elsevier Inc., 360 Park Avenue South, New York, NY 10010-1710. Months of issue are January, April, July, and October. Business and Editorial Offices: 1600 John F. Kennedy Blvd., Suite 1800, Philadelphia, PA 19103-2899. Customer Service Office: 6277 Sea Harbor Drive, Orlando, FL 32887-4800. Periodicals postage paid at New York, NY and additional mailing offices. Subscription prices are $199.00 per year for US individuals, $482.00 per year for US institution, $97.00 per year for US students and residents, $245.00 per year for Canadian individuals, $597.00 per year for Canadian institutions, $287.00 per year for international individuals, $597.00 per year for international institutions and $141.00 per year for Canadian and foreign students/residents. To receive student/resident rate, orders must be accompanied by name of affiliated institution, date of term, and the signature of program/residency coordinator on institution letterhead. Orders will be billed at individual rate until proof of status is received. Foreign air speed delivery is included in all Clinics subscription prices. All prices are subject to change without notice. POSTMASTER: Send address changes to Critical Care Clinics, Elsevier Periodicals Customer Service, 11830 Westline Industrial Drive, St. Louis, MO 63146. **Customer Service: 1-800-654-2452 (US). From outside of the US, call 1-314-447-8871. Fax: 1-314-447-8029. E-mail: journalscustomerservice-usa@elsevier.com (for print support) or journalsonlinesupport-usa@elsevier.com (for online support).**

Reprints. For copies of 100 or more of articles in this publication, please contact the Commercial Reprints Department, Elsevier Inc., 360 Park Avenue South, New York, NY 10010-1710. Tel.: 212-633-3874; Fax: 212-633-3820; E-mail: reprints@elsevier.com.

Critical Care Clinics is also published in Spanish by Editorial Inter-Medica, Junin 917, 1er A, 1113, Buenos Aires, Argentina.

Critical Care Clinics is covered in MEDLINE/PubMed (Index Medicus), EMBASE/Excerpta Medica, Current Concepts/Clinical Medicine, ISI/BIOMED, and Chemical Abstracts.

Printed in the United States of America.

Contributors

CONSULTING EDITOR

RICHARD W. CARLSON, MD, PhD
Chairman Emeritus, Director, Medical Intensive Care Unit, Department of Medicine, Maricopa Medical Center; Professor, University of Arizona College of Medicine; Professor, Department of Medicine, Mayo Graduate School of Medicine, Phoenix, Arizona

EDITOR

ANAND KUMAR, MD, FRCPC
Section of Critical Care, Department of Medicine, University of Manitoba, Winnipeg, Manitoba, Canada

AUTHORS

HASAN M. AL-DORZI, MD
Section Head, Adult ICU and Consultant, Intensive Care Department; Assistant Professor, College of Medicine, King Saud bin Abdulaziz University for Health Sciences, Riyadh, Saudi Arabia

DANIEL A. ANAYA, MD, FACS
Operative Care Line, Michael E. DeBakey Veterans Affairs Medical Center; Houston Veterans Affairs Health Services Research and Development Center of Excellence; Associate Professor of Medicine, Michael E. DeBakey Department of Surgery, Baylor College of Medicine, Houston, Texas

YASEEN M. ARABI, MD, FCCP, FCCM
Medical Director, Respiratory Services; Chairman, Intensive Care Department; Associate Professor, College of Medicine, King Saud bin Abdulaziz University for Health Sciences, Riyadh, Saudi Arabia

RAKESH C. ARORA, MD, PhD
Manitoba Cardiac Sciences Program; Department of Surgery, Anesthesia, and Physiology, University of Manitoba, Manitoba, Canada

THOMAS P. BLECK, MD, FCCM
Professor of Neurological Sciences, Neurosurgery, Internal Medicine, and Anesthesiology, Rush Medical College; Associate Chief Medical Officer (Critical Care), Rush University Medical Center, Chicago, Illinois

MATTHEW P. CHENG, MD
Physician, Department of Medicine, University of British Columbia, Vancouver, Canada

GLORIA OBLOUK DAROVIC, RN
Section of Critical Care Medicine, University of Manitoba, Winnipeg, Manitoba, Canada

CHARLES DE MESTRAL, MD, PhD
Division of General Surgery, Sunnybrook Health Sciences Center, Sunnybrook Research Institute, University of Toronto, Toronto, Ontario, Canada

STEPHEN R. EATON, MD
Section of Acute and Critical Care Surgery, Department of Surgery, Washington University School of Medicine, St Louis, Missouri

HENRY FRAIMOW, MD
Associate Professor of Medicine, Department of Medicine, Cooper Medical School of Rowan University; Hospital Epidemiologist, Cooper University Hospital, Camden, New Jersey

ATUL HUMAR, MD, MSc, FRCPC
Transplant Infectious Diseases, Alberta Transplant Institute, University of Alberta, Edmonton, Alberta, Canada

QAALI A. HUSSEIN, MD
Surgical Resident, Michael E. DeBakey Department of Surgery, Baylor College of Medicine, Houston, Texas

SHRAVAN KETHIREDDY, MD
Department of Critical Care and Infectious Diseases, Geisinger Health System, Danville, Pennsylvania

YOAV KEYNAN, MD
Assistant Professor, Section of Infectious Diseases, Department of Internal Medicine, Medical Microbiology, and Community Health Sciences, University of Manitoba, Winnipeg, Manitoba, Canada

RAYMOND KHAN, MD
Consultant, Intensive Care Department; Assistant Professor, College of Medicine, King Saud bin Abdulaziz University for Health Sciences, Riyadh, Saudi Arabia

ANAND KUMAR, MD, FRCPC
Section of Critical Care, Department of Medicine, University of Manitoba, Winnipeg, Manitoba, Canada

KANWAL KUMAR, MD
Department of Surgery, University of Manitoba, Manitoba, Canada

MICHEL LAVERDIERE, MD, FRCP(c)
Department of Medicine, Hopital Maisonneuve Rosemont; Professor of Microbiology and Infectious Diseases, Université de Montréal, Montréal, Québec, Canada

NELSON LEE, MD, FRCP (Lond. Edin.)
Professor, Division of Infectious Diseases, Department of Medicine and Therapeutics, Faculty of Medicine, Prince of Wales Hospital, The Chinese University of Hong Kong, Shatin, New Territories, Hong Kong, China

JOHN E. MAZUSKI, MD, PhD
Section of Acute and Critical Care Surgery, Department of Surgery, Washington University School of Medicine, St Louis, Missouri

ALLISON MCGEER, MD, FRCPC
Microbiologist and Infectious Disease Consultant; Director, Infectious Diseases Epidemiology Research Unit; Principal Investigator, Toronto Invasive Bacterial Diseases Network; Director of Infection Control, Mount Sinai Hospital, Toronto, Ontario, Canada

RAQUEL NAHRA, MD
Associate Professor of Medicine, Department of Medicine, Cooper Medical School of Rowan University, Camden, New Jersey

AVERY B. NATHENS, MD, PhD, MPH
Division of General Surgery and Critical Care, Sunnybrook Health Sciences Center, Sunnybrook Research Institute, University of Toronto; Li Ka Shing Knowledge Institute, St. Michael's Hospital, University of Toronto, Toronto, Ontario, Canada

DAIRE T. O'SHEA, MB BCh, MSc, MRCPI
Transplant Infectious Diseases, Alberta Transplant Institute, University of Alberta, Edmonton, Alberta, Canada

SALMAN T. QURESHI, MD, FRCPC
Associate Professor, Department of Medicine, McGill University; Division of Respirology, Department of Critical Care Medicine, McGill University Health Centre, Montréal, Québec, Canada

CLARE D. RAMSEY, MD, MSc, FRCPC
Sections of Respiratory Medicine and Critical Care, Department of Medicine; Department of Community Health Sciences, University of Manitoba, Winnipeg, Manitoba, Canada

JOAO B. REZENDE-NETO, MD
Associate Professor of Surgery, University of Toronto; Department of Surgery, St. Michael's Hospital, Toronto, Ontario, Canada

ORI D. ROTSTEIN, MD
Professor of Surgery, University of Toronto; Department of Surgery, St. Michael's Hospital, Toronto, Ontario, Canada

ETHAN RUBINSTEIN, MD
Professor, Section of Infectious Diseases, Department of Internal Medicine and Medical Microbiology, University of Manitoba, Winnipeg, Manitoba, Canada

ROHIT SINGAL, MD
Manitoba Cardiac Sciences Program; Department of Surgery, University of Manitoba, Manitoba, Canada

YOANNA SKROBIK, MD, FRCP(c)
Chair, Lise and Jean Saine Chair in Critical Care; Professor of Medicine, Université de Montréal; Respiratory Critical Care Group, Respiratory Health Network of the FRQS, Montréal, Québec, Canada

CEDRIC P. YANSOUNI, MD, FRCPC
Assistant Professor, Division of Infectious Diseases, Department of Medical Microbiology, J.D. MacLean Centre for Tropical Diseases, McGill University Health Centre, Montreal, Canada

Contents

eradicate. VRE are difficult to treat; therefore, infection control measures in hospitals are of prime importance in preventing the establishment of these pathogens. Most severe VRE infections will need combination therapy because many of the effective antimicrobial agents, when used alone, have only a bacteriostatic effect.

Infective endocarditis has many facets and various expressions depending on the site of infection, microorganism, underlying heart lesion, immune status of the host, and remote effects such as emboli, organ dysfunction, and the condition of the host. Diagnosis depends on meticulous clinical examination, blood cultures results, and echocardiographic findings. The management of the patient with endocarditis in the intensive care unit is complex and needs a multidisciplinary team, including an intensivist, cardiologist, experienced echocardiologist, infectious diseases specialist, and cardiac surgeon. The medical and surgical management of such patients is complex, and timely decisions are important.

Modern post-transplant care pathways commonly encompass periods of critical care support. Infectious events account for many of these interactions making critical care physicians integral members of multidisciplinary transplant teams. Despite continuing advances in clinical care and infection prophylaxis, the morbidity and mortality attributable to infection post-transplant remains considerable. Emerging entities constantly add to the breadth of potential opportunistic pathogens. Individualized risk assessments, rapid and thorough diagnostic evaluation, and prompt initiation of appropriate antimicrobial therapies are essential. The approach to managing transplant recipients with infection in critical care is discussed and common and emerging opportunistic pathogens are reviewed.

Bacteria and fungi, owing to their intrinsic properties and the host responses they produce, result in relatively specific clinical syndromes when they infect the central nervous system. The infecting organism may produce symptoms and signs by interfering with the function of the nervous system tissue being invaded or compressed. The definitive treatment of central nervous system infection depends on correct identification and antimicrobial treatment of the infecting organism, relief of excessive pressure or mass effect that it exerts, and modulation of the host's immune response to allow clearance of the organism while minimizing excessive inflammation.

This article focuses on the pathogenesis, diagnosis, prevention, and management of infectious complications of intravascular cannulation and fluid infusion. Although continuous vascular access is one of the most essential modalities in modern-day medicine, there is a substantial and underappreciated potential for producing iatrogenic complications, the most important

CRITICAL CARE CLINICS

In Memoriam

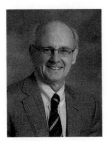

Donald E. Low—Colleague, Mentor, Friend

It is with great sadness that we remember here Dr Donald Low, a legend in Canadian microbiology practice, research, teaching, administration, and advocacy, who died shortly after submitting his article on "Toxic Shock Syndrome," published in the July issue of *Critical Care Clinics*. Dr Low was an infectious diseases physician and clinical microbiologist who was for many years a professor of laboratory medicine and pathobiology at the University of Toronto and the director of clinical microbiology at the Mount Sinai Hospital/University Health Network. He was also the director of the Ontario Public Health Laboratory from 2005 to 2012.

In the changing world of clinical microbiology, Don was a visionary. His laboratory was a leader in innovation, and in his research he described novel human pathogens, new mechanisms of antibiotic resistance, and new approaches to clinical diagnosis. He had an infectious passion for discovery, for excellence in everything, and for translating new discovery into benefit for patients. He also had a talent for translating science to policy-makers and to the general public, which led to an important role in the management of the SARS outbreak in Toronto in 2003. He was a frequent presence and voice for science and medical education in the media.

Without a doubt, however, his most important scientific legacy will be the generation of Canadian microbiologists and infectious disease physicians—and the many other clinicians, researchers, and policy-makers around the world—whom he mentored and inspired. He is greatly missed.

Allison McGeer, MD, FRCPC
Infectious Diseases Epidemiology Research Unit
Toronto Invasive Bacterial Diseases Network
Mount Sinai Hospital
600 University Avenue, Room 210
Toronto, Ontario M5G 1X5, Canada

Crit Care Clin 29 (2013) xiii–xiv
http://dx.doi.org/10.1016/j.ccc.2013.09.001
0749-0704/13/$ – see front matter © 2013 Published by Elsevier Inc.

criticalcare.theclinics.com

Anand Kumar, MD, FRCPC
Section of Critical Care
Department of Medicine
University of Manitoba
Winnipeg, Manitoba R3A 1R9, Canada

E-mail addresses:
amcgeer@mtsinai.on.ca (A. McGeer)
akumar61@yahoo.com (A. Kumar)

Necrotizing Soft Tissue Infections

Qaali A. Hussein, MD[a], Daniel A. Anaya, MD[a,b,c],*

KEYWORDS

- Necrotizing soft tissue infections • NSTI • Necrotizing fasciitis • Gangrene
- Clostridial infection • Group A streptococcal infection

KEY POINTS

- A standardized nomenclature for necrotizing soft tissue infection will improve early diagnosis and treatment.
- Early diagnosis and treatment is key in managing necrotizing soft tissue infections.
- Repeated surgical debridement until adequate source control is the primary means of treating necrotizing soft tissue infections.
- Adjunct treatment for necrotizing soft tissue infections include close monitoring of patients for other system organ failure.
- Long-term support and rehabilitation is essential for optimal recovery.

BACKGROUND

Hippocrates gave the first description of necrotizing soft tissue infection (NSTI) circa 500 BC when he wrote, "Many were attacked by the erysipelas all over the body when the exciting cause was a trivial accident flesh, sinews, and bones fell away in large quantities there were many deaths."[1] Joseph Jones, a Confederate Army surgeon, described NSTI in further detail in 1871 when he reported 2642 cases of "hospital gangrene" with a mortality rate of 46%.[2,3] Despite many advances in understanding the pathophysiology of this disease process and improvements in medical care, the mortality associated with NSTI remains high at 25% to 35%, and is directly

Funding Source: This material is the result of work supported with resources and the use of facilities at the Houston VA Health Services Research and Development Center of Excellence at the Michael E. DeBakey Veterans Affairs Medical Center (HFP90-020). None of the funding agencies played a role in the design and conduct of the study, analysis and interpretation of the data, or preparation and approval of the article. The views expressed are those of the authors and do not necessarily reflect those of the Department of Veterans Affairs, the US government, or Baylor College of Medicine.
Conflict of Interest: The authors have no financial conflict of interest to disclose.
[a] Michael E. DeBakey Department of Surgery, Baylor College of Medicine, One Baylor Plaza (BCM390), Houston, TX 77030, USA; [b] Operative Care Line, Michael E. DeBakey Veterans Affairs Medical Center, 2002 Holcombe Boulevard (OCL 112), Houston, TX 77030, USA; [c] Michael E. DeBakey Veterans Affairs Medical Center, Houston Veterans Affairs Health Services Research and Development Center of Excellence, Houston, TX, USA
* Corresponding author. 2002 Holcombe Boulevard (OCL 112), Houston, TX 77030.
E-mail address: danaya@bcm.edu

Crit Care Clin 29 (2013) 795–806
http://dx.doi.org/10.1016/j.ccc.2013.06.001
0749-0704/13/$ – see front matter Published by Elsevier Inc.

impacted by delays in time to intervention.[1,4] Lack of physician familiarity with NSTIs because of its low prevalence contributes to this high mortality and delay to diagnosis and intervention. Another contributing factor is the various terms used to describe this disease process: *necrotizing fasciitis*, *myonecrosis*, *gangrene*, *clostridial infection*, and *streptococcal infection*. The term *necrotizing fasciitis* was proposed by Wilson in 1951, who stated that the fascial necrosis is the sine qua non of this disease process.[5] Currently, the term *necrotizing soft tissue infection* is advocated to encompass all forms of the disease process, because necrotizing infection involving any level of the soft tissues requires a similar approach to diagnosis and treatment regardless of anatomic location or depth of infection.[6] This article provides a review of NSTIs and the current recommendations for diagnosis and treatment, and emphasizes the need for long-term support and rehabilitation for optimal recovery.

EPIDEMIOLOGY

The incidence of NSTI is approximately 500 to 1500 cases per year in United States.[6] A recent study using insurance databases from various states in the United States determined the incidence of NSTI to be approximately 0.04 cases per 1000 person-years.[7] Intravenous drug use and diabetes mellitus have been identified as the conditions more commonly associated with the development of NSTI.[8] Although no epidemiologic association between any specific factor and NSTI incidence seems to be applicable to all populations, specific populations with a high proportion of intravenous drug use have been found to present with outbreaks of NSTI. A recent report noted that approximately 1% of patients (30/3560) who presented to San Francisco General Hospital and required incision and drainage for injection-related cutaneous abscesses needed wide debridement for NSTI.[9] It has also been documented that, although NSTIs are uncommon, they seem, at least in certain geographic areas with a high incidence of intravenous drug use, to have increased during the past decade.[9,10] A retrospective survey of risk factors for NSTI in an urban community serving an indigent population found that diabetes mellitus (44%), obesity (33%), alcohol abuse (31%), and malnutrition (serum albumin <30.0 g/L, 31%) were other major preexisting risk factors.[11]

DIAGNOSIS

One challenge in managing NSTI remains establishing early diagnosis. Because of nonspecific findings on physical examination and variable time course to fulminant disease, one must have a high index of suspicion whenever evaluating a patient with soft tissue infection in order to pursue early intervention. Although true risk factors for NSTI have not been identified, some conditions have been found to be commonly associated and are important to consider when evaluating patients, including injection drug use and comorbid conditions, such as diabetes mellitus, immune suppression, and obesity.[6]

The clinical presentation of NSTI can vary from minimal skin changes to frank necrosis. The initial signs and symptoms may include cellulitis (80%), skin discoloration or gangrene (70%), and anesthesia of involved skin (frequent but unknown incidence).[12] These symptoms may progress fairly quickly to the more typical signs of tense edema, ecchymosis, blisters/bullae, crepitus, and necrosis.[1] Systemic findings include fever, tachycardia, hypotension, and shock. Although these findings are typical of NSTI, their sensitivity remains low. A retrospective single-center review showed that 35% of cases were initially misdiagnosed as simple cellulitis or severe, nonnecrotizing skin infection.[13] The only signs that were present in greater than 50% of patients were erythema, tenderness, or edema beyond the confines of clinically apparent infection.[14,15] This finding is contrary to the standard teaching that shock, fever, and mental status changes are frequent findings.[1]

Specific Clinical Clues

Because of the difficulty of differentiating NSTIs from non-NSTIs and the morbidity associated with delayed diagnosis of NSTI, certain clinical findings can help increase the suspicion for NSTI and prompt surgical debridement before further laboratory testing (**Table 1**). These hard signs of NSTI, which include hemodynamic instability, crepitance, bullae, and skin necrosis, although helpful are often late findings of NSTI, and are present only in a small percentage of patients.[9] However, presence of these signs should trigger expeditious emergent surgical debridement.[8] Soft signs such as pain disproportionate to examination and tense edema may be present in other infections, such as cellulitis, and require further assessment with laboratory testing.

The need for more accurate and expeditious diagnosis of NSTI has prompted the search for a variety of diagnostic tools. The diagnosis may not be completely accurate even in the most experienced hands, and both clinical clues and diagnostic tools should be used in combination to help make an early diagnosis.[16] High suspicion for NSTI should prompt early surgical evaluation. When the diagnosis of NSTI is confirmed, surgical debridement is indicated. When suspicion remains high but laboratory and imaging studies have remained inconclusive, some researchers have recommended surgery as a means to evaluate for macroscopic findings consistent with NSTI.[6]

Laboratory Findings

To help differentiate between necrotizing and nonnecrotizing infections, different studies have examined the role of laboratory parameters at initial evaluation/admission. When comparing 359 patients with necrotizing and nonnecrotizing soft tissue infections, Wall and colleagues[17] found that having a white blood cell (WBC) count greater than 15,400 cells/mm^3 or a serum sodium level less than 135 mmol/L was associated with NSTI, and that a combination of these increased the likelihood of NSTI significantly. This method proved to be a very sensitive tool, with a negative predictive value (NPV) of 99%, but not very specific, with a positive predictive value (PPV) of only 26%. In conclusion, this method is a good tool to rule out NSTI, but is less helpful for confirming diagnosis.

Wong and colleagues[18] expanded on this concept and in a similar study compared a set of laboratory variables between patients with and without NSTI. They found 6 independent variables to be associated with NSTI, and used these to develop a diagnostic tool/score (Laboratory Risk Indicator for Necrotizing Fasciitis [LRINEC] score) (**Table 2**). The total score ranged from 0 to 13 points, and helped stratify patients into low-, intermediate-, and high-risk groups (**Table 3**). Wong and colleagues[18]

Table 1	
Clinical signs of NSTI	
Hard Signs	**Soft Signs**
Hemodynamic instability	Tense edema
Crepitance	Pain disproportionate to examination
Skin necrosis	Ecchymosis
Bullae	
Gas on radiographic imaging	

Table 2
Laboratory risk indicator for necrotizing fasciitis

Value	LRINEC Points
WBC count (cells/mm^3)	
<15	0
15–25	1
>25	2
Hemoglobin (g/dL)	
>13.5	0
11.0–13.5	1
<11.0	2
Sodium (mmol/L)	
≥135	0
<135	2
Creatinine (mg/dL)	
≤1.6	0
>1.6	2
Glucose (mg/dL)	
≤180	0
>180	1
C-reactive protein (mg/L)	
<150	0
>150	4

Abbreviation: WBC, white blood cell.

internally validated this diagnostic tool, finding that a score greater than 6 (intermediate- and high-risk patients) had a PPV of 92% and an NPV of 96%. This score is an important tool for confirming and ruling out NSTI. Furthermore, since its initial publication in 2004, a variety of studies have examined the accuracy of the LRINEC score and validated it externally, proving its role in helping diagnose NSTI early during its course. However, some limitations of the score highlighted by these studies include the small sample size on which the score was devised (89 patients with NSTI and 225 control cases); overreliance on C-reactive protein level, which can be increased in any form of inflammatory process, not necessarily an infectious process; and the fact that some of these biochemical derangements can be seen in chronic disease, such as in patients with diabetes with renal insufficiency.[19]

Table 3
Risk stratification based on LRINEC score

Risk Category	LRINEC Score	Probability of NSTI (%)
Low	≤5	<50
Intermediate	6–7	50–75
High	≥8	>75

Adapted from Wong CH, Khin LW, Heng KS, et al. The LRINEC (Laboratory Risk Indicator for Necrotizing Fasciitis) score: a tool for distinguishing necrotizing fasciitis from other soft tissue infections. Crit Care Med 2004;32(7):1535–41; with permission.

In summary, this score is a valuable tool that adds data when suspecting NSTI, but additional information is often needed to confirm the diagnosis.

Imaging Studies

Plain radiography is often used as the first imaging study and can help identify subcutaneous gas, when present. However, this finding is often associated with late phases of NSTI and is not as common in earlier stages of the infection. Computed tomography (CT) has higher accuracy and the additional advantage of identifying other causes of infection, particularly deep abscesses. Studies comparing ultrasonography, CT, and magnetic resonance imaging (MRI) evaluation have shown that increased thickness of the fascial layer with or without enhancement can be associated with NSTI.[20,21] The primary limitation of these studies is that they tend to compare the involved site (usually a limb) with the contralateral or an uninvolved site, rather than comparing it with non-necrotizing infections imaging findings. Despite the high sensitivity of this additional workup, the main limitation of these imaging studies is their low specificity, which limit their use for confirming NSTI, particularly early during its course.[22]

Frozen Section Biopsy

To achieve an earlier diagnosis of NSTI, frozen section analysis of a biopsy specimen from the compromised site, including deep fascia and possibly muscle, has been recommended. Two studies evaluating this method have shown decreased mortality based on historical comparisons.[23,24] However, this finding may be related to the fact that an earlier diagnosis can be accomplished if clinicians are suspicious enough to perform the biopsy. Moreover, if enough suspicion exists to perform a biopsy, the diagnosis is usually evident at gross inspection without histologic slides.[12]

Operative Exploration to Confirm Diagnosis

Another option, preferred in the authors' practice, is to explore the compromised area during an operation, rather than examine a frozen biopsy specimen. Their experience has shown that frozen biopsy is not very practical, because it requires availability and experience from the pathologists. The authors are usually able to explore the site and identify macroscopic findings consistent with NSTI during an operation, and intervene without further delay. These findings include gray necrotic tissue, lack of bleeding, thrombosed vessels, "dishwater" pus, noncontracting muscle, and a positive "finger test" result, which is characterized by lack of resistance to finger dissection in normally adherent tissues (**Table 4**).[6] If no necrosis is seen on exploratory incision, the procedure can be terminated with very little risk or morbidity to the patient.[12] If NSTI is confirmed, however, catastrophic consequences can be minimized through extending the incision and performing additional debridement.[6]

Table 4 Microscopic and operative findings of NSTI	
Microscopic Findings	**Operative Findings**
Tissue necrosis	Gray necrotic tissue
Thrombosed vessels	"Dishwater" pus
Leukocyte infiltration	Lack of bleeding
Gram-positive rods[a]	Noncontracting muscle
	Positive "finger test"

[a] In the setting of clostridial infections.

ANTIMICROBIAL MANAGEMENT

In most cases, NSTIs are polymicrobial, with both gram-positive and gram-negative pathogens causing infections of this nature, the most common being group A *Streptococcus*, *Clostridium* spp, community-acquired methicillin-resistant *Staphylococcus aureus* (MRSA), *Vibrio* spp, *Aeromonas hydrophila*, and *Pasteurella* spp.[25] In a relatively recent series, approximately two-thirds of cases of NSTI were polymicrobial, and one-third were monomicrobial, with most monomicrobial cases being a result of gram-positive cocci.[6] In more recent reports, MRSA soft tissue infections seem to have gained an important role as causative organisms of community-acquired NSTI.[26]

Although antimicrobial therapy is an essential adjunctive therapy, the principles of treatment for any kind of surgical infection apply in particular to NSTI: source control, antimicrobial therapy, support, and monitoring. The importance of source control cannot be overemphasized in the treatment of NSTIs.[27] The natural history of NSTIs treated with only antimicrobial therapy and support, and without surgical debridement, results in progression to sepsis and organ dysfunction, which often leads to the high risk of mortality.[6] Source control must be obtained early and completely. Adjunct therapy with appropriate broad-spectrum antibiotics combined with adequate organ support and close monitoring is an important part of the resuscitation process that should be provided simultaneously.

According to the Infectious Diseases Society of America (IDSA), antimicrobial therapy must be directed at the pathogens expected to be causing the infection and used in appropriate doses until: (1) repeated operative procedures are no longer needed, (2) the patient has shown obvious clinical improvement, and (3) fever has been absent for 48 to 72 hours.[12] Prolonged courses or an arbitrary duration of antimicrobial therapy are not necessary and may predispose the patient to wound colonization with drug-resistant organisms.[6] **Table 5** lists IDSA recommendations for antibiotic regimens to be used in the treatment of NSTIs.

Specific circumstances are worth mentioning in which, given the suspected microorganisms and the aggressive nature of the infection, more focused or aggressive antimicrobial regimens are recommended. Specifically, antimicrobial agents for treating group A streptococcal infections associated with streptococcal toxic shock syndrome should include high-dose penicillin and clindamycin.[12] The Eagle effect is named after Harry Eagle, who demonstrated in the mouse that penicillin therapy was effective in treating myositis caused by *Streptococcus pyogenes* only if it was given early or after a low organism inoculum.[28] In a similar mouse model, Stevens and colleagues[29] showed that clindamycin and erythromycin were more effective under the conditions in which penicillin fails. These animal studies and at least 2 observational studies[30,31] have shown that clindamycin may have an exotoxin suppression effect, modulates cytokine production (ie, tumor necrosis factor), and has superior efficacy versus that of penicillin alone in these types of infections.[12] These effects are thought to be crucial for controlling the inflammatory response in patients with NSTI, particularly those with streptococcal infections.[32] Similar regimens are recommended for clostridial infection, in which exotoxin production greatly mediates the physiologic derangement observed in these patients. In addition to the benefits of clindamycin as described earlier, high-dose penicillin provides excellent coverage for anaerobic infections, such as those related to *Clostridium* species.

SURGICAL INDICATIONS AND THERAPY

High suspicion for NSTI should prompt early surgical evaluation. When the diagnosis of NSTI is confirmed, surgical debridement is indicated. When suspicion remains high

Table 5
Treatment of necrotizing infections of the skin, fascia, and muscle

First-line Antimicrobial Agent by Infection Type	Adult Dosage	Antimicrobial Agents for Patients with Severe Penicillin Hypersensitivity
Mixed infection		
Ampicillin/sulbactam	1.5–3.0 g IV every 6–8 h	Clindamycin or metronidazole[a] with an aminoglycoside or fluoroquinolone
or		
Piperacillin/tazobactam plus	3.3 g IV every 6–8 h	
Clindamycin plus	600–900 mg/kg IV every 8 h	
Ciprofloxacin	400 mg IV every 12 h	
Imipenem/cilastatin	1 g IV every 6–8 h	
Meropenem	1 g IV every 8 h	
Ertapenem	1 g every day IV	
Cefotaxime plus	2 g IV every 6 h	
Metronidazole or	500 mg IV every 6 h	
Clindamycin	600–900 mg/kg IV every 8 h	
Streptococcus infection		
Penicillin	2–4 mU IV every 4–6 h (adults)	Vancomycin, linezolid, quinupristin/dalfopristin or daptomycin
plus		
Clindamycin	600–900 mg/kg IV every 8 h	
Staphylococcus aureus infection		
Nafcillin	1–2 g IV every 4 h	Vancomycin, linezolid, quinupristin/dalfopristin, daptomycin
Oxacillin	1–2 g IV every 4 h	
Cefazolin	1 g IV every 8 h	
Vancomycin (for resistant strains)	30 mg/kg/d IV in 2 divided doses	
Clindamycin	600–900 mg/kg IV every 8 h	Bacteriostatic; potential of cross-resistance and emergence of resistance in erythromycin-resistant strains; inducible resistance in methicillin-resistant *S aureus*
Clostridium infection		
Clindamycin	600–900 mg/kg IV every 8 h	
Penicillin	2–4 mU IV every 4–6 h	

Abbreviation: IV, intravenously.

[a] If *Staphylococcus* infection is present or suspected, add an appropriate agent.

From Stevens DL, Bisno AL, Chambers HF, et al. Practice guidelines for the diagnosis and management of skin and soft-tissue infections. Clin Infect Dis 2005;41(10):1373–406; with permission.

but laboratory and imaging studies have remained inconclusive, surgery has been recommended by some researchers as a means to evaluate for macroscopic findings consistent with NSTI.[6] Surgical debridement should be accomplished as early as possible, because this has been shown to have a significant impact on final outcome in patients with NSTI.[33–35] The operation should include a generous incision with complete debridement of infected and necrotic tissue. The limits of dissection should be healthy, viable, bleeding tissue. Occasionally, amputation of a limb is necessary to achieve this goal and can be a life-saving measure in patients with severe and extensive NSTI of the corresponding limb.[6]

Once the initial debridement has been performed, supportive management in an intensive care unit (ICU) is recommended with aggressive resuscitation. Scheduled debridements at intervals of 6 to 48 hours should be performed until no further necrosis or infected tissue is seen.[12] The physiology of the patient should be closely monitored and serial WBC counts should be performed every 6 to 12 hours. Any additional physiologic derangement or increase in the WBC count occurring earlier than planned redebridement should prompt more frequent reoperations.[6]

SUPPORTIVE CARE

As part of the adjunct treatment of patients with NSTI, close monitoring in an ICU with physiologic support is encouraged. Depending on the severity of the infectious process, patients may develop organ failure, such as acute renal failure and acute respiratory distress syndrome, which require replacement therapies. Given the metabolic demand of the physiologic response to this aggressive infection, the nutritional status of these patients must be optimized. Early enteral nutritional support helps the catabolic response of these patients.[6,36] However, parenteral nutrition can be used when the enteral route is not possible or practical.[37] Appropriate vitamins (A, C, and D) and minerals such as zinc should be provided because these can promote wound healing.[37] Aggressive fluid resuscitation and blood component therapy guided by invasive monitoring is often required during the perioperative period. Judicious control of glucose and novel therapeutic approaches for severe sepsis or septic shock should be considered for better optimization.

A series of experimental adjunct therapies have been reported in select groups of patients with NSTI. Investigators arguing for a decreased number of debridements and decreased mortality have advocated hyperbaric oxygen.[38,39] Results from this strategy are contradictory, and no appropriate epidemiologically based studies have been performed to elucidate the effect of hyperbaric oxygen in these patients. Additionally, hyperbaric oxygen is often not readily available, requiring daily hospital transfers, jeopardizing the appropriate ICU care for the sickest patients. The authors do not recommend the routine use of hyperbaric oxygen, particularly if it is not readily available, and outside of a clinical trial.

Another adjunct treatment is intravenous immune globulin (IVIG), which is thought to halt the infectious/systemic inflammatory response syndrome process through neutralizing the destructive toxins, especially in NSTIs associated with group A streptococcal infection.[36] These studies are also controversial and difficult to compare, given the small number of patients and the different methodologies used.[6] According to the IDSA, a recommendation to use IVIG to treat streptococcal toxic shock syndrome cannot be made with certainty (grade B-II).[12] This decision was attributed to the idea that different batches of IVIG contain variable quantities of neutralizing antibodies to some of the toxins, and definitive clinical data are lacking.[12] Although some retrospective and prospective studies show a potential benefit with IVIG,[40–42] additional studies are required before it can be recommended for routine use in NSTI.[36]

Once surgical debridement is no longer required, wound care becomes an important aspect of the recovery process. Perineal wounds are especially difficult to manage, because fecal and urinary soilage of the wound occurs frequently.[36] However, stool diversion by colostomy is rarely required. Meticulous wound care is all that is required even with the most difficult wounds. When the wound is clean, use of a vacuum wound dressing is an option to facilitate wound granulation. For most wounds, closure is achieved with simple split-thickness skin grafts. More-complex wounds should be managed in conjunction with the plastic surgery team.[36]

REHABILITATION

Once a patient survives NSTI, return to function becomes a critical outcome.[43] Because of the paucity of research on the factors associated with favorable and unfavorable NSTI functional outcome, Pham and colleagues[43] in the Burn Center in Seattle adapted the impairment rating scale previously validated in burn patients to attempt to quantify physical limitation in NSTI survivors. A significant number of patients (30%) were found to have at least mild to severe functional limitation, and the involvement of an extremity was clearly associated with a higher functional limitation class.[43] The investigators hypothesized that the physical status may change significantly over time and that serial measurements would more accurately describe the impact of rehabilitation on this outcome.[43] Data are also scarce on the impact of this life-threatening disease on quality of life and emotional well-being throughout the process and during recovery. Because of the prolonged hospitalization and multiple procedures, some of which may be disfiguring, this disease process often becomes life-altering in survivors, and a new diagnosis of depression and anxiety is not uncommon. Studies assessing the changes in NSTI survivors' ability to return to previous functional status and work, and assessment of new psychiatric diagnoses will shed light on the impact of this disease.

OUTCOMES

Although some improvements in overall outcomes of NSTI have been seen, mortality remains high. Jones[2] first reported a mortality rate of 46% in his large series of more than 2000 patients, and a recent pooled analysis revealed mortality rates ranging 16% to 34%.[33] Multiple studies have focused on identifying predictors of mortality, finding a wide number of prognostic factors. However, these are not universal and vary from series to series. In an effort to develop a standardized prognostic tool, Anaya and colleagues[3] used a robust multi-institutional database to identify the most important predictors of mortality found at initial admission. In their study of 350 patients with NSTI, a prognostic score was developed and validated using the following independent predictors of mortality (**Table 6**): age older than 50 years, WBC count greater than 40,000 cells/mm^3, hematocrit greater than 50%, heart rate greater than 110 beats per minute, temperature lower than 36°C, and serum creatinine level greater than 1.5 mg/dL. This tool allows stratification of patients into 3 groups according to the risk of mortality, with a score of 6 or greater associated with a mortality of 88%. Although this tool has proven useful in the authors' experience, it lacks external validation, calling into question its role for predicting mortality in patients with NSTI of different characteristics. Further validation of this and similar tools should help identify high-risk patients who may benefit from novel therapeutic strategies and patients eligible for future trials.[3]

Table 6		
Clinical score predictive of death in patients with NSTI		
Variables on Admission		**Points**
Heart rate >110 beats per minute		1
Temperature <36°C		1
Serum creatinine >1.5 mg/dL		1
White blood cell count >40,000/μL		3
Hematocrit >50%		3
Age >50 y		3
Group Category	**Number of Points**	**Mortality (%)**
1	0–2	6
2	3–5	24
3	≥6	88

COST

Patients with NSTI require multidisciplinary care and extensive use of ICU resources.[36] The mean ICU stay for patients with NSTI is 21 days, with a mean hospital stay of 32 days for survivors and 12 days for nonsurvivors.[44] This condition has a significant cost of care, ranging from $71,000 to $83,000.[44] Most NSTIs are treated by surgeons in the community, but patients are increasingly being referred to tertiary care hospitals and burn centers for specialized wound and critical care management,[36] contributing to the increased burden to the health care system.

SUMMARY

NSTIs are infrequent but highly lethal infections. One of the greatest challenges in managing NSTIs is establishing early diagnosis. A high index of suspicion is critical in making the diagnosis. Accuracy of early diagnosis increases with familiarity with clinical findings and knowledge of laboratory and imaging tools. Once the diagnosis is made, surgical debridement until adequate and complete source control is achieved is the primary means of treating NSTIs. Antimicrobial therapy together with physiologic monitoring and support constitute adjuvant therapies. Diagnostic scores that identify high-risk patients help guide novel therapeutic strategies and determine eligibility for future trials.

REFERENCES

1. Sarani B, Strong M, Pascual J, et al. Necrotizing fasciitis: current concepts and review of the literature. J Am Coll Surg 2009;208(2):279–88.
2. Jones J. Surgical memoirs of the War of the Rebellion. In: Hamilton FH, editor. Investigation upon the nature, causes and treatment of hospital gangrene as prevailed in the Confederate Armies 1861-1865. New York: U.S. Sanitary Commission; 1871.
3. Anaya DA, Bulger EM, Kwon YS, et al. Predicting death in necrotizing soft tissue infections: a clinical score. Surg Infect (Larchmt) 2009;10(6):517–22.
4. Anaya DA, McMahon K, Nathens AB, et al. Predictors of mortality and limb loss in necrotizing soft tissue infections. Arch Surg 2005;140(2):151–7.
5. Wilson B. Necrotizing fasciitis. Am Surg 1952;18(4):416–31.

6. Anaya DA, Dellinger EP. Necrotizing soft-tissue infection: diagnosis and management. Clin Infect Dis 2007;44(5):705–10.

7. Ellis Simonsen SM, van Orman ER, Hatch BE, et al. Cellulitis incidence in a defined population. Epidemiol Infect 2006;134(2):293–9.

8. Anaya DA, Dellinger EP. Necrotizing soft-tissue infection. In: Jong EC, Stevens DL, editors. Netter's infectious disease. 1st edition. Philadelphia: Saunders; 2012. p. 273–8.

9. Callahan TE, Schecter WP, Horn JK. Necrotizing soft tissue infection masquerading as cutaneous abscess following illicit drug injection. Arch Surg 1998;133(8): 812–7.

10. Chen JL, Fullerton KE, Flynn NM. Necrotizing fasciitis associated with injection drug use. Clin Infect Dis 2001;33(1):6–15.

11. Bosshardt TL, Henderson VJ, Organ CH Jr. Necrotizing soft-tissue infections. Arch Surg 1996;131(8):846–52.

12. Stevens DL, Bisno AL, Chambers HF, et al. Practice guidelines for the diagnosis and management of skin and soft-tissue infections. Clin Infect Dis 2005;41(10): 1373–406.

13. Haywood CT, McGeer A, Low DE. Clinical experience with 20 cases of group A streptococcus necrotizing fasciitis and myonecrosis: 1995 to 1997. Plast Reconstr Surg 1999;103(6):1567–73.

14. Elliott DC, Kufera JA, Myers RA. Necrotizing soft tissue infections. Risk factors for mortality and strategies for management. Ann Surg 1996;224(5):672–83.

15. Wong CH, Chang HC, Pasupathy S, et al. Necrotizing fasciitis: clinical presentation, microbiology, and determinants of mortality. J Bone Joint Surg Am 2003; 85-A(8):1454–60.

16. Wong CH, Wang YS. The diagnosis of necrotizing fasciitis. Curr Opin Infect Dis 2005;18(2):101–6.

17. Wall DB, Klein SR, Black S, et al. A simple model to help distinguish necrotizing fasciitis from nonnecrotizing soft tissue infection. J Am Coll Surg 2000;191(3):227–31.

18. Wong CH, Khin LW, Heng KS, et al. The LRINEC (Laboratory Risk Indicator for Necrotizing Fasciitis) score: a tool for distinguishing necrotizing fasciitis from other soft tissue infections. Crit Care Med 2004;32(7):1535–41.

19. Holland MJ. Application of the Laboratory Risk Indicator in Necrotising Fasciitis (LRINEC) score to patients in a tropical tertiary referral centre. Anaesth Intensive Care 2009;37(4):588–92.

20. Wysoki MG, Santora TA, Shah RM, et al. Necrotizing fasciitis: CT characteristics. Radiology 1997;203(3):859–63.

21. Struk DW, Munk PL, Lee MJ, et al. Imaging of soft tissue infections. Radiol Clin North Am 2001;39(2):277–303.

22. Arslan A, Pierre-Jerome C, Borthne A. Necrotizing fasciitis: unreliable MRI findings in the preoperative diagnosis. Eur J Radiol 2000;36(3):139–43.

23. Stamenkovic I, Lew PD. Early recognition of potentially fatal necrotizing fasciitis. The use of frozen-section biopsy. N Engl J Med 1984;310(26):1689–93.

24. Majeski J, Majeski E. Necrotizing fasciitis: improved survival with early recognition by tissue biopsy and aggressive surgical treatment. South Med J 1997; 90(11):1065–8.

25. May AK. Skin and soft tissue infections: the new surgical infection society guidelines. Surg Infect (Larchmt) 2011;12(3):179–84.

26. Miller LG, Perdreau-Remington F, Rieg G, et al. Necrotizing fasciitis caused by community-associated methicillin-resistant Staphylococcus aureus in Los Angeles. N Engl J Med 2005;352(14):1445–53.

27. Marshall JC, Maier RV, Jimenez M, et al. Source control in the management of severe sepsis and septic shock: an evidence-based review. Crit Care Med 2004; 32(Suppl 11):S513–26.

28. Eagle H. Experimental approach to the problem of treatment failure with penicillin. I. Group A streptococcal infection in mice. Am J Med 1952;13(4):389–99.

29. Stevens DL, Gibbons AE, Bergstrom R, et al. The Eagle effect revisited: efficacy of clindamycin, erythromycin, and penicillin in the treatment of streptococcal myositis. J Infect Dis 1988;158(1):23–8.

30. Zimbelman J, Palmer A, Todd J. Improved outcome of clindamycin compared with beta-lactam antibiotic treatment for invasive Streptococcus pyogenes infection. Pediatr Infect Dis J 1999;18(12):1096–100.

31. Mulla ZD, Leaverton PE, Wiersma ST. Invasive group A streptococcal infections in Florida. South Med J 2003;96(10):968–73.

32. Stevens DL, Bryant AE, Hackett SP. Antibiotic effects on bacterial viability, toxin production, and host response. Clin Infect Dis 1995;20(Suppl 2):S154–7.

33. McHenry CR, Piotrowski JJ, Petrinic D, et al. Determinants of mortality for necrotizing soft-tissue infections. Ann Surg 1995;221(5):558–63.

34. Bilton BD, Zibari GB, McMillan RW, et al. Aggressive surgical management of necrotizing fasciitis serves to decrease mortality: a retrospective study. Am Surg 1998;64(5):397–400.

35. Lille ST, Sato TT, Engrav LH, et al. Necrotizing soft tissue infections: obstacles in diagnosis. J Am Coll Surg 1996;182(1):7–11.

36. Phan HH, Cocanour CS. Necrotizing soft tissue infections in the intensive care unit. Crit Care Med 2010;38(Suppl 9):S460–8.

37. Ustin JS, Malangoni MA. Necrotizing soft-tissue infections. Crit Care Med 2011; 39(9):2156–62.

38. Riseman JA, Zamboni WA, Curtis A, et al. Hyperbaric oxygen therapy for necrotizing fasciitis reduces mortality and the need for debridements. Surgery 1990; 108(5):847–50.

39. Jallali N, Withey S, Butler PE. Hyperbaric oxygen as adjuvant therapy in the management of necrotizing fasciitis. Am J Surg 2005;189(4):462–6.

40. Kaul R, McGeer A, Norrby-Teglund A, et al. Intravenous immunoglobulin therapy for streptococcal toxic shock syndrome–a comparative observational study. The Canadian Streptococcal Study Group. Clin Infect Dis 1999;28(4):800–7.

41. Darenberg J, Ihendyane N, Sjolin J, et al. Intravenous immunoglobulin G therapy in streptococcal toxic shock syndrome: a European randomized, double-blind, placebo-controlled trial. Clin Infect Dis 2003;37(3):333–40.

42. Norrby-Teglund A, Muller MP, McGeer A, et al. Successful management of severe group A streptococcal soft tissue infections using an aggressive medical regimen including intravenous polyspecific immunoglobulin together with a conservative surgical approach. Scand J Infect Dis 2005;37(3):166–72.

43. Pham TN, Moore ML, Costa BA, et al. Assessment of functional limitation after necrotizing soft tissue infection. J Burn Care Res 2009;30(2):301–6.

44. Endorf FW, Klein MB, Mack CD, et al. Necrotizing soft-tissue infections: differences in patients treated at burn centers and non-burn centers. J Burn Care Res 2008;29(6):933–8.

Life-threatening Infections in Medically Immunocompromised Patients

Hasan M. Al-Dorzi, MD[a], Raymond Khan, MD[a],
Yaseen M. Arabi, MD[b],*

KEYWORDS

- Critical illness • Chronic kidney failure • Chronic obstructive pulmonary disease
- Diabetes mellitus • Heart failure

KEY POINTS

- Chronic illnesses, such as diabetes mellitus, chronic obstructive pulmonary disease, chronic kidney disease, cirrhosis, and heart failure, are often associated with immune abnormalities that make affected patients prone to specific life-threatening infections.
- Although encountered in patients without chronic illnesses, the presentation and prognosis of these infections are frequently different making physicians' awareness about them crucial for appropriate management.
- Further studies on the management of life-threatening infections in these patients are needed to understand their special characteristics and determine the specific diagnostic and therapeutic approaches.

INTRODUCTION

Life-threatening infections occur frequently in patients with chronic diseases, which are increasing by approximately 1.5% per year.[1] A large cohort study (n = 192,980) found that 56% of patients with severe sepsis have at least one chronic comorbidity, with complicated diabetes mellitus (DM) present in 3.2%, chronic obstructive pulmonary disease (COPD) in 12.3%, chronic kidney disease (CKD) in 5.4%, and chronic liver disease in 4.5%.[1] Although patients with these conditions do not have primary defects in the immune system, they often have various immune abnormalities that make them prone to specific infections. In this review, we describe the

Disclosures: All authors declare no conflicts of interest and do not have any direct financial interest in the subject matter or materials discussed in the article or with a company making a competing product.
[a] Intensive Care Department, College of Medicine, King Saud bin Abdulaziz University for Health Sciences, PO Box 22490, MC 1425, Riyadh 11426, Saudi Arabia; [b] Respiratory Services, Intensive Care Department, College of Medicine, King Saud bin Abdulaziz University for Health Sciences, PO Box 22490, MC 1425, Riyadh 11426, Saudi Arabia
* Corresponding author.
E-mail address: yaseenarabi@yahoo.com

Crit Care Clin 29 (2013) 807–826
http://dx.doi.org/10.1016/j.ccc.2013.06.002
criticalcare.theclinics.com

life-threatening infections that occur in patients with chronic medical diseases, namely DM, COPD, CKD, cirrhosis, and heart failure (HF), and discuss their management and reported outcomes.

PATHOGENESIS

Various changes in the innate, cell-medicated, and humoral immunity have been described in patients with these chronic medical conditions. Reduced neutrophil chemotaxis after stimulation[2] and blunted inflammatory response to endotoxemia[3] have been shown in DM and functional abnormalities of neutrophils, monocytes, dendritic cells, and lymphocytes[4–6] in uremia. In cirrhosis, several abnormalities have been described, including reduced numbers and function of Kupffer cells,[7] impaired phagocytotic function of neutrophils,[8] and downregulation of proinflammatory cytokine production after lipopolysaccharide stimulation.[9] In patients with HF, natural killer cells have been shown to have decreased sensitivity to activation by interleukin (IL)-2 and interferon-γ.[10]

Additionally, soft tissue breakage in DM and edema in cirrhosis and HF increase the risk of skin and soft tissue infections (SSTIs). Glucosuria promotes bacterial growth in the urinary tract. The presence of hemodialyis or peritoneal dialysis access may lead to bacterial invasion into the blood or peritoneal space. Injury to the respiratory epithelial cells, ciliary dysfunction, and corticosteroid therapy predispose patients with COPD to recurrent respiratory tract infections. In cirrhosis, translocation of bacteria into ascitic fluid leads to spontaneous bacterial peritonitis (SBP) and the presence of intrahepatic shunts predisposes to endotipsitis.

LIFE-THREATENING INFECTIONS IN DIABETIC PATIENTS
Epidemiology

DM is a global health problem. In 2010, the prevalence of DM among adults was 6.4% worldwide, 10.3% in the United States and 9.2% in Canada.[11] The prevalence was generally lower in Europe[11] and higher in the Middle East.[11] The worldwide DM prevalence is expected to increase to 7.7% by 2030.[11] Studies from intensive care units (ICUs) have consistently shown higher DM prevalence than population-based studies, suggesting that DM predisposes to critical illness. DM prevalence among critically ill patients in the United States was 22.6% in the University Health System Consortium cohort[12] and 16.3% of the Mayo cohort.[12] However, it was less prevalent (7.2%) in a European cohort of critically ill patients with sepsis.[13]

DM is associated with increased risk of specific infections. In a 12-month prospective Dutch cohort study, which compared diabetic patients with hypertensive nondiabetic patients, DM was associated with increased risk of urinary tract infections (UTIs), SSTIs, and lower respiratory tract infections.[14]

Specific Infections

UTIs
UTIs are among the most common infections that affect diabetic patients and are often complicated. Emphysematous cystitis is a rare but serious complication of lower UTI and occurs mainly in individuals with DM.[15] It most commonly occurs due to *Escherichia coli,* but other pathogens, including *Enterobacter, Proteus, Klebsiella,* and *Candida* species, have also been implicated.[15] Emphysematous pyelonephritis almost exclusively occurs in patients with diabetes. It results from a severe form of acute multifocal bacterial nephritis. *E coli* is the most commonly implicated pathogen, followed by other enteric gram-negative bacilli.[15]

SSTIs

A 2-year longitudinal prospective outpatient study showed that 9.1% of diabetic patients developed foot infections.[16] SSTIs are composed of heterogeneous conditions, including simple cellulitis, infected foot ulcer with or without cellulitis, necrotizing fasciitis, deep abscesses, osteomyelitis, and septic arthritis. Causative pathogens vary depending on the condition. Among pathogens, β-hemolytic streptococci and *Staphylococcus aureus* predominate in cellulitis and acute infected foot ulcers. Methicillin-resistant *S aureus* (MRSA) prevalence has been increasing in infected foot ulcers.[17] A multicenter study of hospitalized diabetic patients with SSTI and positive cultures showed that MRSA was the only isolate with a significantly increased prevalence from 11.6% to 21.9%.[17] Studies from India have also showed increasing prevalence of other multidrug-resistant gram-negative organisms.[18,19] Gram-negative bacteria and anaerobes should be considered in chronic and deeper infections and polymicrobial infection should be considered in severe situations.[20] Fournier gangrene represents a severe form of SSTI that involves the perineal, perianal, or genital regions, with 40% to 60% of patients having DM.[21] Infecting microorganisms are usually mixed aerobic and anaerobic bacteria.

Fungal infections

DM is also a risk factor for fungal infections, including candidiasis and mucormycosis. A population-based surveillance for candidemia found that among diabetic adults, the average annual incidence of candidemia was 28 per 100,000 population.[22] Approximately 50% of rhinocerebral mucormycosis cases occur in patients with DM.[23]

Other infections

DM also increases the morbidity associated with certain viral infections. DM has been associated with increased hospitalization and ICU admission after H1N1 infection.[24]

In the ICU, DM has been found to be a predictor of central line–associated bloodstream infections caused by gram-negative bacteria.[25]

Antimicrobial Therapy

Early and appropriate antimicrobial therapy has been shown to be associated with lower mortality in patients with severe sepsis and septic shock.[26,27] DM is considered a risk factor for infections with resistant microorganisms. Hence, empiric therapy is should be broad and directed against the suspected causative agents taking into consideration local susceptibility patterns.

Surgical Indications and Therapy

Current evidence suggests that the treatment of choice for emphysematous pyelonephritis is medical management combined with percutaneous drainage.[28] However, nephrectomy may be needed in patients with extensive diffuse gas and renal destruction.[28] Debridement and amputation may be necessary in diabetic foot ulcers with deep infection and gangrene. Necrotizing fasciitis and Fournier gangrene frequently require surgical intervention. Immediate debridement of necrotic tissues is one of the principles of treatment and the most important for improved survival.[29] For mucormycosis, aggressive surgery and long-term therapy with amphotericin B may lead to improved outcomes.[30]

Supportive Therapy

Insulin therapy is essential in the management of infected diabetic patients with hyperglycemia. A meta-analysis of 29 randomized controlled trials totaling 8432 critically ill adult patients found that tight glucose control for diabetic and nondiabetic patients was associated with significantly decreased risk of septicemia.[31] However, intensive insulin therapy has not been shown to reduce mortality in critically ill diabetic and nondiabetic patients.[32]

Agents used for reducing cardiovascular risk have been evaluated in infected diabetic patients. In a retrospective case-control study of 142,175 diabetic patients, van de Garde and colleagues[33] found that statin use was associated with reducing pneumonia risk.

Outcome

Certain DM-associated infections are known for their aggressive course and poor prognosis, especially if not treated promptly. Examples include Fournier gangrene and mucormycosis. DM is also associated with increased risk of death after H1N1 infection.[34] In a prospective multicenter cohort study of invasive candidiasis, type 1 DM was independently associated with increased mortality.[35] Analysis of 2 multicenter cohorts found that DM was associated with increased mortality risk within the first year after community-acquired pneumonia (CAP).[36] Pittet and colleagues[37] found that DM was significantly associated with increased mortality from septicemia in surgical ICU patients.

LIFE-THREATENING INFECTIONS IN PATIENTS WITH COPD
Epidemiology

In 2011, the Centers for Disease Control and Prevention reported that 6.3% (15 million) of American adults had COPD, with prevalence increasing from 3.2% among people aged 18 to 44 years to more than 11.6% among those aged 65 years or older.[38] The main causes of hospitalization are COPD exacerbation and cardiovascular disease.[39,40]

Specific Infections

Acute exacerbation of COPD

Even with therapy, patients with COPD have 1.4 acute exacerbations, on average, each year.[41] Most COPD exacerbations are due to recurrent infections with viral or bacterial pathogens. Viruses may account for more than 50% of exacerbations.[42] A meta-analysis of 8 studies found that picornavirus was the most commonly detected virus (17.3%), followed by influenza (7.4%), respiratory syncytial virus (5.3%), corona viruses (3.1%), and parainfluenza (2.6%).[43] Viral COPD exacerbations appear to be more severe and last longer than those without a viral trigger.[44] Although bacteria frequently colonize the airways in COPD, bacterial exacerbations are usually associated with acquiring new bacterial strains of nontypeable *Haemophilus influenzae, Streptococcus pneumoniae, Moraxella catarrhalis,* and *Pseudomonas aeruginosa.*[45]

CAP

COPD course is frequently complicated by CAP.[46] A cohort study of 40,414 patients with COPD aged 45 years or older found a CAP incidence rate of 22.4 per 1000 person-years.[47] A population-based Spanish study of 1336 CAP cases and 1326 controls found that chronic bronchitis was present in 16.2% of cases versus 6.1% of controls and was an independent risk factor for CAP.[48] The use of inhaled corticosteroids in patients with COPD has been implicated in the increased CAP risk as shown in a meta-analysis of 11 studies of combination preparations (fluticasone/salmeterol and budesonide/formoterol).[49] When having CAP, patients with COPD usually present with more severe respiratory failure and higher Pneumonia Severity Index (PSI).[50]

S pneumoniae is the most common isolated pathogen, followed by *H influenzae, P aeruginosa, S aureus, M catarrhalis,* and atypical pathogens.[51,52] One study found that COPD was associated with increased pneumococcal bacteremia[53] and another one found that *Legionella pneumophila* occurred predominantly in patients without COPD.[51] Having repeated severe COPD exacerbations is a risk factor for CAP due to *Pseudomonas* species.[54]

COPD is also a risk factor for ventilator-associated pneumonia (VAP).[55–57] *P aeruginosa, Acinetobacter* species, and *S aureus* are the usual causative organisms.[58,59] Systemic corticosteroid use increases the risk of infections with multidrug-resistant organisms.[60]

Invasive pulmonary aspergillosis

Patients with severe COPD who are receiving broad-spectrum antibiotics and corticosteroids have an increased incidence of invasive pulmonary aspergillosis (IPA).[61,62] Guinea and colleagues[61] found that *Aspergillus* was isolated from the lower respiratory tract of 16.3 patients per 1000 COPD admissions, but only 22.1% of them had probable IPA. IPA risk factors were ICU admission, receiving antibiotics in the prior 3 months, and accumulated corticosteroid doses (>700 mg) in the prior 3 months.[61] A study of 96 episodes of severe hospital-acquired pneumonia at 2 Spanish ICUs found that 13 episodes were thought to be due to *Aspergillus* species (8 cases were classified as definite), most of which were in patients with COPD (84%) and on steroids (69%).[63] One prospective study evaluated 55 consecutive patients with severe COPD, moderate to severe persistent bronchial asthma, or bronchiectasis who were admitted to a respiratory ICU in China and found that 13 (23.6%) patients had IPA.[62] Cumulative prednisone doses greater than 350 mg before ICU admission was an independent risk factor.[62]

Other infections

Pneumocystis jiroveci causes opportunistic fungal respiratory tract infections in immunocompromised patients. However, it is a frequent colonizer of the lungs and was detected in the bronchoalveolar lavage of 20% of 169 immunocompetent patients in one study.[64] Patients with COPD are at increased risk for *Pneumocystis* colonization.[65,66] Infection with this organism should be considered in patients with COPD, especially those on corticosteroids or with nonresolving pneumonias.

Patients with COPD are at risk for influenza infections. Additionally, COPD was a risk factor for bacterial coinfection, as shown during the 2009 to 2010 influenza A H1N1 pandemic at 2 Spanish hospitals.[67]

Antimicrobial Management

Management of acute COPD exacerbation includes the administration of antibiotics, usually in the presence of increased sputum volume and purulence. A systematic review found that antibiotics significantly reduced the treatment failure risk, although the evidence was of low quality.[68]

The Infectious Diseases Society of America/American Thoracic Society has outlined evidence-based clinical practice guidelines for CAP management, which are stratified based on pneumonia severity.[69] For non-ICU inpatients, a respiratory fluoroquinolone or β-lactam plus a macrolide are recommended.[69] For ICU patients, a β-lactam (cefotaxime, ceftriaxone, or ampicillin-sulbactam) plus either azithromycin or a fluoroquinolone are recommended. When *Pseudomonas* risk exists, an antipneumococcal, antipseudomonal β-lactam (piperacillin-tazobactam, cefepime, imipenem, or meropenem) plus either ciprofloxacin, levofloxacin, or aminoglycoside are recommended.[69] When MRSA risk exists, vancomycin or linezolid should be added.[69]

Voriconazole is the primary IPA treatment, as in a randomized trial that showed a survival benefit in patients with IPA who received voriconazole compared with amphotericin B.[70] However, most of the enrolled patients had allogeneic hematopoietic-cell transplantation, acute leukemia, or other hematologic diseases.[70] The use of combination therapy remains controversial with some evidence supporting combination antifungal therapy for salvage or failed monotherapy.[71]

Influenza is usually treated with the neuraminidase inhibitors, oseltamivir and zanamivir. For severe cases, it is recommended to increase oseltamivir dosage from 75 mg to 150 mg twice daily.[72] In 2009, the Food and Drug Administration approved the use of peramivir, an intravenous neuraminidase inhibitor, for the treatment of patients with severe influenza.[73]

Supportive Care

Systemic corticosteroids are used in acute COPD exacerbations, but their role in the management of patients with COPD with pneumonia is less defined.[74] Hyperglycemia may develop and blood glucose control may be needed. Evaluation for adrenal insufficiency and corticosteroid replacement should be considered in severe COPD with frequent exacerbation and corticosteroid use.

There is emerging literature about the effect of cardioprotective medications in hospitalized patients with COPD exacerbation, including those with infection. Patients with COPD are at increased risk for specific cardiovascular conditions: arrhythmia, angina, acute myocardial infarction, HF, stroke, and pulmonary embolism.[40] One retrospective study of 825 patients hospitalized for COPD exacerbation found that β-blocker use was associated with reduced mortality.[75] A nested case-control study found that more than 2 years of statin use was associated with 39% reduction in mortality risk in COPD.[76] A retrospective cohort study of elderly patients hospitalized with COPD exacerbation, current statin use, and angiotensin-converting enzyme inhibitor/angiotensin receptor blocker use were significantly associated with decreased 90-day mortality.[77]

Outcomes

Infections in patients with COPD are usually associated with significant morbidity and mortality. Acute COPD exacerbations requiring hospitalization are associated with a 30-day all-cause mortality of 4% to 30%.[78] Mortality predictors include higher values of acute physiology scoring systems, low Glasgow Coma Scale on ICU admission, cardiac dysrhythmia, and length of hospital stay before ICU admission.[79] The relationship between mortality and COPD in CAP is inconsistent with one study showing no increase in mortality risk, and other ones finding higher mortality,[80] and other studies found increased mortality in hospitalized patients with COPD with CAP.[52,81] In general, the mortality ascribed to CAP in this population is 4% to 34%.[50–52,81] One prospective observational study of patients with VAP found COPD to be an independent predictor of ICU mortality.[58] Another study of mechanically ventilated patients with COPD found that VAP was independently associated with ICU mortality.[59] The mortality associated with IPA in patients with COPD is extremely high, reaching 91%.[82]

LIFE-THREATENING INFECTIONS IN PATIENTS WITH CKD
Epidemiology

CKD is a global public health problem. In the United States, 9.6% of noninstitutionalized adults are estimated to have CKD.[83] It is predicted that by 2015 there will be 136,166 patients with incident end-stage renal disease (ESRD) per year and 712,290 prevalent patients in the United States.[84]

Patients with CKD have high sepsis prevalence and severity.[85,86] Evaluation of the ESRD program in the United States found that for new patients on hemodialysis, infection-related hospitalizations within the first year increased almost 100% from 1993 to 2005, especially in the first 2 months.[86] A study of 433 patients on hemodialysis found 2412 episodes of bacterial or fungal infections, with infection rate of 5.7 episodes per 1000 dialysis-days.[87] Dialysis-related infections were responsible for 24% of the episodes,[87] followed by below-the-knee SSTI (19%), pneumonia (13%), and other SSTIs (9%).[87] Most (82%) infections were acquired in the community.[87] Almost half (48%) of cultured organisms were gram-positive cocci and 35% were aerobic gram-negative bacilli.[87] Fifty percent of the total infection episodes occurred in the final year of life.[87]

Specific Infections

Catheter-related bloodstream infections

Central venous catheters are the most frequent vascular access for dialysis initiation among patients with incident ESRD.[88] Incidence of catheter-related blood stream infection (CRBSI) ranges between 0.6 and 6.5 episodes per 1000 catheter-days.[89–91] CRBSI diagnosis is usually confirmed by isolation of the same microorganism from quantitative cultures of both the catheter and the peripheral blood in a septic patient without any other apparent source. Most CRBSI-causative agents are gram-positive organisms (52%–64%), most commonly *S aureus* and *Staphylococcus epidermidis*.[89,90]

Peritonitis

Peritonitis is a complication of peritoneal dialysis (PD). One Australian study showed a peritonitis rate of 0.60 episodes per patient-year.[92] Gram-positive organisms are the most common causative organisms, followed by gram-negative bacteria.[92] Cultures can be polymicrobial and may be negative.[92] Evaluation of 990 patients with incident PD from 1997 to 2009 identified 90 of them who required ICU admission and found that sepsis was the second (23%) most common reason for ICU admission after cardiac problems, with peritonitis accounting for 69% of the sepsis admissions.[93]

CAP

Patients with CKD usually have more severe CAP, as reflected by higher PSI compared with other patients.[94] The microbiology is similar to non-CKD, with *S pneumoniae* being the most frequent pathogen.[94]

Antimicrobial Therapy

Empiric antimicrobial therapy for CRBSI should include broad-spectrum coverage for both gram-positive and gram-negative organisms. Owing to the high MRSA prevalence in the hemodialysis setting, empiric therapy should include anti-MRSA coverage[95] with deescalation when culture results become available. Antimicrobial therapy is usually administered for 7 to 14 days.[96] The duration is extended to 4 to 6 weeks if there is persistent bacteremia or fungemia occurring more than 72 hours after hemodialysis catheter removal and for patients with endocarditis or suppurative thrombophlebitis and to 6 to 8 weeks for the treatment of osteomyelitis.[96] The use of antibiotic catheter lock has been suggested to be instituted when catheter salvage is desired in the absence of exit site and tunnel infection.[96] For the management of peritonitis associated with PD, a systematic review found similar primary response and relapse rate for intraperitoneal glycopeptide-based regimens compared with first-generation cephalosporin regimens.[97] Nevertheless, glycopeptide-based regimens were more likely to achieve complete cure.[97] The review also found that intraperitoneal antibiotics were superior to intravenous antibiotics in reducing treatment failure based on one study.[97]

Surgical Indications and Therapy

Patients with tunnel infection or port abscess require removal of the catheter, and incision and drainage if indicated.[96] For CRBSI associated with tunneled hemodialysis access, the catheter should be surgically removed when any of the following conditions is present: severe complications (such as severe sepsis, endocarditis, and suppurative thrombophlebitis), persistent bacteremia or persistent clinical infection signs despite 48 to 72 hours of appropriate antimicrobial therapy, infection with S aureus, P aeruginosa, multidrug-resistant organisms, fungi, or mycobacetria.[96] For patients on PD, surgical removal of the PD catheter should be performed in the presence of refractory peritonitis, defined as failure of the effluent to clear after 5 days of appropriate antibiotics.[98]

Supportive Therapy

Early arteriovenous fistula planning and institution may reduce access-related infections. A meta-analysis of 11 trials found that antibiotic catheter lock solutions significantly reduced CRBSI and catheter removal.[99] As such, clinical practice guidelines recommended the prophylactic use of antimicrobial lock solution in patients with long-term catheters who have a history of multiple CRBSIs despite optimal maximal adherence to aseptic technique.[100]

Cardiovascular medications in patients with CKD have been studied in relationship to sepsis. A prospective multicenter cohort study of 1041 incident dialysis patients (1995–1998) with follow-up to 2005 found that sepsis-related hospitalizations were less frequent in patients receiving statins than in those not receiving statins.[101]

Outcome

A population-based study from the United States found that infections accounted for 20% of ESRD deaths, the second most after cardiovascular disease, and that sepsis-related mortality in ESRD was approximately 100-fold to 300-fold higher compared with the general population.[85] In a systematic review of 16 studies, comprising 6591 ICU admissions in which cardiovascular disease and sepsis accounted for most admissions, hospital mortality of patients with ESRD was high compared with matched patients with mild acute kidney injury.[102] In a study of 619 patients with ESRD admitted to 11 Canadian ICUs mostly for sepsis, the mortality was 13.3% in the ICU and 38% and 48% at 6 and 12 months of follow-up.[103] Among patients with CKD with CAP, mortality rates are markedly higher in dialysis patients compared with the general population[104] and prior pneumococcal vaccination is associated with reduced mortality risk.[94] In a retrospective study of 565 PD patients with infectious peritonitis, the mortality rate was 5.9% with peritonitis directly implicated in 15.2% of deaths and 68.5% of the infectious deaths.[105] Another study of critically ill PD patients, with sepsis due to peritonitis as the most common admitting diagnosis, found a 1-year mortality of 53.3%.[93]

LIFE-THREATENING INFECTIONS IN PATIENTS WITH CIRRHOSIS
Epidemiology

In the United States, approximately 15% of the population has chronic liver disease, with cirrhosis being a major cause of death worldwide. Life-threatening infections are a major reason for admissions to the hospital and ICU.[106–108] Cirrhosis-related infections are unique in terms of presentation, outcome, and therapeutic options.

Specific Infections

Patients with cirrhosis may have a different presentation of infections compared with other patients. Studies have shown that up to one-third of patients with cirrhosis fail to develop leukocytosis or a temperature higher than 38°C or lower than 36°C.[109] Patients with cirrhosis have lower baseline blood pressure, and higher heart rate and respiratory rate.[110] Therefore, a complete workup, including a diagnostic paracentesis and ascitic fluid culture, urine and blood cultures, and chest radiograph, should be done soon when sepsis is suspected.

Spontaneous bacterial peritonitis

SBP is the most frequent infection in cirrhosis, accounting for 10% to 30% of all documented bacterial infections in hospitalized patients with cirrhosis.[111–113] The European Association for the Study of the Liver (EASL) recommends that SBP diagnosis be based on neutrophil count in ascitic fluid of higher than $250/mm^3$.[114] EASL defines bacterascites when an ascitic neutrophil count is lower than $250/mm^3$ but with a positive ascitic fluid culture and recommends antimicrobial therapy if the patient exhibits signs of systemic inflammation or infection.[114]

The most frequently isolated organisms in SBP are *E coli*, *Klebsiella* species, and other Enterobacteriaceae.[115] The microbiological etiology of SBP has changed in recent years. In particular, there is an upsurge in isolation in quinolone-resistant gram-negative bacteria (up to 30%),[111] extended-spectrum β-lactamase (from 7.9%–33%)[116,117] and multidrug-resistant gram-positive bacteria.[118] A recent study has shown an increase in *Enterococcus* species, *S aureus* and *Candida* species, attributed to nosocomial infections and recent antibiotic treatment.[119]

CAP

Bacterial CAP is common in patients with cirrhosis.[107,120] In fact, cirrhosis is a minor criterion in defining severe CAP.[69] Compared with other patients, patients with cirrhosis more frequently presented with impaired consciousness, septic shock, higher PSI scores (classes IV–V) and bacteremia.[121] *S pneumoniae* was the most common microorganism, followed by *H influenzae* and *L pneumophila*.[121]

Skin and SSTIs

SSTIs constitute approximately 11% of infections in patients with cirrhosis.[122] These infections are caused by both gram-positive *(S aureus* and group A streptococci*)* and gram-negative bacteria (*Klebsiella* species, *Aeromonas* species, and *Vibrio vulnificus*). Cellulitis is the most frequently observed SSTI. Necrotizing fasciitis is less common[123] and is predominantly caused by gram-negative bacilli. Necrotizing fasciitis from *V vulnificus,* attributed to contaminated shellfish, has been reported in patients with cirrhosis.[124]

Community-acquired bacterial meningitis

Community-acquired bacterial meningitis in patients with cirrhosis is an uncommon but a serious infection. In a Danish cohort study of 22,743 patients with cirrhosis, bacterial meningitis incidence was 54.4 per 100,000 person-years, and was highest in alcoholic cirrhosis, 65.3 per 100,000 person-years.[125] Unfortunately, the diagnosis is often delayed. Su and colleagues[126] showed that among 25 meningitis cases in patients with cirrhosis, meningitis was the initial tentative diagnosis in only 10 patients, whereas the other were given alternative diagnoses, such as hepatic encephalopathy, seizure, and alcohol withdrawal. In contrast, only 14 of the 192 patients without cirrhosis were labeled with alternative diagnoses.[126] Patients with cirrhosis with meningitis presented with lower Glasgow Coma Scale and were more likely to have seizure and septic shock. Signs of meningeal irritation may be delayed or absent and mental status changes are often confused with hepatic encephalopathy.[127]

Data on microbiology are based on small series but show distinct pathogens. Su and colleagues[126] showed that *K pneumoniae* was responsible for 19 of 25 cases. Other cases were caused by *Salmonella*, *Listeria monocytogenes,* and *P aeruginosa*. In another series of 29 cases, *E coli* and *L monocytogenes* were statistically more common in patients with cirrhosis than those without cirrhosis.[128]

Endotipsitis

Endotipsitis refers to transjugular intrahepatic portosystemic shunt (TIPS) infection. Its definition is still debated, but involves persistent bacteremia and fever together with either shunt occlusion, or vegetation, or bacteremia in the presence of a patent shunt, when other sources of bacteremia have been ruled out.[129] Based on 4 small case series, endotipsitis incidence was approximately 1.5% (range 0.6%–5.5%).[129] Patients present with fever and chills.[129] Bacteremia can either occur early (<120 days) or late (>120 days) after stent insertion.[129] The causative organisms were Enterobacteriaceae species (24%), *Enterococcus* species (21%), *Staphylococcus* species (18%), *Streptococcus* species (9%), anaerobic species (5%), *Lactobacillus* species (5%), fungal organisms (5%), and other organisms in 14%.[129]

Antimicrobial Management

Empiric antibiotics should be started immediately following the diagnosis of SBP. Because the most common causative organisms of SBP are gram-negative aerobic bacteria, EASL recommended third-generation cephalosporins as the first-line antibiotic treatment with amoxicillin/clavulanic acid and quinolones as alternative options.[114] However, quinolones are not recommended if they are used for SBP prophylaxis, in areas where there is a high prevalence of quinolone-resistance, or in nosocomial SBP.[114] In nosocomial SBP, the incidence of ESBL-producing bacteria, as well as multidrug-resistant gram-positive bacteria such as *Enterococcus faecium* and MRSA, is increasing.[130] Empiric therapy with carbapenems and glycopeptides is suggested in nosocomial infections in which there is high suspicion of multidrug-resistant organisms, with deescalation as soon as possible.

The management of CAP in patients with cirrhosis follows the same guidelines outlined previously in the COPD section. Clinical practice guidelines of the Infectious Diseases Society of America[131] and the European Federation of the Neurologic Societies[132] did not specifically address bacterial meningitis in patients with cirrhosis. Given the unique microbiology in this population, it is important for empiric antimicrobial therapy to cover *K pneumoniae, E coli, Listeria monocytogenes,* and pneumococcus. SSTIs should be treated with broad-spectrum antimicrobials with timely surgical intervention for necrotizing fasciitis. The treatment of endotipsitis relies mainly on antimicrobial therapy because infected stent removal is impractical. Broad-spectrum antibiotics to cover both gram-positive and gram-negative bacteria should be initiated. Vancomycin plus third-generation cephalosporins have been the most common regimen reported in some series.[129] Carbapenems may be used if there is increased risk of multidrug-resistant organisms. If fungal infection is suspected, antifungal therapy should be started.[129]

In patients with cirrhosis presenting with septic shock, a recent multinational cohort study revealed that the use of inappropriate initial antimicrobials was related to increased mortality. Additionally, a single rather than 2 or more appropriate antimicrobials was also associated with higher mortality.[120]

Supportive Therapy

Intravenous albumin

A randomized, controlled study in SBP patients treated with cefotaxime showed that albumin significantly reduced mortality from 29% to 10% compared with cefotaxime alone.[133] Awaiting further evidence, the EASL recommends that that all patients who develop SBP should be treated with broad-spectrum antibiotics and intravenous albumin.[114]

Low-dose Hydrocortisone Therapy

Relative adrenal insufficiency is very common (77%) in patients with cirrhosis in septic shock.[134] In a randomized controlled trial of 75 patients with cirrhosis presenting with septic shock, hydrocortisone therapy resulted in a significant hemodynamic improvement compared to placebo.[134] However, there was no mortality benefit and hydrocortisone therapy was associated with increase shock relapse and gastrointestinal bleeding.[134]

Granulocyte Colony-stimulating Factor

A recent randomized controlled trial compared 5 µg/kg granulocyte colony-stimulating factor (G-CSF) with placebo in 47 patients with acute-on-chronic liver failure and found significant improvement of survival at day 60 (66% vs 26%) and reduction in sepsis incidence.[135] However, a recent meta-analysis of the use G-CSF in patients with severe sepsis and septic shock showed no benefit.[136] Whether G-CSF has a special benefit in patients with cirrhosis remains unknown.

Outcome

Infections in patients with cirrhosis generally carry a poor prognosis. In-hospital mortality for the first episode of SBP ranges from 10% to 37%[113,137] and 1-year mortality has been reported to be 31% to 93%.[130] Similarly, CAP in cirrhosis is associated with 14% to 30% mortality.[112,121] Factors associated with mortality include impaired consciousness, multilobar pneumonia, ascites, acute renal failure, bacteremia, ICU admission, and high Model For End-Stage Liver Disease score.[121] Meningitis has a reported mortality of 38% to 63% in patients with cirrhosis.[126,127] In patients with cirrhosis who develop septic shock, the mortality reaches 75.6%.[120] Further research in this important group of patients is needed with special focus on system-based interventions to improve the delivery of timely and appropriate management.

LIFE-THREATENING INFECTIONS IN PATIENTS WITH HF
Epidemiology

An estimated 23 million people have HF worldwide[138] including 5.7 million people in the United States alone.[139] Patients with HF are at increased risk for CAP, a common reason for their hospitalization.[48] Additionally, HF is a risk factor for admission of patients with CAP into the ICU.[34] Patients with HF are at increased risk for influenza infection, including H1N1, as documented with the 2009 H1N1 influenza infection.[140]

Specific Infections

The diagnostic approach to patients with severe CAP has been outlined earlier (COPD section).[69] If viral pneumonia is suspected, respiratory samples for viral pathogens, including H1N1 polymerase chain reaction (PCR), should be obtained. CAP diagnosis in acute HF may be difficult because of similarity of the 2 conditions on physical examination and chest radiography. Serum B-type natriuretic peptide and N-terminal pro-B-type natriuretic peptide may help to differentiate between these 2 entities in patients presenting with acute dyspnea. A recent trial in patients presenting to the emergency department with dyspnea found that a model using procalcitonin was more accurate than any other individual clinical variable for pneumonia diagnosis in all patients, and in those with acute HF.[141] The study found that patients with acute HF and an elevated procalcitonin concentration (>0.21 ng/mL) had a worse outcome if not treated with antibiotics.[141] Thoracic ultrasound demonstrating B-lines that suggests thickened interstitial or fluid-filled alveoli, seen most commonly in patients with HF, have been suggested to further aid in differentiating pneumonia from HF.[142]

Antimicrobial Management

Management of CAP in patients with HF follows the Infectious Diseases Society of America/American Thoracic Society consensus guidelines as summarized in the COPD section.[69] Patients with suspected severe influenza, including H1N1, should be treated with oseltamivir as soon as possible.

Outcome

A population-based cohort study of adult patients hospitalized for pneumonia found a 30-day mortality of 24.4% among patients with HF compared with 14.4% among other patients[143] and that the severity of HF substantially increased mortality.[143] Similarly, HF is independently associated with increased mortality risk in patients with H1N1 infections.[34]

SUMMARY

Physicians who care for patients with life-threatening infections should know about the associated chronic illnesses, as these illnesses may affect immune function and predispose patients to specific infections that could be caused by multidrug-resistant or opportunistic organisms. This knowledge is crucial for proper care and management. Additionally, further prospective studies on the management of life-threatening infections in patients with DM, COPD, HF, CKD, or cirrhosis are needed to further understand the special characteristics and the specific diagnostic and therapeutic approaches.

REFERENCES

1. Angus DC, Linde-Zwirble WT, Lidicker J, et al. Epidemiology of severe sepsis in the United States: analysis of incidence, outcome, and associated costs of care. Crit Care Med 2001;29(7):1303–10.
2. Delamaire M, Maugendre D, Moreno M, et al. Impaired leucocyte functions in diabetic patients. Diabet Med 1997;14(1):29–34.
3. Andreasen AS, Pedersen-Skovsgaard T, Berg RM, et al. Type 2 diabetes mellitus is associated with impaired cytokine response and adhesion molecule expression in human endotoxemia. Intensive Care Med 2010;36(9):1548–55.
4. Ando M, Shibuya A, Yasuda M, et al. Impairment of innate cellular response to in vitro stimuli in patients on continuous ambulatory peritoneal dialysis. Nephrol Dial Transplant 2005;20(11):2497–503.
5. Lim WH, Kireta S, Leedham E, et al. Uremia impairs monocyte and monocyte-derived dendritic cell function in hemodialysis patients. Kidney Int 2007;72(9): 1138–48.

6. Cendoroglo M, Jaber BL, Balakrishnan VS, et al. Neutrophil apoptosis and dysfunction in uremia. J Am Soc Nephrol 1999;10(1):93–100.

7. Rimola A, Soto R, Bory F, et al. Reticuloendothelial system phagocytic activity in cirrhosis and its relation to bacterial infections and prognosis. Hepatology 1984; 4(1):53–8.

8. Mookerjee RP, Stadlbauer V, Lidder S, et al. Neutrophil dysfunction in alcoholic hepatitis superimposed on cirrhosis is reversible and predicts the outcome. Hepatology 2007;46(3):831–40.

9. Xing T, Li L, Cao H, et al. Altered immune function of monocytes in different stages of patients with acute on chronic liver failure. Clin Exp Immunol 2007; 147(1):184–8.

10. Vredevoe DL, Moser DK, Gan XH, et al. Natural killer cell anergy to cytokine stimulants in a subgroup of patients with heart failure: relationship to norepinephrine. Neuroimmunomodulation 1995;2(1):16–24.

11. Shaw JE, Sicree RA, Zimmet PZ. Global estimates of the prevalence of diabetes for 2010 and 2030. Diabetes Res Clin Pract 2010;87(1):4–14.

12. Graham BB, Keniston A, Gajic O, et al. Diabetes mellitus does not adversely affect outcomes from a critical illness. Crit Care Med 2010;38(1):16–24.

13. Vincent JL, Preiser JC, Sprung CL, et al. Insulin-treated diabetes is not associated with increased mortality in critically ill patients. Crit Care 2010;14(1):R12.

14. Muller LM, Gorter KJ, Hak E, et al. Increased risk of common infections in patients with type 1 and type 2 diabetes mellitus. Clin Infect Dis 2005;41(3):281–8.

15. Patterson JE, Andriole VT. Bacterial urinary tract infections in diabetes. Infect Dis Clin North Am 1997;11(3):735–50.

16. Lavery LA, Armstrong DG, Wunderlich RP, et al. Risk factors for foot infections in individuals with diabetes. Diabetes Care 2006;29(6):1288–93.

17. Lipsky BA, Tabak YP, Johannes RS, et al. Skin and soft tissue infections in hospitalised patients with diabetes: culture isolates and risk factors associated with mortality, length of stay and cost. Diabetologia 2010;53(5):914–23.

18. Ramakant P, Verma AK, Misra R, et al. Changing microbiological profile of pathogenic bacteria in diabetic foot infections: time for a rethink on which empirical therapy to choose? Diabetologia 2011;54(1):58–64.

19. Gadepalli R, Dhawan B, Sreenivas V, et al. A clinico-microbiological study of diabetic foot ulcers in an Indian tertiary care hospital. Diabetes Care 2006;29(8): 1727–32.

20. Pellizzer G, Strazzabosco M, Presi S, et al. Deep tissue biopsy vs. superficial swab culture monitoring in the microbiological assessment of limb-threatening diabetic foot infection. Diabet Med 2001;18(10):822–7.

21. Sentochnik DE. Deep soft-tissue infections in diabetic patients. Infect Dis Clin North Am 1995;9(1):53–64.

22. Kao AS, Brandt ME, Pruitt WR, et al. The epidemiology of candidemia in two United States cities: results of a population-based active surveillance. Clin Infect Dis 1999;29(5):1164–70.

23. Joshi N, Caputo GM, Weitekamp MR, et al. Infections in patients with diabetes mellitus. N Engl J Med 1999;341(25):1906–12.

24. Allard R, Leclerc P, Tremblay C, et al. Diabetes and the severity of pandemic influenza A (H1N1) infection. Diabetes Care 2010;33(7):1491–3.

25. Sreeramoju PV, Tolentino J, Garcia-Houchins S, et al. Predictive factors for the development of central line-associated bloodstream infection due to gram-negative bacteria in intensive care unit patients after surgery. Infect Control Hosp Epidemiol 2008;29(1):51–6.

26. Kumar A, Ellis P, Arabi Y, et al. Initiation of inappropriate antimicrobial therapy results in a fivefold reduction of survival in human septic shock. Chest 2009; 136(5):1237–48.

27. Kumar A, Roberts D, Wood KE, et al. Duration of hypotension before initiation of effective antimicrobial therapy is the critical determinant of survival in human septic shock. Crit Care Med 2006;34(6):1589–96.

28. Somani BK, Nabi G, Thorpe P, et al. Is percutaneous drainage the new gold standard in the management of emphysematous pyelonephritis? Evidence from a systematic review. J Urol 2008;179(5):1844–9.

29. Ustin JS, Malangoni MA. Necrotizing soft-tissue infections. Crit Care Med 2011; 39(9):2156–62.

30. Fairley C, Sullivan TJ, Bartley P, et al. Survival after rhino-orbital-cerebral mucormycosis in an immunocompetent patient. Ophthalmology 2000;107(3):555–8.

31. Wiener RS, Wiener DC, Larson RJ. Benefits and risks of tight glucose control in critically ill adults: a meta-analysis. J Am Med Assoc 2008;300(8):933–44.

32. Griesdale DE, de Souza RJ, van Dam RM, et al. Intensive insulin therapy and mortality among critically ill patients: a meta-analysis including NICE-SUGAR study data. CMAJ 2009;180(8):821–7.

33. van de Garde EM, Hak E, Souverein PC, et al. Statin treatment and reduced risk of pneumonia in patients with diabetes. Thorax 2006;61(11):957–61.

34. Hanslik T, Boelle PY, Flahault A. Preliminary estimation of risk factors for admission to intensive care units and for death in patients infected with A(H1N1)2009 influenza virus, France, 2009-2010. PLoS Curr 2010;2:RRN1150.

35. Leroy O, Gangneux JP, Montravers P, et al. Epidemiology, management, and risk factors for death of invasive Candida infections in critical care: a multicenter, prospective, observational study in France (2005-2006). Crit Care Med 2009; 37(5):1612–8.

36. Yende S, van der Poll T, Lee M, et al. The influence of pre-existing diabetes mellitus on the host immune response and outcome of pneumonia: analysis of two multicentre cohort studies. Thorax 2010;65(10):870–7.

37. Pittet D, Thievent B, Wenzel RP, et al. Importance of pre-existing co-morbidities for prognosis of septicemia in critically ill patients. Intensive Care Med 1993; 19(5):265–72.

38. Centers for Disease Control and Prevention (CDC). Chronic obstructive pulmonary disease among adults—United States, 2011. MMWR Morb Mortal Wkly Rep 2012;23(61):938–43.

39. Holguin F, Folch E, Redd SC, et al. Comorbidity and mortality in COPD-related hospitalizations in the United States, 1979 to 2001. Chest 2005;128(4):2005–11.

40. Curkendall SM, DeLuise C, Jones JK, et al. Cardiovascular disease in patients with chronic obstructive pulmonary disease, Saskatchewan Canada cardiovascular disease in COPD patients. Ann Epidemiol 2006;16(1):63–70.

41. Aaron SD, Vandemheen KL, Fergusson D, et al. Tiotropium in combination with placebo, salmeterol, or fluticasone-salmeterol for treatment of chronic obstructive pulmonary disease: a randomized trial. Ann Intern Med 2007;146(8): 545–55.

42. Rohde G, Wiethege A, Borg I, et al. Respiratory viruses in exacerbations of chronic obstructive pulmonary disease requiring hospitalisation: a case-control study. Thorax 2003;58(1):37–42.

43. Mohan A, Chandra S, Agarwal D, et al. Prevalence of viral infection detected by PCR and RT-PCR in patients with acute exacerbation of COPD: a systematic review. Respirology 2010;15(3):536–42.

44. Papi A, Bellettato CM, Braccioni F, et al. Infections and airway inflammation in chronic obstructive pulmonary disease severe exacerbations. Am J Respir Crit Care Med 2006;173(10):1114–21.
45. Sethi S, Evans N, Grant BJ, et al. New strains of bacteria and exacerbations of chronic obstructive pulmonary disease. N Engl J Med 2002;347(7): 465–71.
46. Chatila WM, Thomashow BM, Minai OA, et al. Comorbidities in chronic obstructive pulmonary disease. Proc Am Thorac Soc 2008;5(4):549–55.
47. Mullerova H, Chigbo C, Hagan GW, et al. The natural history of community-acquired pneumonia in COPD patients: a population database analysis. Respir Med 2012;106(8):1124–33.
48. Almirall J, Bolibar I, Serra-Prat M, et al. New evidence of risk factors for community-acquired pneumonia: a population-based study. Eur Respir J 2008;31(6):1274–84.
49. Nannini L, Cates CJ, Lasserson TJ, et al. Combined corticosteroid and long-acting beta-agonist in one inhaler versus placebo for chronic obstructive pulmonary disease. Cochrane Database Syst Rev 2007;(4):CD003794.
50. Liapikou A, Polverino E, Ewig S, et al. Severity and outcomes of hospitalised community-acquired pneumonia in COPD patients. Eur Respir J 2012;39(4): 855–61.
51. Molinos L, Clemente MG, Miranda B, et al. Community-acquired pneumonia in patients with and without chronic obstructive pulmonary disease. J Infect 2009;58(6):417–24.
52. Rello J, Rodriguez A, Torres A, et al. Implications of COPD in patients admitted to the intensive care unit by community-acquired pneumonia. Eur Respir J 2006; 27(6):1210–6.
53. Marrie TJ. Bacteraemic pneumococcal pneumonia: a continuously evolving disease. J Infect 1992;24(3):247–55.
54. Arancibia F, Bauer TT, Ewig S, et al. Community-acquired pneumonia due to gram-negative bacteria and Pseudomonas aeruginosa: incidence, risk, and prognosis. Arch Intern Med 2002;162(16):1849–58.
55. Rello J, Ausina V, Ricart M, et al. Risk factors for infection by Pseudomonas aeruginosa in patients with ventilator-associated pneumonia. Intensive Care Med 1994;20(3):193–8.
56. Al-Dorzi HM, El-Saed A, Rishu AH, et al. The results of a 6-year epidemiologic surveillance for ventilator-associated pneumonia at a tertiary care intensive care unit in Saudi Arabia. Am J Infect Control 2012;40(9):794–9.
57. Celis R, Torres A, Gatell JM, et al. Nosocomial pneumonia. A multivariate analysis of risk and prognosis. Chest 1988;93(2):318–24.
58. Makris D, Desrousseaux B, Zakynthinos E, et al. The impact of COPD on ICU mortality in patients with ventilator-associated pneumonia. Respir Med 2011; 105(7):1022–9.
59. Nseir S, Di Pompeo C, Soubrier S, et al. Impact of ventilator-associated pneumonia on outcome in patients with COPD. Chest 2005;128(3):1650–6.
60. American Thoracic Society, Infectious Diseases Society of America. Guidelines for the management of adults with hospital-acquired, ventilator-associated, and healthcare-associated pneumonia. Am J Respir Crit Care Med 2005;171(4): 388–416.
61. Guinea J, Torres-Narbona M, Gijon P, et al. Pulmonary aspergillosis in patients with chronic obstructive pulmonary disease: incidence, risk factors, and outcome. Clin Microbiol Infect 2010;16(7):870–7.

62. He H, Ding L, Li F, et al. Clinical features of invasive bronchial-pulmonary aspergillosis in critically ill patients with chronic obstructive respiratory diseases: a prospective study. Crit Care 2011;15(1):R5.

63. Valles J, Mesalles E, Mariscal D, et al. A 7-year study of severe hospital-acquired pneumonia requiring ICU admission. Intensive Care Med 2003; 29(11):1981–8.

64. Nevez G, Jounieaux V, Linas MD, et al. High frequency of *Pneumocystis carinii* sp.f. hominis colonization in HIV-negative patients. J Eukaryot Microbiol 1997; 44(6):36S.

65. Probst M, Ries H, Schmidt-Wieland T, et al. Detection of *Pneumocystis carinii* DNA in patients with chronic lung diseases. Eur J Clin Microbiol Infect Dis 2000;19(8):644–5.

66. Morris A, Sciurba FC, Lebedeva IP, et al. Association of chronic obstructive pulmonary disease severity and *Pneumocystis* colonization. Am J Respir Crit Care Med 2004;170(4):408–13.

67. Cilloniz C, Ewig S, Menendez R, et al. Bacterial co-infection with H1N1 infection in patients admitted with community acquired pneumonia. J Infect 2012;65(3): 223–30.

68. Vollenweider DJ, Jarrett H, Steurer-Stey CA, et al. Antibiotics for exacerbations of chronic obstructive pulmonary disease. Cochrane Database Syst Rev 2012;(12):CD010257.

69. Mandell LA, Wunderink RG, Anzueto A, et al. Infectious Diseases Society of America/American Thoracic Society consensus guidelines on the management of community-acquired pneumonia in adults. Clin Infect Dis 2007;44(Suppl 2): S27–72.

70. Herbrecht R, Denning DW, Patterson TF, et al. Voriconazole versus amphotericin B for primary therapy of invasive aspergillosis. N Engl J Med 2002;347(6):408–15.

71. Singh N, Limaye AP, Forrest G, et al. Combination of voriconazole and caspofungin as primary therapy for invasive aspergillosis in solid organ transplant recipients: a prospective, multicenter, observational study. Transplantation 2006; 81(3):320–6.

72. Rello J, Rodriguez A, Ibanez P, et al. Intensive care adult patients with severe respiratory failure caused by Influenza A (H1N1)v in Spain. Crit Care 2009; 13(5):R148.

73. Birnkrant D, Cox E. The emergency use authorization of peramivir for treatment of 2009 H1N1 influenza. N Engl J Med 2009;361(23):2204–7.

74. Confalonieri M, Urbino R, Potena A, et al. Hydrocortisone infusion for severe community-acquired pneumonia: a preliminary randomized study. Am J Respir Crit Care Med 2005;171(3):242–8.

75. Dransfield MT, Rowe SM, Johnson JE, et al. Use of beta blockers and the risk of death in hospitalised patients with acute exacerbations of COPD. Thorax 2008; 63(4):301–5.

76. Lahousse L, Loth DW, Joos GF, et al. Statins, systemic inflammation and risk of death in COPD: the Rotterdam study. Pulm Pharmacol Ther 2012;26:212–7.

77. Mortensen EM, Copeland LA, Pugh MJ, et al. Impact of statins and ACE inhibitors on mortality after COPD exacerbations. Respir Res 2009;10:45.

78. Donaldson GC, Wedzicha JA. COPD exacerbations. 1: epidemiology. Thorax 2006;61(2):164–8.

79. Messer B, Griffiths J, Baudouin SV. The prognostic variables predictive of mortality in patients with an exacerbation of COPD admitted to the ICU: an integrative review. QJM 2012;105(2):115–26.

80. Fine MJ, Auble TE, Yealy DM, et al. A prediction rule to identify low-risk patients with community-acquired pneumonia. N Engl J Med 1997;336(4):243–50.
81. Restrepo MI, Mortensen EM, Pugh JA, et al. COPD is associated with increased mortality in patients with community-acquired pneumonia. Eur Respir J 2006; 28(2):346–51.
82. Samarakoon P, Soubani A. Invasive pulmonary aspergillosis in patients with COPD: a report of five cases and systematic review of the literature. Chron Respir Dis 2008;5(1):19–27.
83. Coresh J, Byrd-Holt D, Astor BC, et al. Chronic kidney disease awareness, prevalence, and trends among U.S. adults, 1999 to 2000. J Am Soc Nephrol 2005; 16(1):180–8.
84. Gilbertson DT, Liu J, Xue JL, et al. Projecting the number of patients with end-stage renal disease in the United States to the year 2015. J Am Soc Nephrol 2005;16(12):3736–41.
85. Sarnak MJ, Jaber BL. Mortality caused by sepsis in patients with end-stage renal disease compared with the general population. Kidney Int 2000;58(4): 1758–64.
86. Collins AJ, Foley RN, Gilbertson DT, et al. The state of chronic kidney disease, ESRD, and morbidity and mortality in the first year of dialysis. Clin J Am Soc Nephrol 2009;4(Suppl 1):S5–11.
87. Berman SJ, Johnson EW, Nakatsu C, et al. Burden of infection in patients with end-stage renal disease requiring long-term dialysis. Clin Infect Dis 2004; 39(12):1747–53.
88. Astor BC, Eustace JA, Powe NR, et al. Type of vascular access and survival among incident hemodialysis patients: the Choices for Healthy Outcomes in Caring for ESRD (CHOICE) Study. J Am Soc Nephrol 2005;16(5):1449–55.
89. Tanriover B, Carlton D, Saddekni S, et al. Bacteremia associated with tunneled dialysis catheters: comparison of two treatment strategies. Kidney Int 2000; 57(5):2151–5.
90. Saad TF. Bacteremia associated with tunneled, cuffed hemodialysis catheters. Am J Kidney Dis 1999;34(6):1114–24.
91. Solomon LR, Cheesbrough JS, Ebah L, et al. A randomized double-blind controlled trial of taurolidine-citrate catheter locks for the prevention of bacteremia in patients treated with hemodialysis. Am J Kidney Dis 2010;55(6):1060–8.
92. Ghali JR, Bannister KM, Brown FG, et al. Microbiology and outcomes of peritonitis in Australian peritoneal dialysis patients. Perit Dial Int 2011;31(6):651–62.
93. Khan A, Rigatto C, Verrelli M, et al. High rates of mortality and technique failure in peritoneal dialysis patients after critical illness. Perit Dial Int 2012; 32(1):29–36.
94. Viasus D, Garcia-Vidal C, Cruzado JM, et al. Epidemiology, clinical features and outcomes of pneumonia in patients with chronic kidney disease. Nephrol Dial Transplant 2011;26(9):2899–906.
95. Stryjewski ME, Szczech LA, Benjamin DK Jr, et al. Use of vancomycin or first-generation cephalosporins for the treatment of hemodialysis-dependent patients with methicillin-susceptible *Staphylococcus aureus* bacteremia. Clin Infect Dis 2007;44(2):190–6.
96. Mermel LA, Allon M, Bouza E, et al. Clinical practice guidelines for the diagnosis and management of intravascular catheter-related infection: 2009 update by the Infectious Diseases Society of America. Clin Infect Dis 2009;49(1):1–45.
97. Wiggins KJ, Craig JC, Johnson DW, et al. Treatment for peritoneal dialysis-associated peritonitis. Cochrane Database Syst Rev 2008;(1):CD005284.

98. Li PK, Szeto CC, Piraino B, et al. Peritoneal dialysis-related infections recommendations: 2010 update. Perit Dial Int 2010;30(4):393–423.

99. Yahav D, Rozen-Zvi B, Gafter-Gvili A, et al. Antimicrobial lock solutions for the prevention of infections associated with intravascular catheters in patients undergoing hemodialysis: systematic review and meta-analysis of randomized, controlled trials. Clin Infect Dis 2008;47(1):83–93.

100. O'Grady NP, Alexander M, Burns LA, et al. Summary of recommendations: guidelines for the Prevention of Intravascular Catheter-related Infections. Clin Infect Dis 2011;52(9):1087–99.

101. Gupta R, Plantinga LC, Fink NE, et al. Statin use and sepsis events [corrected] in patients with chronic kidney disease. J Am Med Assoc 2007;297(13): 1455–64.

102. Arulkumaran N, Annear NM, Singer M. Patients with end-stage renal disease admitted to the intensive care unit: systematic review. Br J Anaesth 2013;110: 13–20.

103. Sood MM, Miller L, Komenda P, et al. Long-term outcomes of end-stage renal disease patients admitted to the ICU. Nephrol Dial Transplant 2011;26(9): 2965–70.

104. Sarnak MJ, Jaber BL. Pulmonary infectious mortality among patients with end-stage renal disease. Chest 2001;120(6):1883–7.

105. Perez Fontan M, Rodriguez-Carmona A, Garcia-Naveiro R, et al. Peritonitis-related mortality in patients undergoing chronic peritoneal dialysis. Perit Dial Int 2005;25(3):274–84.

106. Arabi Y, Ahmed QA, Haddad S, et al. Outcome predictors of cirrhosis patients admitted to the intensive care unit. Eur J Gastroenterol Hepatol 2004;16(3): 333–9.

107. Borzio M, Salerno F, Piantoni L, et al. Bacterial infection in patients with advanced cirrhosis: a multicentre prospective study. Dig Liver Dis 2001;33(1): 41–8.

108. Cheruvattath R, Balan V. Infections in patients with end-stage liver disease. J Clin Gastroenterol 2007;41(4):403–11.

109. Rolando N, Harvey F, Brahm J, et al. Prospective study of bacterial infection in acute liver failure: an analysis of fifty patients. Hepatology 1990;11(1):49–53.

110. Canabal JM, Kramer DJ. Management of sepsis in patients with liver failure. Curr Opin Crit Care 2008;14(2):189–97.

111. Fernandez J, Navasa M, Gomez J, et al. Bacterial infections in cirrhosis: epidemiological changes with invasive procedures and norfloxacin prophylaxis. Hepatology 2002;35(1):140–8.

112. Caly WR, Strauss E. A prospective study of bacterial infections in patients with cirrhosis. J Hepatol 1993;18(3):353–8.

113. Pinzello G, Simonetti RG, Craxi A, et al. Spontaneous bacterial peritonitis: a prospective investigation in predominantly nonalcoholic cirrhotic patients. Hepatology 1983;3(4):545–9.

114. European Association for the Study of the Liver. EASL clinical practice guidelines on the management of ascites, spontaneous bacterial peritonitis, and hepatorenal syndrome in cirrhosis. J Hepatol 2010;53(3):397–417.

115. Wiest R, Garcia-Tsao G. Bacterial translocation (BT) in cirrhosis. Hepatology 2005;41(3):422–33.

116. Park YH, Lee HC, Song HG, et al. Recent increase in antibiotic-resistant microorganisms in patients with spontaneous bacterial peritonitis adversely affects the clinical outcome in Korea. J Gastroenterol Hepatol 2003;18(8):927–33.

117. Angeloni S, Leboffe C, Parente A, et al. Efficacy of current guidelines for the treatment of spontaneous bacterial peritonitis in the clinical practice. World J Gastroenterol 2008;14(17):2757–62.

118. Cholongitas E, Papatheodoridis GV, Lahanas A, et al. Increasing frequency of gram-positive bacteria in spontaneous bacterial peritonitis. Liver Int 2005; 25(1):57–61.

119. Reuken PA, Pletz MW, Baier M, et al. Emergence of spontaneous bacterial peritonitis due to enterococci—risk factors and outcome in a 12-year retrospective study. Aliment Pharmacol Ther 2012;35(10):1199–208.

120. Arabi YM, Dara SI, Memish Z, et al. Antimicrobial therapeutic determinants of outcomes from septic shock among patients with cirrhosis. Hepatology 2012; 56(6):2305–15.

121. Viasus D, Garcia-Vidal C, Castellote J, et al. Community-acquired pneumonia in patients with liver cirrhosis: clinical features, outcomes, and usefulness of severity scores. Medicine (Baltimore) 2011;90(2):110–8.

122. Rongey C, Lim NH, Runyon BA. Cellulitis in patients with cirrhosis and edema: an under-recognized complication currently more common than spontaneous bacterial peritonitis. Open Gastroenterol J 2008;2:24–7.

123. Lee CC, Chi CH, Lee NY, et al. Necrotizing fasciitis in patients with liver cirrhosis: predominance of monomicrobial gram-negative bacillary infections. Diagn Microbiol Infect Dis 2008;62(2):219–25.

124. Muldrew KL, Miller RR, Kressin M, et al. Necrotizing fasciitis from *Vibrio vulnificus* in a patient with undiagnosed hepatitis and cirrhosis. J Clin Microbiol 2007; 45(3):1058–62.

125. Molle I, Thulstrup AM, Svendsen N, et al. Risk and case fatality rate of meningitis in patients with liver cirrhosis. Scand J Infect Dis 2000;32(4): 407–10.

126. Su CM, Chang WN, Tsai NW, et al. Clinical features and outcome of community-acquired bacterial meningitis in adult patients with liver cirrhosis. Am J Med Sci 2010;340(6):452–6.

127. Pauwels A, Pines E, Abboura M, et al. Bacterial meningitis in cirrhosis: review of 16 cases. J Hepatol 1997;27(5):830–4.

128. Cabellos C, Viladrich PF, Ariza J, et al. Community-acquired bacterial meningitis in cirrhotic patients. Clin Microbiol Infect 2008;14(1):35–40.

129. Mizrahi M, Adar T, Shouval D, et al. Endotipsitis-persistent infection of transjugular intrahepatic portosystemic shunt: pathogenesis, clinical features and management. Liver Int 2010;30(2):175–83.

130. Wiest R, Krag A, Gerbes A. Spontaneous bacterial peritonitis: recent guidelines and beyond. Gut 2012;61(2):297–310.

131. Tunkel AR, Hartman BJ, Kaplan SL, et al. Practice guidelines for the management of bacterial meningitis. Clin Infect Dis 2004;39(9):1267–84.

132. Chaudhuri A, Martinez-Martin P, Kennedy PG, et al. EFNS guideline on the management of community-acquired bacterial meningitis: report of an EFNS Task Force on acute bacterial meningitis in older children and adults. Eur J Neurol 2008;15(7):649–59.

133. Sort P, Navasa M, Arroyo V, et al. Effect of intravenous albumin on renal impairment and mortality in patients with cirrhosis and spontaneous bacterial peritonitis. N Engl J Med 1999;341(6):403–9.

134. Arabi YM, Aljumah A, Dabbagh O, et al. Low-dose hydrocortisone in patients with cirrhosis and septic shock: a randomized controlled trial. CMAJ 2010; 182(18):1971–7.

135. Garg V, Garg H, Khan A, et al. Granulocyte colony-stimulating factor mobilizes CD34(+) cells and improves survival of patients with acute-on-chronic liver failure. Gastroenterology 2012;142(3):505–512 e1.
136. Mohammad RA. Use of granulocyte colony-stimulating factor in patients with severe sepsis or septic shock. Am J Health Syst Pharm 2010;67(15):1238–45.
137. Nobre SR, Cabral JE, Gomes JJ, et al. In-hospital mortality in spontaneous bacterial peritonitis: a new predictive model. Eur J Gastroenterol Hepatol 2008; 20(12):1176–81.
138. McMurray JJ, Petrie MC, Murdoch DR, et al. Clinical epidemiology of heart failure: public and private health burden. Eur Heart J 1998;19(Suppl P):P9–16.
139. Roger VL, Go AS, Lloyd-Jones DM, et al. Heart disease and stroke statistics—2012 update: a report from the American Heart Association. Circulation 2012;125(1):e2–220.
140. Cui W, Zhao H, Lu X, et al. Factors associated with death in hospitalized pneumonia patients with 2009 H1N1 influenza in Shenyang, China. BMC Infect Dis 2010;10:145.
141. Maisel A, Neath SX, Landsberg J, et al. Use of procalcitonin for the diagnosis of pneumonia in patients presenting with a chief complaint of dyspnoea: results from the BACH (Biomarkers in Acute Heart Failure) trial. Eur J Heart Fail 2012; 14(3):278–86.
142. Liteplo AS, Marill KA, Villen T, et al. Emergency thoracic ultrasound in the differentiation of the etiology of shortness of breath (ETUDES): sonographic B-lines and N-terminal pro-brain-type natriuretic peptide in diagnosing congestive heart failure. Acad Emerg Med 2009;16(3):201–10.
143. Thomsen RW, Kasatpibal N, Riis A, et al. The impact of pre-existing heart failure on pneumonia prognosis: population-based cohort study. J Gen Intern Med 2008;23(9):1407–13.

Overview of Severe *Clostridium difficile* Infection

Stephen R. Eaton, MD, John E. Mazuski, MD, PhD*

KEYWORDS

- *Clostridium difficile* • *Clostridium difficile* colitis • Pseudomembranous colitis
- Nosocomial infection

KEY POINTS

- *Clostridium difficile* infection constitutes a significant burden both to the individual patient as well as to the health care system in general.
- In recent years, there has been an increase not only in the incidence but also the severity of *C difficile*-associated disease.
- The management of patients with severe and fulminant *C difficile* infection presents a challenge for the critical care practitioner.
- Surgical intervention may be necessary for severe, and particularly for fulminant *C difficile* colitis.

BACKGROUND

Complications associated with the use of antibiotics began to be recognized soon after their introduction into clinical practice. Antibiotic-associated diarrhea was noted to be a relatively common complication. A distinct type of antibiotic-associated diarrhea, characterized by colonic mucosal necrosis and the development of pseudomembranes came to be recognized as pseudomembranous colitis. In 1978, the bacterial-pathogen causing, antibiotic-associated pseudomembranous colitis was identified as *Clostridium difficile*.[1]

C difficile is an anaerobic, spore-forming, gram-positive bacillus. It is capable of causing a wide spectrum of disease, ranging from asymptomatic colonization to fulminant colitis requiring surgical intervention.[2–5] Morbidity rates associated with *C difficile* infection have been reported to be as high as 80%, with mortality rates of up to 8%.[6,7]

Disclosures: S.R. Eaton has nothing to disclose. Research grants: Astra-Zeneca, Cubist, Merck; advisory boards: Bayer, Cubist, Forest Laboratories, Pfizer; consultant: Astra-Zeneca, Pfizer; speaker: Merck, Pfizer (J.E. Mazuski).
Section of Acute and Critical Care Surgery, Department of Surgery, Washington University School of Medicine, Campus Box 8109, 660 South Euclid Avenue, St Louis, MO 63110-1093, USA
* Corresponding author.
E-mail address: mazuskij@wustl.edu

Crit Care Clin 29 (2013) 827–839
http://dx.doi.org/10.1016/j.ccc.2013.06.004
0749-0704/13/$ – see front matter © 2013 Elsevier Inc. All rights reserved.

The problem of C difficile-associated disease is growing worse rather than better. Of particular note, the severity of illness also seems to be increasing. Thus, knowledge of this disease, including its clinical manifestations, diagnosis, and potential treatment options is imperative in managing the critically ill patient population. Treatment is multifaceted, including pharmacologic therapy; supportive care; and, in a small number of patients, surgical intervention. Surgical consultation is particularly important in critically ill patients who have severe or fulminant C difficile colitis.

EPIDEMIOLOGY

C difficile is the most common pathogen associated with nosocomial infectious diarrhea in hospitalized patients.[8] The overall incidence and severity of C difficile-associated disease seems to be increasing. From 1990 to 2000, the reported incidence of severe or fulminant C difficile colitis increased from 0% to 3.2%.[9] The increase in the number and severity of infections can likely be attributed to the emergence of more pathogenic strains, particularly the B1/NAP1/O27 strain.[2–5] This strain produces large amounts of C difficile toxins A and B, which are thought to mediate the disease process. In addition to significant morbidity and mortality, C difficile infection is associated with significant increases in hospital lengths of stay and costs.[5,10] In the United States, the costs were estimated to be approximately $3.7 billion in 2003[11] and $4.8 billion in 2008.[12]

C difficile-associated disease is usually a health care-associated infection, typically acquired during hospitalization.[13,14] The most common risk factor for acquisition of this disease is prior antibiotic exposure. The antibiotics most strongly implicated in this acquisition are clindamycin, cephalosporins, some penicillins, and fluoroquinolones; the latter are particularly associated with acquisition of the highly toxigenic B1/NAP1/O27 strain.[3,6,15–19] Other risk factors for C difficile-associated disease include age, immunosuppression, and possibly use of gastric acid–suppressing medications.[16,20,21]

CLINICAL MANIFESTATIONS

Infection with C difficile can range from asymptomatic colonization to fulminant disease. The most common symptom of patients with C difficile infection is diarrhea; the number of bowel movements may be highly variable.[22,23] Patient may also have more acute symptoms, such as abdominal pain and cramping, which usually indicates somewhat more severe disease. Systemic signs of infection, such as fever and leukocytosis are also evidence of more severe disease. Some of these more severely ill patients manifest signs of severe sepsis, with evidence of organ dysfunction due to hypoperfusion, or frank septic shock, with evidence of hypotension.[3,22,24] In critically ill patients with severe sepsis or septic shock without an obvious source, infection with C difficile should be included in the differential diagnosis. It is important to realize that many of these critically ill patients will not present with diarrhea as a predominant symptom, because of severe colonic dysmotility induced by the infection.[8]

Because of the wide spectrum of clinical manifestations of C difficile-associated disease, several systems have been developed to stratify disease severity and provide some rationale for directing therapy. For the intensivist, it may be particularly important to recognize symptoms and signs of severe disease so that patients who would benefit from the care provided in an ICU are appropriately admitted to that facility. As mentioned above, greater severity of disease is associated with evidence of increasing hypovolemia and systemic signs of infection, with the greatest severity of disease (classified as fulminant or life-threatening) found in patients with catastrophic abdominal emergencies or signs of severe sepsis or septic shock. A stratification scheme for symptomatic *C difficile*-associated disease, based on that used at the authors' institution, is shown in **Table 1**. This scheme is largely based on expert opinion and the best available evidence for differentiating severity of disease in *C difficile* colitis.[25–30]

DIAGNOSIS

Laboratory examinations are used to confirm the diagnosis of suspected *C difficile*-associated disease. However, these examinations should only be obtained in symptomatic patients. Random testing for *C difficile* will lead to significant numbers of false-positive tests as well as identification of patients for whom no treatment is needed. There is also generally no need for follow-up testing in patients who are asymptomatic after treatment of *C difficile* infection.

The most common test used by clinical laboratories in the United States is the stool ELISA or enzyme immunoassay for *C difficile* toxins A and/or B. These tests are used because of their speed and technical ease.[31,32] The sensitivity of these tests varies somewhat, although it seems to be improving as technical improvements in the assays are made. Clinicians should be aware of the rates of false-negative results at their institutions; if these are relatively high, it may be prudent to test more than one sample in a symptomatic patient.[33,34] However, with most current generation of tests having a sensitivity greater than 95%, the value of repeat testing is questionable.

Polymerase chain reaction (PCR) testing is becoming more common for the detection of *C difficile* infection. These tests identify the presence of DNA encoding

Table 1
Grading of severity of *C difficile* infection

C difficile Infection Severity	Any of the Following
Mild	• Diarrhea with minimal constitutional symptoms
Moderate	• Need for IV fluid administration to maintain intravascular volume • Abdominal pain • Mucus or blood in the stool • White blood cell count of 10,000–20,000 cells/mm^3, in the absence of another cause of leukocytosis • Fever to 38.0°–38.5°C • Endoscopic evidence of pseudomembranous colitis
Severe	• Severe fluid deficits with a need for large amounts of IV fluids to restore intravascular volume (if the patient has prolonged hypotension or if vasopressors are used, the disease is considered fulminant) • Ileus • Peritoneal signs • White blood cell >20,000 cells/mm^3 in the absence of another cause • Fever >38.5°C
Fulminant (life-threatening)	• Perforation • Toxic megacolon • Colonic ischemia • Significant colonic bleeding requiring ongoing transfusion • Severe sepsis (evidence of organ dysfunction due to sepsis) • Septic shock (hypotension with use of vasopressors despite adequate fluid resuscitation) in the absence of another cause

the *C difficile* toxins. A theoretical disadvantage is that the test could identify microorganisms that do not express the toxins. Older PCR analyses were labor intensive and required significant sample preparation. Current generation PCR testing seems to be highly sensitive and specific for toxigenic strains of *C difficile*, and may eventually supplant immunologic tests for toxins.[35]

In some patients, particularly those with more fulminant disease who may not produce significant amounts of stool, radiological examinations and endoscopic visualization may be important tools to establish the diagnosis of *C difficile* colitis. Endoscopic visualization of the colonic mucosa may show pseudomembrane formation, which is virtually pathognomonic for *C difficile* infection. A significant number of patients (20%–33%) have pseudomembranes proximal to the sigmoid colon and cannot be diagnosed using flexible sigmoidoscopy; thus, full colonoscopy may be a better option to improve sensitivity. Nonetheless, the overall false-negative rate for endoscopic visualization of pseudomembranes is estimated to be approximately 10% to 25%.[15] There are also risks with this study because many patients will have a dilated colon susceptible to perforation. This test is typically reserved for patients who are severely ill and need rapid assessment to determine if they have a potential infection due to *C difficile*.[6,33,36–39]

Radiologic tests, chiefly CT scan of the abdomen and pelvis may be used to support a diagnosis of *C difficile* colitis. Radiological findings suggestive of *C difficile* colitis include pericolonic stranding, an accordion sign (high-attenuation oral contrast in the colonic lumen alternating with low-attenuating inflamed mucosa), and the double-halo or target sign (varying degrees of attenuation of the intravenous [IV] contrast material in the mucosa caused by submucosal inflammation and hyperemia). This imaging modality may also be used to diagnose complications related to *C difficile* colitis, such as pneumatosis or perforation.[12,26,27]

GENERAL MANAGEMENT AND SUPPORTIVE CARE

The treatment of *C difficile* infection generally involves supportive care and antimicrobial therapy directed against the causative organism. The need for significant medical intervention in patients with *C difficile*-associated disease is dictated to a large degree by the acuity of the disease. In asymptomatic patients who are incidentally found to be carriers of the organism, antibiotic therapy is generally not indicated. In patients who have only mild symptoms, dietary modification and discontinuation of prior antimicrobial therapy may be all that is needed. However, for patients with more severe disease, supportive care and pathogen-directed antimicrobial therapy are generally indicated.

In patients with moderate disease, supportive care usually includes IV fluid administration to replace intravascular and extravascular fluid deficits, which may be sizable depending on the degree of diarrheal fluid losses. Electrolyte disturbances should be corrected as well. Patients with severe disease may need to be observed and treated in an ICU. Virtually every patient with fulminant disease will meet criteria for admission to an ICU. Appropriate fluid resuscitation is the mainstay of supportive therapy in patients with severe or fulminant disease. For patients meeting criteria of severe sepsis or septic shock, early goal-directed therapy should be provided, as outlined in the recently updated Surviving Sepsis Campaign guidelines.[40] Volume deficits may be massive in patients with septic shock due to fulminant *C difficile* infection, and large quantities of IV fluids may need to be administered to restore intravascular volume and permit a decrease in the amounts of vasopressors being administered. Patients who continue to show signs of inadequate tissue perfusion despite restoration of intravascular volume should be considered for surgical treatment of the disease (see later discussion).

ANTIMICROBIAL MANAGEMENT

In patients with presumed or confirmed *C difficile* infection, the first treatment modality is to limit antibiotic exposure. If a patients is receiving empiric antimicrobial therapy other than for the *C difficile* infection, those agents should be discontinued if no other source of infection has been identified. If it is considered necessary to continue antibiotics for treatment of another infection, it is reasonable to select a regimen that does not include agents considered high-risk for inducing *C difficile*-associated disease, such as ampicillin, cephalosporins, clindamycin, or fluoroquinolones. It should be noted that this hypothesis has not been verified clinically.

Metronidazole and oral vancomycin are the mainstays of specific antibiotic therapy for *C difficile* infection. The dosing regimens are listed in **Table 2**. Oral vancomycin has been approved by the Food and Drug Administration for this indication, but oral metronidazole has not.[41] However, oral metronidazole was shown to have similar efficacy to oral vancomycin in the treatment of patients with primarily mild or moderate disease.[42] Oral vancomycin is not appreciably absorbed from the gastrointestinal tract and generally reaches relatively high concentrations in the colonic lumen, which are sufficient to treat this microorganism. However, IV vancomycin, which does not reach significant luminal concentrations, has little use in the treatment of *C difficile*-associated disease. Both IV and oral metronidazole reach relatively high concentration within the colonic mucosa, so use of the IV formulation may be justified, although it has not been tested in prospective trials for this indication.[43]

For severe or fulminant *C difficile* colitis, oral vancomycin seems to be preferable to metronidazole.[44–46] However, in patients who have a paralytic ileus or poor gastrointestinal motility, it is uncertain if oral vancomycin will actually reach the colon and achieve therapeutic concentrations in the colonic lumen. Alternatives ways of introducing vancomycin directly into the colon have been suggested. Vancomycin can be introduced into the distal colon via enema. However, very little drug will likely reach the proximal colon with this approach, unless a large volume (500–1000 mL) is administered. There is also likely little value in administration of vancomycin via enema to patients who have significant diarrhea because the drug is unlikely to be retained.[41,47] An alternative method of achieving high vancomycin concentrations within the colon is infusion through a catheter placed colonoscopically into the cecum[48] or via the distal limb of a loop ileostomy placed surgically.[49] However, there is a risk of iatrogenic

Table 2		
Antibiotic therapy for severe *C difficile* infection		
Pharmacologic Therapy	**Indication**	**Dose**
Vancomycin po	Severe *C difficile* infection	125–500 mg po q 6 h × 10–14 d
Vancomycin enema	Severe *C difficile* infection with colonic ileus and no improvement with po vancomycin	500 mg in 100 mL q 6–8 h
Metronidazole IV	Potential adjunctive therapy in severe *C difficile* infection with colonic ileus	500 mg IV p8 h × 10–14 d
Fidaxomicin	For patients with recurrent *C difficile* infection or patients who fail to respond to vancomycin	200 mg po bid

perforation of the severely inflamed colon with colonoscopy and ileostomy placement requires a surgical procedure. Unfortunately, there is not yet high-quality evidence supporting these methods of direct delivery of vancomycin into the colon.

In patients with severe or fulminant disease, metronidazole, usually IV, is frequently added to the regimen. There is no evidence supporting an additive or synergistic effect of metronidazole with vancomycin for the treatment of C difficile colitis. However, if there are concerns that adequate luminal concentrations of vancomycin might not be achieved, use of this additional agent seems rational. However, as with alternative methods of vancomycin delivery, high-quality evidence demonstrating the benefit of this approach is lacking.

A new agent now available with activity against Clostridium difficile is fidaxomicin, a macrolide antibiotic.[50] Fidaxomicin (200 mg twice daily) was shown to be as effective as oral vancomycin (125 mg every 6 hours) in phase III studies.[34] In one study of subjects with C difficile infection who were also being treated with systemic antibiotics for a concomitant infection, fidaxomicin cure rates were higher and recurrence rates were lower when compared with vancomycin therapy.[51] This expensive agent has not been evaluated in critically ill patients with severe or fulminant disease.

SURGICAL INDICATIONS AND THERAPY

Severe C difficile colitis, and even some fulminant disease, is generally treated with supportive care and antibiotics. Only a small number of patients with this disease (0.4%–3.5%) undergo operative interventions.[32] Nonetheless, most patients with severe or fulminant disease should undergo evaluation by a surgeon relatively early in their course, for consideration of potential operative treatment should medical therapy prove ineffective.

The most common operative procedure performed for treatment of C difficile colitis is subtotal colectomy. This usually results in control of the source of the infection. However, this large and morbid operative procedure is performed in quite ill patients. Thus, mortality and complication rates are high. In a series of studies, the operative mortality of subjects undergoing surgical intervention for C difficile colitis was approximately 50%.[48,52,53]

The indications for surgical treatment of patients with C difficile colitis are ambiguous. The unpredictability of the clinical course of the disease, as well as the desire to avoid a highly morbid and potentially lethal procedure, frequently leads to delays in surgical intervention. This may lead to an attempt to perform an operation on a patient whose overall prognosis is poor due to progressive disease.[54]

In general, the decision to pursue surgical therapy should be based on an assessment of the acuity of the disease, as well as its trajectory. For a few patients with fulminant or life-threatening colitis, the decision to carry out operative management is straightforward.[48,49,52] Patients presenting with toxic megacolon, colonic perforation, refractory bleeding, or colonic necrosis as a result of colonic ischemia are unlikely to survive with medical management alone. If operative therapy is deferred, institution of patient comfort measures is generally appropriate. In patients with septic shock or severe sepsis due to of C difficile colitis, early surgical intervention should also be considered. The authors' recommendation is to proceed with operative treatment if there is no improvement in systemic perfusion after 24 hours of aggressive medical treatment of sepsis and institution of appropriate antibiotic management of the C difficile infection.

In patients with severe, but not fulminant disease, failure to improve with optimal medical treatment is a further indication for surgical therapy. However, there is no consensus on what constitutes a failure to improve or how long medical therapy should be undertaken before declaring the patient a failure of medical management. Many clinicians continue medical therapy for a minimum of 3 to 5 days before considering surgical treatment, as long as the patient is not deteriorating.

Nonetheless, there are studies that also suggest that earlier colectomy is associated with an overall decrease in the mortality of patients with severe *C difficile* colitis.[46,54–58] Various investigators have attempted to use risk factor analyses to identify patients with severe or fulminant *C difficile* colitis who are appropriate candidates for early surgical intervention. Based on a review of several studies, Osman and colleagues described a set of clinical characteristics, including older age, which that they thought could be used in selecting appropriate patients with *C difficile* colitis for earlier surgical intervention.[59] Older age predicts a poorer outcome, as shown in data by Gash and colleagues[60] who favored earlier operative intervention in such patients. In their series, only 29% of their patients undergoing operative intervention for *C difficile* colitis were younger than the age of 65. Greenstein and colleagues[25] also described a list of criteria that portended a poor prognosis in patients with fulminant *C difficile* colitis and that could be used as potential criteria to select patients for operative intervention. In this multivariate analysis, a white blood cell count greater than 16,000 cells/mm^3, operative intervention within the past 30 days, a history of inflammatory bowel disease, and past treatment with intravenous immunoglobulin were found to be significant risk factors predicting an adverse outcome. Unfortunately, there are no prospective multicenter trials validating use of these or other criteria for selection of patients for surgical treatment of *C difficile*-associated disease.

As noted above, standard operative intervention for *C difficile* colitis is usually subtotal colectomy with end ileostomy. Older studies indicated that survival was higher in patients this procedure than in those who undergoing a lesser procedure, such as segmental resection of the colon or catheter drainage of the colon.[61–67] Recently, however, some investigators have revisited the use of less invasive and morbid procedures for the surgical treatment of severe or fulminant disease. There are reports now on the use of laparoscopic loop ileostomy with colonic lavage and subsequent vancomycin infusion for the treatment of severe *C difficile*-associated disease. In 2011, Neal and colleagues[68] published a report on 42 subjects who were treated with diverting loop ileostomy and colonic lavage. Thirty-five of these procedures were done laparoscopically. Mortality in these subjects was 19%, compared with 50% in matched historical controls. The colon was preserved in 39 of these subjects. At the University of Pittsburgh, Carchman and colleagues[69] outlined the current practice in which exploratory laparoscopy, loop ileostomy, and colonic lavage is used as the primary treatment of patients with severe, complicated *C difficile* infections. The confirmation that less morbid procedures are effective for the treatment of patients with this disease could help resolve some of the ambiguity regarding appropriate indications for surgical management of *C difficile* colitis.

OTHER TREATMENTS

In addition to the acute problems associated with the initial *C difficile* infection, it has been increasingly recognized that many patients develop recurrent episodes of the disease. A recurrence rate of 15% to 35% is commonly reported.[70–72] Initial recurrences are usually treated with antibiotic therapy similar to that used for the initial episode because resistance of the microorganism to antibiotics does not seem to lead to recurrence.[29] Subsequent recurrences tend to be much more refractory to treatment. Use of prolonged and pulse therapy with vancomycin has been advocated for some of these patients. The administration of probiotics has been proposed as a measure to prevent recurrent *C difficile*. In prospective trials, however, only *Saccharomyces boulardii* has shown to be effective in this regard.[73–75] There is also renewed interest in the use of fecal microbiota transplantation for the treatment of recurrent *C difficile* infection.[76–78] Anecdotal data and case series suggest a decrease in the recurrence of *C difficile* infection using this approach. There is a case report by Neemann and colleagues[7] that describes the use fecal transplantation in a severely ill, immunocompromised patient who had resolution of symptoms without needing operative intervention. IV immunoglobulin has also been studied as a treatment adjunct for patients with recurrent or severe *C difficile* infections[79]; however, its overall role in therapy remains obscure.

PREVENTION

Preventing the spread of *C difficile* to susceptible patients is the key to reducing the morbidity and mortality of *C difficile* infections. Adherence to standard infection control practices will greatly help to avoid further dissemination of the disease within an institution. Practices generally recommended for prevention of spread of *C difficile* include strict isolation of patients with the disease and cleaning of contaminated environmental surfaces using bleach or other sporicidal solutions.[80–82] It is also important to acknowledge that following the principles of antimicrobial stewardship should reduce the risk of collateral damage, such as infection with *C difficile*.[83–85] Thus, reducing unnecessary use of antibiotics is also an important measure in reducing the incidence of this disease. Ultimately, primary prevention using such measures will be the most effective and least expensive manner in which to limit the burden of this disease.

SUMMARY

Severe *C difficile* colitis is associated with a high morbidity and mortality. Overall mortality is reported to be approximately 8%,[6,7] with much higher mortality rates reported in patients with fulminant disease who are typically treated in the ICU setting. For patients undergoing operative treatment, mortality rates have ranged from 34% to 80%.[48,52,55,59,60,86–89]

In recent years, there has been an increase not only in the incidence of *C difficile* infection but also in the severity of the disease.[17,89–91] A major contributing factor is the emergence of hypervirulent strains of the microorganism, particularly the BI/NAP1/O27 strain. This particular variant has been isolated in several outbreaks in the United States and Europe, and now seems endemic in many facilities.[2–5]

The management of patients with severe and fulminant *C difficile* infection presents a challenge for the critical care practitioner. The mainstay of treatment remains supportive measures, particularly maintenance of adequate intravascular volume and treatment of sepsis when needed, and pathogen-directed antibiotic therapy. For severe *C difficile* infections, oral or luminal vancomycin is generally the preferred agent. IV metronidazole may be used as a supplement to this in selected patients, particularly when it is uncertain if oral or enteral vancomycin will actually reach the site of infection in the colon. Other antimicrobial agents have now been released or are in investigation, but none of these agents has been evaluated for patients with severe or fulminant disease. Adjuncts to antimicrobial therapy have also been proposed, but there is no clear role for these agents at this time.

A key question for the intensivist is if and when surgical intervention should be considered for a patient with severe or fulminant *C difficile* colitis. This decision is quite complex. Opting for early therapy may subject large numbers of patients to an unnecessary operation. On the other hand, waiting until the disease is clearly refractory to treatment can lead to high mortality rates. The confirmation that procedures less morbid than subtotal colectomy, such as laparoscopic exploration and loop ileostomy placement, could provide adequate source control for this disease would make this decision somewhat less difficult and potentially lead to early surgical intervention, with a reduction in the morbidity and mortality of severe disease.

Overall, *C difficile* infection constitutes a significant burden on the health care system, both in terms of the disease it inflicts on individual patients as well as the appreciable costs it places on the system. This certainly applies to the ICU, as the number of critically ill patients with this disease has increased significantly. Ultimately, primary prevention is the key to reducing this burden. Adherence to the principles of infection control and antibiotic stewardship could go a long way in furthering the goal of primary prevention. Thus, the critical care practitioner should not only be prepared to treat patients with this potentially lethal disease, but also to advocate for appropriate measures designed to reduce the dissemination of this nosocomially acquired microorganism.

REFERENCES

1. Bartlett JG, Chang TW, Gurwith M, et al. Antibiotic-associated pseudomembranous colitis due to toxin-producing clostridia. N Engl J Med 1978;298(10):531–4.
2. McDonald LC, Killgore GE, Thompson A, et al. An epidemic, toxin gene-variant strain of *Clostridium difficile*. N Engl J Med 2005;353(23):2433–41.
3. Sunenshine RH, McDonald LC. *Clostridium difficile*-associated disease: new challenges from an established pathogen. Cleve Clin J Med 2006;73(2):187–97.
4. Bartlett JG, Perl TM. The new *Clostridium difficile*—what does it mean? N Engl J Med 2005;353(23):2503–5.
5. Hubert B, Loo VG, Bourgault AM, et al. A portrait of the geographic dissemination of the *Clostridium difficile* North American pulsed-field type 1 strain and the epidemiology of *C. difficile*-associated disease in Quebec. Clin Infect Dis 2007; 44(2):238–44.
6. Kelly CP, Pothoulakis C, LaMont JT. *Clostridium difficile* colitis. N Engl J Med 1994;330(4):257–62.
7. Neemann K, Eichele DD, Smith PW, et al. Fecal microbiota transplantation for fulminant *Clostridium difficile* infection in an allogeneic stem cell transplant patient. Transpl Infect Dis 2012;14(6):E161–5.
8. Bartlett JG, Gerding DN. Clinical recognition and diagnosis of *Clostridium difficile* infection. Clin Infect Dis 2008;46(Suppl 1):S12–8.
9. Gould CV, McDonald LC. Bench-to-bedside review: *Clostridium difficile* colitis. Crit Care 2008;12(1):203.
10. Drudy D, Calabi E, Kyne L, et al. Human antibody response to surface layer proteins in *Clostridium difficile* infection. FEMS Immunol Med Microbiol 2004;41(3): 237–42.
11. Wilkins TD, Lyerly DM. *Clostridium difficile* testing: after 20 years, still challenging. J Clin Microbiol 2003;41(2):531–4.
12. Dubberke ER, Olsen MA. Burden of *Clostridium difficile* on the healthcare system. Clin Infect Dis 2012;55(Suppl 2):S88–92.
13. McFarland LV, Mulligan ME, Kwok RY, et al. Nosocomial acquisition of *Clostridium difficile* infection. N Engl J Med 1989;320(4):204–10.
14. Simor AE, Bradley SF, Strausbaugh LJ, et al. Clostridium difficile in long-term-care facilities for the elderly. Infect Control Hosp Epidemiol 2002;23(11): 696–703.

15. Reinke CM, Messick CR. Update on *Clostridium difficile*-induced colitis, Part 1. Am J Hosp Pharm 1994;51(14):1771–81.
16. Bignardi GE. Risk factors for *Clostridium difficile* infection. J Hosp Infect 1998; 40(1):1–15.
17. Loo VG, Poirier L, Miller MA, et al. A predominantly clonal multi-institutional outbreak of *Clostridium difficile*-associated diarrhea with high morbidity and mortality. N Engl J Med 2005;353(23):2442–9.
18. Gaynes R, Rimland D, Killum E, et al. Outbreak of *Clostridium difficile* infection in a long-term care facility: association with gatifloxacin use. Clin Infect Dis 2004; 38(5):640–5.
19. Pepin J, Saheb N, Coulombe MA, et al. Emergence of fluoroquinolones as the predominant risk factor for *Clostridium difficile*-associated diarrhea: a cohort study during an epidemic in Quebec. Clin Infect Dis 2005;41(9):1254–60.
20. Aronsson B, Mollby R, Nord CE. Diagnosis and epidemiology of *Clostridium difficile* enterocolitis in Sweden. J Antimicrob Chemother 1984;14(Suppl D): 85–95.
21. Yolken RH, Bishop CA, Townsend TR, et al. Infectious gastroenteritis in bone-marrow-transplant recipients. N Engl J Med 1982;306(17):1010–2.
22. Mogg GA, Keighley MR, Burdon DW, et al. Antibiotic-associated colitis—a review of 66 cases. Br J Surg 1979;66(10):738–42.
23. Bartlett JG, Taylor NS, Chang T, et al. Clinical and laboratory observations in *Clostridium difficile* colitis. Am J Clin Nutr 1980;33(Suppl 11):2521–6.
24. Tedesco FJ, Barton RW, Alpers DH. Clindamycin-associated colitis. A prospective study. Ann Intern Med 1974;81(4):429–33.
25. Greenstein AJ, Byrn JC, Zhang LP, et al. Risk factors for the development of fulminant *Clostridium difficile* colitis. Surgery 2008;143(5):623–9.
26. Ananthakrishnan AN. *Clostridium difficile* infection: epidemiology, risk factors and management. Nat Rev Gastroenterol Hepatol 2010;8(1):17–26.
27. Butala P, Divino CM. Surgical aspects of fulminant *Clostridium difficile* colitis. Am J Surg 2010;200(1):131–5.
28. Fekety R, Shah AB. Diagnosis and treatment of *Clostridium difficile* colitis. JAMA 1993;269(1):71–5.
29. Gerding DN, Muto CA, Owens RC Jr. Treatment of *Clostridium difficile* infection. Clin Infect Dis 2008;46(Suppl 1):S32–42.
30. Cohen SH, Gerding DN, Johnson S, et al. Clinical practice guidelines for *Clostridium difficile* infection in adults: 2010 update by the Society for Healthcare Epidemiology of America (SHEA) and the infectious diseases society of America (IDSA). Infect Control Hosp Epidemiol 2010;31(5):431–55.
31. Ticehurst JR, Aird DZ, Dam LM, et al. Effective detection of toxigenic *Clostridium difficile* by a two-step algorithm including tests for antigen and cytotoxin. J Clin Microbiol 2006;44(3):1145–9.
32. Fekety R. Guidelines for the diagnosis and management of *Clostridium difficile*-associated diarrhea and colitis. American College of Gastroenterology, Practice Parameters Committee. Am J Gastroenterol 1997;92(5):739–50.
33. Manabe YC, Vinetz JM, Moore RD, et al. *Clostridium difficile* colitis: an efficient clinical approach to diagnosis. Ann Intern Med 1995;123(11):835–40.
34. National Clostridium difficile Standards Group. National *Clostridium difficile* Standards Group: report to the Department of Health. J Hosp Infect 2004; 56(Suppl 1):1–38.
35. Wren MW, Sivapalan M, Kinson R, et al. Laboratory diagnosis of clostridium difficile infection. An evaluation of tests for faecal toxin, glutamate dehydrogenase,

lactoferrin and toxigenic culture in the diagnostic laboratory. Br J Biomed Sci 2009;66(1):1–5.

36. Mylonakis E, Ryan ET, Calderwood SB. *Clostridium difficile*-associated diarrhea: a review. Arch Intern Med 2001;161(4):525–33.

37. Tedesco FJ, Corless JK, Brownstein RE. Rectal sparing in antibiotic-associated pseudomembranous colitis: a prospective study. Gastroenterology 1982;83(6): 1259–60.

38. Tedesco FJ. Antibiotic associated pseudomembranous colitis with negative proctosigmoidoscopy examination. Gastroenterology 1979;77(2):295–7.

39. Kirkpatrick ID, Greenberg HM. Evaluating the CT diagnosis of *Clostridium difficile* colitis: should CT guide therapy? AJR Am J Roentgenol 2001;176(3):635–9.

40. Dellinger RP, Levy MM, Rhodes A, et al. Surviving sepsis campaign: international guidelines for management of severe sepsis and septic shock: 2012. Crit Care Med 2013;41(2):580–637.

41. Shetler K, Nieuwenhuis R, Wren SM, et al. Decompressive colonoscopy with intracolonic vancomycin administration for the treatment of severe pseudomembranous colitis. Surg Endosc 2001;15(7):653–9.

42. Teasley DG, Gerding DN, Olson MM, et al. Prospective randomised trial of metronidazole versus vancomycin for *Clostridium-difficile*-associated diarrhoea and colitis. Lancet 1983;2(8358):1043–6.

43. Bolton RP, Culshaw MA. Faecal metronidazole concentrations during oral and intravenous therapy for antibiotic associated colitis due to *Clostridium difficile*. Gut 1986;27(10):1169–72.

44. Bartlett JG. The case for vancomycin as the preferred drug for treatment of *Clostridium difficile* infection. Clin Infect Dis 2008;46(10):1489–92.

45. Zar FA, Bakkanagari SR, Moorthi KM, et al. A comparison of vancomycin and metronidazole for the treatment of *Clostridium difficile*-associated diarrhea, stratified by disease severity. Clin Infect Dis 2007;45(3):302–7.

46. Louie TJ, Gerson M, Johnson L, et al. Results of a phase III trial comparing tolevamer, vancomycin and metronidazole for the treatment of *Clostridium difficile*-associated diarrhea (CDAD) [abstract K-425a]. In: 47th Interscience Conference on Antimicrobial Agents and Chemotherapy. Washington, DC: ASM Press; 2007.

47. Haaga JR, Bick RJ, Zollinger RM Jr. CT-guided percutaneous catheter cecostomy. Gastrointest Radiol 1987;12(2):166–8.

48. Longo WE, Mazuski JE, Virgo KS, et al. Outcome after colectomy for *Clostridium difficile* colitis. Dis Colon Rectum 2004;47(10):1620–6.

49. Olivas AD, Umanskiy K, Zuckerbraun B, et al. Avoiding colectomy during surgical management of fulminant *Clostridium difficile* colitis. Surg Infect (Larchmt) 2010;11(3):299–305.

50. Gerber M, Ackermann G. OPT-80, a macrocyclic antimicrobial agent for the treatment of *Clostridium difficile* infections: a review. Expert Opin Investig Drugs 2008;17(4):547–53.

51. Mullane KM, Miller MA, Weiss K, et al. Efficacy of fidaxomicin versus vancomycin as therapy for *Clostridium difficile* infection in individuals taking concomitant antibiotics for other concurrent infections. Clin Infect Dis 2011;53(5):440–7.

52. Dallal RM, Harbrecht BG, Boujoukas AJ, et al. Fulminant *Clostridium difficile*: an underappreciated and increasing cause of death and complications. Ann Surg 2002;235(3):363–72.

53. Lamontagne F, Labbe AC, Haeck O, et al. Impact of emergency colectomy on survival of patients with fulminant *Clostridium difficile* colitis during an epidemic caused by a hypervirulent strain. Ann Surg 2007;245(2):267–72.

54. Pepin J, Vo TT, Boutros M, et al. Risk factors for mortality following emergency colectomy for fulminant *Clostridium difficile infection*. Dis Colon Rectum 2009; 52(3):400–5.

55. Byrn JC, Maun DC, Gingold DS, et al. Predictors of mortality after colectomy for fulminant *Clostridium difficile* colitis. Arch Surg 2008;143(2):150–4 [discussion: 155].

56. Markelov A, Livert D, Kohli H. Predictors of fatal outcome after colectomy for fulminant *Clostridium difficile* Colitis: a 10-year experience. Am Surg 2011; 77(8):977–80.

57. Ali SO, Welch JP, Dring RJ. Early surgical intervention for fulminant pseudomembranous colitis. Am Surg 2008;74(1):20–6.

58. Sailhamer EA, Carson K, Chang Y, et al. Fulminant *Clostridium difficile* colitis: patterns of care and predictors of mortality. Arch Surg 2009;144(5):433–9 [discussion: 439–40].

59. Osman KA, Ahmed MH, Hamad MA, et al. Emergency colectomy for fulminant *Clostridium difficile colitis*: Striking the right balance. Scan J Gastroenterol 2011; 46(10):1222–7.

60. Gash K, Brown E, Pullyblank A. Emergency subtotal colectomy for fulminant *Clostridium difficile* colitis—is a surgical solution considered for all patients? Ann R Coll Surg Engl 2010;92(1):56–60.

61. Morris JB, Zollinger RM Jr, Stellato TA. Role of surgery in antibiotic-induced pseudomembranous enterocolitis. Am J Surg 1990;160(5):535–9.

62. Drapkin MS, Worthington MG, Chang TW, et al. *Clostridium difficile* colitis mimicking acute peritonitis. Arch Surg 1985;120(11):1321–2.

63. Lipsett PA, Samantaray DK, Tam ML, et al. Pseudomembranous colitis: a surgical disease? Surgery 1994;116(3):491–6.

64. Synnott K, Mealy K, Merry C, et al. Timing of surgery for fulminating pseudomembranous colitis. Br J Surg 1998;85(2):229–31.

65. Medich DS, Lee KK, Simmons RL, et al. Laparotomy for fulminant pseudomembranous colitis. Arch Surg 1992;127(7):847–52 [discussion: 852–3].

66. Bradbury AW, Barrett S. Surgical aspects of *Clostridium difficile* colitis. Br J Surg 1997;84(2):150–9.

67. Grundfest-Broniatowski S, Quader M, Alexander F, et al. *Clostridium difficile* colitis in the critically ill. Dis Colon Rectum 1996;39(6):619–23.

68. Neal MD, Alverdy JC, Hall DE, et al. Diverting loop ileostomy and colonic lavage: An alternative to total abdominal colectomy for the treatment of severe, complicated Clostridium difficile associated disease. Ann Surg 2011;254(3):423–9.

69. Carchman EH, Peitzman AB, Simmons RL, et al. The role of acute care surgery in the treatment of severe, complicated Clostridium difficile-associated disease. J Trauma Acute Care Surg 2012;73(4):789–800.

70. McFarland LV, Surawicz CM, Rubin M, et al. Recurrent *Clostridium difficile* disease: epidemiology and clinical characteristics. Infect Control Hosp Epidemiol 1999;20(1):43–50.

71. Barbut F, Richard A, Hamadi K, et al. Epidemiology of recurrences or reinfections of *Clostridium difficile*-associated diarrhea. J Clin Microbiol 2000;38(6): 2386–8.

72. Pepin J, Alary ME, Valiquette L, et al. Increasing risk of relapse after treatment of *Clostridium difficile* colitis in Quebec, Canada. Clin Infect Dis 2005;40(11):1591–7.

73. McFarland LV, Surawicz CM, Greenberg RN, et al. A randomized placebo-controlled trial of *Saccharomyces boulardii* in combination with standard antibiotics for *Clostridium difficile* disease. JAMA 1994;271(24):1913–8.

74. Surawicz CM, McFarland LV, Greenberg RN, et al. The search for a better treatment for recurrent *Clostridium difficile* disease: use of high-dose vancomycin combined with *Saccharomyces boulardii*. Clin Infect Dis 2000;31(4):1012–7.

75. McFarland LV. Meta-analysis of probiotics for the prevention of antibiotic associated diarrhea and the treatment of *Clostridium difficile* disease. Am J Gastroenterol 2006;101(4):812–22.

76. Brandt LJ. American Journal of Gastroenterology lecture: intestinal microbiota and the role of fecal microbiota transplant (FMT) in treatment of *C. difficile* infection. Am J Gastroenterol 2013;108(2):177–85.

77. Postigo R, Kim JH. Colonoscopic versus nasogastric fecal transplantation for the treatment of *Clostridium difficile* infection: a review and pooled analysis. Infection 2012;40(6):643–8.

78. van Nood E, Vrieze A, Nieuwdorp M, et al. Duodenal infusion of donor feces for recurrent *Clostridium difficile*. N Engl J Med 2013;368(5):407–15.

79. Leav BA, Blair B, Leney M, et al. Serum anti-toxin B antibody correlates with protection from recurrent *Clostridium difficile* infection (CDI). Vaccine 2010; 28(4):965–9.

80. Samore MH, Venkataraman L, DeGirolami PC, et al. Clinical and molecular epidemiology of sporadic and clustered cases of nosocomial Clostridium difficile diarrhea. Am J Med 1996;100(1):32–40.

81. Garner JS. Guideline for isolation precautions in hospitals. The Hospital Infection Control Practices Advisory Committee. Infect Control Hosp Epidemiol 1996; 17(1):53–80.

82. Sehulster L, Chinn RY. Guidelines for environmental infection control in health-care facilities. Recommendations of CDC and the Healthcare Infection Control Practices Advisory Committee (HICPAC). MMWR Recomm Rep 2003; 52(RR-10):1–42.

83. Raymond DP, Kuehnert MJ, Sawyer RG. Preventing antimicrobial-resistant bacterial infections in surgical patients. Surg Infect (Larchmt) 2002;3(4):375–85.

84. Paterson DL. "Collateral damage" from cephalosporin or quinolone antibiotic therapy. Clin Infect Dis 2004;38(Suppl 4):S341–5.

85. Rice LB. The Maxwell Finland lecture: for the duration-rational antibiotic administration in an era of antimicrobial resistance and *Clostridium difficile*. Clin Infect Dis 2008;46(4):491–6.

86. Klipfel AA, Schein M, Fahoum B, et al. Acute abdomen and *Clostridium difficile* colitis: still a lethal combination. Dig Surg 2000;17(2):160–3.

87. Koss K, Clark MA, Sanders DS, et al. The outcome of surgery in fulminant *Clostridium difficile* colitis. Colorectal Dis 2006;8(2):149–54.

88. Chan S, Kelly M, Helme S, et al. Outcomes following colectomy for *Clostridium difficile* colitis. Int J Surg 2009;7(1):78–81.

89. Khanna S, Pardi DS, Aronson SL, et al. The epidemiology of community-acquired *Clostridium difficile* infection: a population-based study. Am J Gastroenterol 2013;107(1):89–95.

90. Muto CA, Pokrywka M, Shutt K, et al. A large outbreak of *Clostridium difficile*-associated disease with an unexpected proportion of deaths and colectomies at a teaching hospital following increased fluoroquinolone use. Infect Control Hosp Epidemiol 2005;26(3):273–80.

91. Pepin J, Valiquette L, Alary ME, et al. *Clostridium difficile*-associated diarrhea in a region of Quebec from 1991 to 2003: a changing pattern of disease severity. CMAJ 2004;171(5):466–72.

Vancomycin-Resistant Enterococci

Ethan Rubinstein, MD*, Yoav Keynan, MD

KEYWORDS

- Vancomycin • Enterococcus • Resistant pathogen • Gram-positive cocci
- Critical care • Infection

KEY POINTS

- Enterococcal infection can be caused by vancomycin-susceptible strains, mainly *E faecalis*, and vancomycin-resistant strains, mainly *E faecium*.
- In penicillin and/or ampicillin and aminoglycoside-susceptible strains, the treatment of severe infections (eg, bacteremia, endocarditis, meningitis, brain abscess) is based on the combination of a β-lactam or vancomycin with an aminoglycoside to achieve bactericidal activity.

INTRODUCTION

Enterococci, formerly called group D streptococci, have become resistant to many antibiotic agents, including vancomycin. Vancomycin-resistant enterococci (VRE) infections are increasingly common and difficult to treat, appearing usually as long-lasting hospital outbreaks that present tremendous challenges for infection control.

Enterococci are equipped with a variety of intrinsic (ie, naturally occurring) antibiotic resistances, but are also capable of acquiring new resistance genes and/or mutations. The combination of high-level resistance to ampicillin, vancomycin, and aminoglycosides is now common with hospital-acquired *Enterococcus faecium*.

The major infections caused by enterococci in general and VRE in particular include urinary tract infections (UTI), wound infections, intraabdominal infections secondary to a perforated viscous or after surgery, cholecystitis, bacteremia, endocarditis, and rarely meningitis. UTI can be cured with a single (bacteriostatic) agent whereas bacteremia, endocarditis, and meningitis require a bactericidal agent or drug combination. Some acute infections due to VRE may be treated to resolution, although in some cases colonization may persist indefinitely.

Disclosure: Dr Ethan Rubinstein is an advisor to Trius and Bayer.
Section of Infectious Diseases, Department of Internal Medicine and Medical Microbiology, University of Manitoba, 543-645 Bannatyne Ave, Basic Medical Building, Winnipeg, Manitoba R3E 0J9, Canada
* Corresponding author.
E-mail address: rubinste@cc.umanitoba.ca

CLINICAL SYNDROMES
Bacteremia and Endocarditis

Bacteremia due to VRE is rarely primary, common sources are the gastrointestinal tract, the urinary tract, intravascular catheters, and wounds or burns. The relative risk of endocarditis in patients with *E faecalis* bacteremia is higher than with *E faecium*, particularly if the infection is community-acquired and there is an underlying valvulopathy. Septic shock in the setting of enterococcal bacteremia is uncommon and it should raise suspicion for a polymicrobial infection.

On occasion, *Enterococcus* represents a contaminant on blood culture. For that reason, positive blood cultures warrant therapy only when the clinical risk of infection and/or the adverse clinical impact of infection is high. Antimicrobial therapy for enterococcal bacteremia is warranted when there are more than two positive blood cultures, a single positive blood culture accompanied by signs of sepsis, or a single positive blood culture together with a positive enterococcal culture from another usually sterile site. In the setting of a single positive blood culture for an *Enterococcus*, particularly *E faecalis*, in a patient with preexisting prosthetic heart valve, the authors favor initiating treatment while awaiting results of additional blood cultures; other clinicians favor withholding therapy pending these results. The optimal duration of therapy in this setting is not known; 1 to 2 weeks may be appropriate for uncomplicated bacteremia. For circumstances in which an intravascular catheter is the likely source of the bacteremia, catheter removal alone may be sufficient. However, if febrile, most patients should be empirically started on antibiotics and, after additional cultures are obtained, such therapy can generally be discontinued after 5 to 7 days if symptoms have resolved. Although several studies suggest that there is no advantage of combination therapy compared with monotherapy, some investigators favor combination therapy in the setting of valvulopathy and/or critical illness.[1,2] The optimal duration of antimicrobial therapy for treatment of enterococcal bacteremia is uncertain. For uncomplicated infection, 5 to 7 days of therapy is likely adequate. Therapy should be extended in the setting of sustained high-grade bacteremia and in the setting of a prosthetic valve, even in the absence of echocardiography evidence for vegetation.

Meningitis

Enterococci rarely cause meningitis in normal adults. Most cases of enterococcal meningitis occur in patients with head trauma, neurosurgery, intraventricular or intrathecal catheters, or anatomic defects of the central nervous system.[3] Enterococcal meningitis is also seen in the setting of endocarditis, AIDS, hematologic malignancies, and in neonatal sepsis, in association with *Strongyloides* hyperinfection, shunt infection, and so forth.[4,5]

The optimal approach for treatment of enterococcal meningitis is not certain, although most clinicians agree that combination therapy is preferable compared with monotherapy. For patients failing to respond to systemic antibiotics, intraventricular vancomycin, gentamicin, or quinupristin-dalfopristin (if *E faecium*) may be useful. Daptomycin and tigecycline have poor central nervous system penetration and need to be administered intrathecally.[5]

Treatment of enterococcal meningitis caused by VRE *E faecium* is a difficult challenge; intravenous (IV) linezolid or IV plus intraventricular quinupristin-dalfopristin are reasonable choices. Although experience is limited, daptomycin has also been administered by the intraventricular route. If the organism is susceptible, rifampin may also be a useful adjunctive agent.[5-7]

NEWER ANTI-ENTEROCOCCAL ANTIBIOTICS

Newer anti-enterococcal antibiotics include linezolid, a bacteriostatic, synthetic oxazolidinone antibiotic that binds to the peptidyl transferase center of the 50S ribosome, preventing peptide bond formation, and thus the addition of new amino acids (**Table 1**). In one study, linezolid was associated with cure of 81% of 500 subjects with VRE infections[8] and, in another report, the cure rate of VRE bacteremia and other severe infections in organ-transplant subjects was 63%.[9] Resistance development during therapy with linezolid has been reported to result in clinical failure.[10] Adverse effects of linezolid use, particularly in courses exceeding 28 days, include thrombocytopenia (particularly common in the setting of renal failure), anemia, lactic acidosis, peripheral neuropathy, and ocular toxicity. When administered with serotonergic agents, linezolid can induce serotonin syndrome due to its inhibition of monoamine oxidase.[11] Blood counts and serum chemistries should be monitored at least weekly during linezolid therapy.

Daptomycin is a cyclic lipopeptide bactericidal antibiotic that causes depolarization of the bacterial cell membrane. The daily dose for severe infections is 8 to 12 mg/kg IV once daily (for skin and soft tissue infections the dose is 4 mg/kg). Several investigators favor the use of daptomycin for treatment of *E faecium* infections that are vancomycin-resistant. The daptomycin minimal inhibitory concentrations (MICs) for *E faecium* are higher than for *E faecalis*. There are no FDA-approved daptomycin MIC breakpoints for *E faecium*, but it has been suggested that an MIC greater than 4 μg/mL is the cutoff for nonsusceptible isolates. Patients receiving daptomycin should be evaluated regularly for clinical evidence of myopathy, through serial measurements of serum creatine kinase (at least weekly). The drug should be discontinued in patients with symptomatic myopathy and creatine phosphokinase (CPK) greater than or equal to five times the upper limit of normal (ULN) or in asymptomatic patients with CPK greater than or equal to ten times ULN.[12]

Tigecycline is a glycylcycline antibiotic derived from minocycline with in vitro activity against many gram-positive pathogens (ie, methicillin-resistant *Staphylococcus aureus* [MRSA], VRE, and penicillin-resistant *Streptococcus pneumoniae*), many gram-negatives (excluding *Pseudomonas*, *Proteus*, *Providencia*, and *Morganella* species), anaerobes, and atypical species. Although tigecycline is not approved by the Food and Drug Administration (FDA) for VRE infections, it seems that VRE would also be susceptible to tigecycline, based on in vitro and animal model data.[13] The usual dose is 100 mg IV loading dose followed by 50 mg twice a day. Some concerns were raised by clinical trials with tigecycline in skin and soft tissue infections, pneumonia, and intraabdominal infections showing higher mortality in tigecycline-treated patients than in the control arms. Major adverse effects include nausea and vomiting. Tigecycline may be useful for patients with VRE infection who are intolerant of other agents or when VRE are present along with other pathogens that are susceptible to tigecycline. It may also be useful in the setting of renal insufficiency. Tigecycline has been used in combination with high-dose daptomycin for severe nonresponding VRE infections.[14]

Quinupristin-dalfopristin is a mixture of streptogramin antibiotics with FDA approval for the treatment of VRE *E faecium* infections. It has poor activity against *E faecalis*. Central venous access requirements and adverse effects limit the use of quinupristin-dalfopristin. Adverse effects include metabolic interactions, severe myalgias, arthralgias, nausea, and hyperbilirubinemia. The agent should be administered into a central vein at a dose 22.5 mg/kg every 24 hours divided into three equal doses.

Teicoplanin is not available in North America but is in use in Europe and some South American countries. It has in vitro activity against *E gallinarum* and *E casseliflavus*

Table 1
New agents active against VRE

Antibiotic	Activity	Indications	Dose in Patients Without Renal Failure	Common Adverse Effects
Linezolid	Bacteriostatic	HAP or VAP, ABSSI, gram-positive bacteremia	600 mg q 12 h	Anemia, thrombocytopenia, leukopenia, serotonin syndrome, mitochondrial toxicity, peripheral & optic neuropathy
Daptomycin	Bactericidal	ABSSI, bacteremia, endocarditis, not pneumonia	4–12 mg/kg OD	Increase in muscle enzymes, eosinophilic pneumonia
Telavancin	Bactericidal	HAP or VAP, ABSSI	10 mg/kg OD	Renal toxicity
Tedizolid[a]	Bactericidal	ABSSI	200 mg OD either IV or PO	—
Teicoplanin[b]	Bactericidal	Similar to vancomycin	6–12 mg/kg for 3 doses, then OD	Similar to vancomycin except no renal toxicity
Tigecycline	Bacteriostatic	ABSSI, intraabdominal infections, not HAP or VAP	100 mg loading dose, then 50 mg q 12 h	Nausea, vomiting, liver-function abnormalities
Quinupristin-dalfopristin	Bacteriostatic	ABSSI, bacteremia, HAP	7.5 mg/kg q 8 h IV	Thrombophlebitis, myalgia, arthralgia, nausea, hyperbilirubinemia

Abbreviations: ABSSI, acute bacterial skin and soft tissue infection; HAP, hospital-acquired pneumonia; OD, once daily; VAP, ventilator associated-pneumonia.
[a] Not marketed yet.
[b] Not used in North America.

(vanC VRE) as well as most vanB-type VRE, although it is rarely active against vanA-type VRE. Some vanB VRE mutant strains are constitutively resistant to teicoplanin. For patients with normal renal function, teicoplanin should be administered with a loading dose of 6 to 12 mg/kg every 12 hours for three doses (for serious infections), followed by 6 mg/kg to 12 mg/kg every 24 hours (for serious infections). The addition of an aminoglycoside, in the absence of high-level resistance should be considered to reduce the emergence of vanB mutants resistant to teicoplanin.

Telavancin is a lipoglycopeptide that is more potent than vancomycin against enterococci (eg, the MIC_{90} is 0.12 µg/mL), with little to no increase in MICs against vanB strains. For vanA strains, the MIC_{90} has been reported as 4 to 16 µg/mL.

ANTIBIOTIC RESISTANCE
β-Lactam and Aminoglycosides

Serious enterococcal infections, including endocarditis, cannot be treated with penicillin alone because this agent is not for enterococci. An aminoglycoside must be added to make the treatment bactericidal and, therefore, is the optimal clinical response. Recently, enterococci have acquired resistance to these agents because of mutations (eg, causing high-level resistance to streptomycin and/or to fluoroquinolones) or the acquisition of new genes carrying resistance elements. The *Enterococcus* is capable of accepting and donating resistance genes, plasmids, and transposomes by multiple mechanisms.

E faecalis, the more susceptible of the two predominant enterococcal species, is usually inhibited by 1 to 4 µg/mL of ampicillin and 2 to 8 µg/mL of penicillin; the comparable MICs for *E faecium* are 8 to 32 µg/mL. However, *E faecium* strains that are much more highly resistant to ampicillin have emerged. This high-level resistance to ampicillin is due to a nonpenicillinase mechanism. Recently, a trend toward much higher levels of resistance has been observed among nosocomial isolates, with some strains failing to be inhibited by 256 µg/mL of ampicillin or more.[15] The intrinsic resistance of *E faecium* seems to be due to the presence of a cell wall synthesis enzyme that is relatively resistant to inhibition by penicillin. This low-affinity penicillin-binding protein (PBP) is called PBP5. Higher levels of resistance to β-lactam antibiotics seem to involve increased expression of PBP5, further alterations in the PBP5 protein, and use of a β-lactam insensitive transpeptidase for cell wall synthesis.[16,17]

Enterococci are intrinsically resistant to low-to-moderate levels of aminoglycosides. However, synergism is generally seen when enterococci are exposed to a combination of an aminoglycoside with a cell wall active agent, such as penicillin or vancomycin. With the combination, there is a marked increase in killing (ie, synergy) and a bactericidal effect is achieved.

In addition to the usual increased MICs of aminoglycosides for all enterococci, a characteristic of *E faecium* is higher MICs of tobramycin (MICs 64 to 1000 µg/mL) and resistance to synergism with this aminoglycoside but not with gentamicin. Therefore, with minor exceptions, gentamicin and streptomycin, if available, are the only aminoglycosides that should be considered to achieve synergistic therapy. High-level resistance to both streptomycin and gentamicin abolishes the synergism between gentamicin or streptomycin and a cell wall active agent such as penicillin or vancomycin. Ceftriaxone has been shown to have a synergistic effect mediated by saturation of PBP2 and PBP3 when administered together with ampicillin. In high-level resistance strains causing endocarditis, the combination of ampicillin and ceftriaxone showed a clinical cure rate of 67%—better than any other antibiotic combination.[18]

Vancomycin Resistance

High-level and low-level resistance to glycopeptides can occur in enterococci. Low-level vancomycin resistance occurs with MICs 8 to 16 μg/mL. The MIC used for defining vancomycin susceptibility and resistance in enterococci greater than or equal to 32 μg/mL are vancomycin-susceptible (≤4 μg/mL, vancomycin-resistant). An MIC of 8 to 16 μg/mL is considered vancomycin-intermediate, but vancomycin therapy is not recommended for infections caused by such isolates.

High-level vancomycin resistance is the most problematic resistance of enterococci, because it often appears in strains already highly resistant to ampicillin (primarily E faecium). Vancomycin inhibits enterococci by binding to the D-alanyl-D-alanine (D-Ala-D-Ala) terminus of cell wall precursors, compromising the subsequent enzymatic steps in the synthesis of cell wall. High-level resistance to vancomycin is encoded by different clusters of genes referred to as the vancomycin-resistance gene clusters (eg, vanA, B, D, and M). The result is the replacement of D-Ala-D-Ala-terminus precursors with D-alanyl-D-lactate termini, to which vancomycin binds with significantly lower affinity, increasing the MIC of this antibiotic almost 1000-fold.[19] VanA is the most common type of vancomycin-resistance; it usually mediates higher levels of resistance than other types and causes cross-resistance to teicoplanin. The vanA gene cluster is typically found on a transposon identical or related to Tn1546, which, in turn, is often found within a plasmid.[20–23] The vanA cluster has disseminated to other bacterial species, including clinical isolates of MRSA.

Linezolid Resistance

Linezolid resistance has been reported in clinical isolates of both staphylococci and enterococci. Oxazolidinone resistance among enterococcal isolates has been increasingly documented.[24] Associated with prolonged use of the antibiotic, linezolid resistance was initially described sporadically.[25] It is evident that the emergence of linezolid resistance is associated with the heavy use of this antibiotic; however, linezolid-resistant enterococci have also been isolated from patients without previous exposure to the antibiotic.[26]

Daptomycin Resistance

Resistance to daptomycin has been reported in enterococci, including isolates from patients who have never received this antibiotic.[27] In one patient, the development of daptomycin resistance was directly linked to mutations in genes encoding several enzymes involving phospholipid metabolism as well as a membrane protein.[28]

Quinupristin-Dalfopristin Resistance

Resistance to quinupristin-dalfopristin among E faecium can occur by enzymatic modification, active transport, and target modification.[29] In the United States, some 1% to 2% of enterococci are resistant to quinupristin-dalfopristin. Full resistance in clinical isolates appears to require a combination of mechanisms. However, resistance to dalfopristin alone is sufficient to reduce efficacy of the combined antibiotic and decrease the bactericidal effect. The vatD and vatE genes, which encode acetyltransferases that inactivate dalfopristin, are frequently found in resistant E faecium isolates. These genes are found on transposable genetic elements where they are sometimes associated with the erm genes that confer parallel resistance to streptogramin B-class (quinupristin) compounds.[30] Resistance emerged during quinupristin-dalfopristin therapy in 5 out of 396 subjects with E faecium infections; four of these cases resulted in treatment failure.[31]

Tigecycline Resistance

Resistance to tigecycline has been documented in an *E faecalis* isolate recovered from the urine of a patient who received a prolonged course of tigecycline for nosocomial pneumonia.[32]

Resistant enterococcal infections remain difficult to treat. In some cases, the pathogen cannot be eradicated despite the disappearance of infectious symptoms, including in soft tissue infections, biliary disease, pancreatic abscess, and so forth. Many experts take the position that enterococci on their own can cause only a limited number of infections (eg, UTI and endocarditis) but not abdominal abscesses and soft tissue infections. The authors concur with this notion; therefore, the situation remains unresolved.

EPIDEMIOLOGY

The presence of VRE in Europe was driven by the use of glycopeptides, including avoparcin as a food additive for growth promotion in farm animals, which was subsequently banned by the European Union. In North America, VRE followed Europe but with a different relationship. Multiple epidemics of VRE infection have been described in diverse hospital settings. Currently, VRE is endemic in many large hospitals.[33,34] The rate of hospitalization with VRE in the United States doubled during 2003 to 2006 from 4.60 to 9.48 hospitalizations per 100,000 population.[35] A single VRE clone can spread within an institution. In addition, VRE strains can transfer resistance horizontally to unrelated strains. Both methods of spread can occur simultaneously in a single institution. One report using specific typing method found 45 different profiles in a single medical center where VRE had become endemic.[36] Most VRE hospital isolates are *E faecium*. Resistance was found in 60% of *E faecium* isolates compared with 2% of *E faecalis* blood isolates. Data from the United States show that resistance trends are worsening; 80% of the 987 isolates of *E faecium* and 6.9% of the 1497 isolates of *E faecalis* reported in 2006 and 2007 were vancomycin-resistant.[37] In VRE bacteremia, the prognosis is worse than that of vancomycin-susceptible enterococci. In a meta-analysis of nine studies of enterococcal bloodstream infections, 42% were due to VRE. The mortality rate was significantly higher in patients with VRE compared with vancomycin-susceptible enterococcal isolates (summary odds ratio 2.5, 95% CI 1.9–3.4).[38]

Transmission

VRE colonize the gastrointestinal tract and, owing to fecal shedding, they are found on the skin. Colonization with VRE generally precedes infection, but not all patients with colonization become infected. Persons either colonized or infected with VRE can serve as sources for secondary transmission. Transmission is determined by selective pressure due to antimicrobial use, the proportion of colonized patients, the availability of susceptible patients, and adherence to prevention efforts.[39] Transmission can occur by both direct contact (eg, the hands of health care workers) and indirectly from environmental surfaces. Modes of transmission include rectal electronic thermometers, contaminated surfaces, bedrails, telephone handpieces, EKG leads, and so forth. It has been demonstrated that VRE-contaminated hands and/or gloves of health care personnel can transmit VRE in approximately 10% of contacts with noninfected patients or surfaces.[40] Risk factors for colonization and infection include previous antimicrobial therapy. In the ICU setting, particularly, the risks include use of vancomycin and cephalosporins, as well as long-term ceftazidime,[37,41] multiple agents with a broad-spectrum of activity,[42] and administration of antibiotics active against anaerobic organisms.[43] Risk factors from patient characteristics include hospital stay of greater than or equal to 72 hours, significant underlying comorbidities, invasive devices,[44] colonization pressure, exposure to contaminated surfaces,[37] and residence in long-term care facilities.[45]

VRE colonization is identified using rectal or perirectal swab cultures or stool cultures. The overall sensitivity varies directly with VRE density in stool, from 100% high densities ($\geq$7.5 logs per gram feces) to 0% at low densities ($\leq$4.5 logs per gram). Prior antibiotic exposure and skin colonization with VRE are more common in patients with high stool densities.[46]

Infection Control

Because the treatment of VRE infections is so complicated and rarely successful, infection control measures are of prime importance. These include strict hand hygiene, contact precautions, cohorting of colonized patients, decolonization attempts, surveillance cultures, and source control.

Active Surveillance

Active surveillance reduces transmission of VRE when performed in outbreak settings or in high-risk patient units such as ICUs and hematology-oncology wards.[47] Legislation has been introduced in several states in the United States mandating surveillance cultures to screen all patients for carriage of MRSA and/or VRE. These laws also require treating or offering treatment to carriers and, in some states, segregating the patient from those who test negative. However, there are concerns with this approach.

Colonization suppression refers to reducing the burden of bacteria on the patient's skin by regular application of antiseptic agents, particularly daily bathing of patients with chlorhexidine gluconate, which was found to be superior to soap and water baths and led to significant reduction in the rate of VRE bacteremia.[48]

VRE Management

The optimal treatment of enterococcal infection due to VRE is unsettled (**Table 2**). VRE *E faecalis* are usually susceptible to β-lactam, as are *E gallinarum and E casseliflavus* (which are intrinsically vancomycin-resistant). In contrast, VRE *E faecium* isolates often have concurrent high-level resistance to β-lactam and aminoglycosides. Linezolid and quinupristin-dalfopristin are approved in the United States for use for infections caused by VRE. However, the usefulness of these agents for serious infections like endocarditis is uncertain. Linezolid, daptomycin, and tigecycline have activity against both vancomycin-resistant *E faecalis* and *E faecium*, whereas quinupristin-dalfopristin has activity against *E faecium* only. In addition, newer agents currently in clinical trials may also prove efficacious for VRE infections, including telavancin, tedizolid, dalbavancin, and oritavancin.

The authors believe that for severe infections caused by VRE *E faecium*-resistant to β-lactam and aminoglycosides, therapy should consist of telavancin with or without linezolid as long as the patient's renal function is normal. In patients with compromised renal functions, linezolid alone is currently the only solution.

Regimens for treatment of VRE infections are: (1) for ampicillin-susceptible VRE, (MIC <32 μg/mL), ampicillin-sulbactam 6 to 12 g per 24 hours in 6 equally divided doses or (2) for ampicillin-resistant VRE, high-dose ampicillin 8 to 30 g IV daily. Another option is high-dose linezolid 600 mg twice a day, either orally or IV.

Possible combinations for treating severe VRE infections include quinupristin-dalfopristin with doxycycline (or minocycline) and rifampin[49–52] and the combination of daptomycin with tigecycline.[53]

Table 2
Current suggested treatments for VRE infections

Infection	Pathogen	Suggested First-Line Therapy	Alternative Therapy
Severe Infections (eg, endocarditis, bacteremia, meningitis)	VRE β-lactam & aminoglycoside-susceptible (*E faecalis; E gallinarum; E casseliflavus*)	Ampicillin-sulbactam 6–12 g/24 h divided into 4 doses ± aminoglycoside	High-dose ampicillin (8–30 g) day in 6 doses
	VRE β-lactam & aminoglycoside-resistant (*E faecium*)	Telavancin[a] ± linezolid	Quinupristin-dalfopristin + doxycycline 200 mg/24 h + rifampin 600 mg/24 h
Nonsevere infections: UTI, abdominal abscesses, soft tissue infections, gynecologic infections	VRE β-lactam & aminoglycoside-susceptible (*E faecalis, E gallinarum, E casseliflavus*)	Ampicillin + aminoglycoside	Linezolid Teicoplanin Tigecycline Quinupristin-dalfopristin
	VRE β-lactam & aminoglycoside-resistant (*E faecium*)	Linezolid Teicoplanin Quinupristin-dalfopristin	Tigecycline Teicoplanin

[a] In nonrenal compromised patients (creatinine clearance >30 mL/min).

SUMMARY

VRE infections have spread and have become a daily occurrence in many hospitals. Although most VRE isolates are merely colonizers, some infections, particularly in immune-suppressed individuals or postsurgery patients, do occur. The treatment of VRE severe infections is difficult, nonconventional, and demands the use of antibiotic combinations, whereas UTI and wound infections can be treated with a single, even bacteriostatic, agent.

REFERENCES

1. Graninger W, Ragette R. Nosocomial bacteremia due to *Enterococcus faecalis* without endocarditis. Clin Infect Dis 1992;15:49.
2. Gullberg RM, Homann SR, Phair JP. Enterococcal bacteremia: analysis of 75 episodes. Rev Infect Dis 1989;11:74.
3. Stevenson KB, Murray EW, Sarubbi FA. Enterococcal meningitis: report of four cases and review. Clin Infect Dis 1994;18:233.
4. Buchino JJ, Ciambarella E, Light I. Systemic group D streptococcal infection in newborn infants. Am J Dis Child 1979;133:270.
5. Elvy J, Porter D, Brown E. Treatment of external ventricular drain-associated ventriculitis caused by *Enterococcus faecalis* with intraventricular daptomycin. J Antimicrob Chemother 2008;61:461.
6. Zeana C, Kubin CJ, Della-Latta P, et al. Vancomycin-resistant *Enterococcus faecium* meningitis successfully managed with linezolid: case report and review of the literature. Clin Infect Dis 2001;33:477.

7. Tush GM, Huneycutt S, Phillips A, et al. Intraventricular quinupristin/dalfopristin for the treatment of vancomycin-resistant *Enterococcus faecium* shunt infection. Clin Infect Dis 1998;26:1460.

8. Birmingham MC, Rayner CR, Meagher AK, et al. Linezolid for the treatment of multidrug-resistant, gram-positive infections: experience from a compassionate-use program. Clin Infect Dis 2003;36:159.

9. El-Khoury J, Fishman JA. Linezolid in the treatment of vancomycin-resistant *Enterococcus faecium* in solid organ transplant recipients: report of a multi-center compassionate-use trial. Transpl Infect Dis 2003;5:121.

10. Meka VG, Gold HS. Antimicrobial resistance to linezolid. Clin Infect Dis 2004;39:1010.

11. Vinh DC, Rubinstein E. Linezolid: a review of safety and tolerability. J Infect 2009;59(Suppl 1):S59–74.

12. Benvenuto M, Benziger DP, Yankelev S, et al. Pharmacokinetics and tolerability of daptomycin at doses up to 12 milligrams per kilogram of body weight once daily in healthy volunteers. Antimicrob Agents Chemother 2006;50:3245.

13. Waites KB, Duffy LB, Dowzicky MJ. Antimicrobial susceptibility among pathogens collected from hospitalized patients in the United States and in vitro activity of ti-gecycline, a new glycylcycline antimicrobial. Antimicrob Agents Chemother 2006;50:3479.

14. Schutt AC, Bohm NM. Multidrug-resistant *Enterococcus faecium* endocarditis treated with combination tigecycline and high-dose daptomycin. Ann Pharmac-other 2009;43:2108.

15. Grayson ML, Eliopoulos GM, Wennersten CB, et al. Increasing resistance to beta-lactam antibiotics among clinical isolates of *Enterococcus faecium*: a 22-year review at one institution. Antimicrob Agents Chemother 1991;35:2180.

16. Rice LB, Bellais S, Carias LL, et al. Impact of specific pbp5 mutations on expression of beta-lactam resistance in *Enterococcus faecium*. Antimicrob Agents Chemother 2004;48:3028.

17. Mainardi JL, Legrand R, Arthur M, et al. Novel mechanism of beta-lactam resistance due to bypass of DD-transpeptidation in *Enterococcus faecium*. J Biol Chem 2000;275:16490.

18. Gavalda J, Len O, Miro JM, et al. Treatment of *Enterococcus faecalis* endocarditis with ampicillin plus ceftriaxone. Ann Intern Med 2007;146:574.

19. Reynolds PE. Structure, biochemistry and mechanism of action of glycopeptide antibiotics. Eur J Clin Microbiol Infect Dis 1989;8:943.

20. Arthur M, Courvalin P. Genetics and mechanisms of glycopeptide resistance in enterococci. Antimicrob Agents Chemother 1993;37:1563.

21. Reynolds PE, Depardieu F, Dutka-Malen S, et al. Glycopeptide resistance mediated by enterococcal transposon Tn1546 requires production of VanX for hydrolysis of D-alanyl-D-alanine. Mol Microbiol 1994;13(6):1065.

22. Van Bambeke F, Chauvel M, Reynolds PE, et al. Vancomycin-dependent *Enterococcus faecalis* clinical isolates and revertant mutants. Antimicrob Agents Chemother 1999;43:41.

23. Bourgeois-Nicolaos N, Massias L, Couson B, et al. Dose dependence of emergence of resistance to linezolid in *Enterococcus faecalis* in vivo. J Infect Dis 2007;195:1480.

24. Pogue JM, Paterson DL, Pasculle AW, et al. Determination of risk factors associated with isolation of linezolid-resistant strains of vancomycin-resistant *Enterococcus*. Infect Control Hosp Epidemiol 2007;28:1382.

25. Gonzales RD, Schreckenberger PC, Graham MB, et al. Infections due to vancomycin-resistant *Enterococcus faecium* resistant to linezolid. Lancet 2001;357:1179.
26. Rahim S, Pillai SK, Gold HS, et al. Linezolid-resistant, vancomycin-resistant *Enterococcus faecium* infection in patients without prior exposure to linezolid. Clin Infect Dis 2003;36:E146.
27. Munoz-Price LS, Lolans K, Quinn JP. Emergence of resistance to daptomycin during treatment of vancomycin-resistant *Enterococcus faecalis* infection. Clin Infect Dis 2005;41:565.
28. Arias CA, Panesso D, McGrath DM, et al. Genetic basis for in vivo daptomycin resistance in enterococci. N Engl J Med 2011;365:892.
29. Hershberger E, Donabedian S, Konstantinou K, et al. Quinupristin-dalfopristin resistance in gram-positive bacteria: mechanism of resistance and epidemiology. Clin Infect Dis 2004;38:92.
30. Kehoe LE, Snidwongse J, Courvalin P, et al. Structural basis of Synercid (quinupristin-dalfopristin) resistance in Gram-positive bacterial pathogens. J Biol Chem 2003;278:29963.
31. Moellering RC, Linden PK, Reinhardt J, et al. The efficacy and safety of quinupristin/dalfopristin for the treatment of infections caused by vancomycin-resistant *Enterococcus faecium*. Synercid Emergency-Use Study Group. J Antimicrob Chemother 1999;44:251.
32. Werner G, Gfrörer S, Fleige C, et al. Tigecycline-resistant *Enterococcus faecalis* strain isolated from a German intensive care unit patient. J Antimicrob Chemother 2008;61:1182.
33. Karanfil LV, Murphy M, Josephson A, et al. A cluster of vancomycin-resistant *Enterococcus faecium* in an intensive care unit. Infect Control Hosp Epidemiol 1992;13:195.
34. Handwerger S, Raucher B, Altarac D, et al. Nosocomial outbreak due to *Enterococcus faecium* highly resistant to vancomycin, penicillin, and gentamicin. Clin Infect Dis 1993;16:750.
35. Ramsey AM, Zilberberg MD. Secular trends of hospitalization with vancomycin-resistant enterococcus infection in the United States, 2000–2006. Infect Control Hosp Epidemiol 2009;30:184.
36. Uttley AH, George RC, Naidoo J, et al. High-level vancomycin-resistant enterococci causing hospital infections. Epidemiol Infect 1989;103:173.
37. Livornese LL Jr, Dias S, Samel C, et al. Hospital-acquired infection with vancomycin-resistant *Enterococcus faecium* transmitted by electronic thermometers. Ann Intern Med 1992;117:112.
38. DiazGranados CA, Zimmer SM, Klein M, et al. Comparison of mortality associated with vancomycin-resistant and vancomycin-susceptible enterococcal bloodstream infections: a meta-analysis. Clin Infect Dis 2005;41:327.
39. Bonten MJ, Slaughter S, Ambergen AW, et al. The role of "colonization pressure" in the spread of vancomycin-resistant enterococci: an important infection control variable. Arch Intern Med 1998;158:1127.
40. Duckro AN, Blom DW, Lyle EA, et al. Transfer of vancomycin-resistant enterococci via health care worker hands. Arch Intern Med 2005;165:302.
41. Fridkin SK, Edwards JR, Courval JM, et al. The effect of vancomycin and third-generation cephalosporins on prevalence of vancomycin-resistant enterococci in 126 U.S. adult intensive care units. Ann Intern Med 2001;135:175.
42. Weinstein JW, Roe M, Towns M, et al. Resistant enterococci: a prospective study of prevalence, incidence, and factors associated with colonization in a university hospital. Infect Control Hosp Epidemiol 1996;17:36.

43. Donskey CJ, Chowdhry TK, Hecker MT, et al. Effect of antibiotic therapy on the density of vancomycin-resistant enterococci in the stool of colonized patients. N Engl J Med 2000;343:1925.

44. Ostrowsky BE, Trick WE, Sohn AH, et al. Control of vancomycin-resistant enterococcus in health care facilities in a region. N Engl J Med 2001;344:1427.

45. Elizaga ML, Weinstein RA, Hayden MK. Patients in long-term care facilities: a reservoir for vancomycin-resistant enterococci. Clin Infect Dis 2002;34:441.

46. D'Agata EM, Gautam S, Green WK, et al. High rate of false-negative results of the rectal swab culture method in detection of gastrointestinal colonization with vancomycin-resistant enterococci. Clin Infect Dis 2002;34:167.

47. Perencevich EN, Fisman DN, Lipsitch M, et al. Projected benefits of active surveillance for vancomycin-resistant enterococci in intensive care units. Clin Infect Dis 2004;38:1108.

48. Climo MW, Sepkowitz KA, Zuccotti G, et al. The effect of daily bathing with chlorhexidine on the acquisition of methicillin-resistant *Staphylococcus aureus*, vancomycin-resistant *Enterococcus*, and healthcare-associated bloodstream infections: results of a quasi-experimental multicenter trial. Crit Care Med 2009;37:1858.

49. Matsumura S, Simor AE. Treatment of endocarditis due to vancomycin-resistant *Enterococcus faecium* with quinupristin/dalfopristin, doxycycline, and rifampin: a synergistic drug combination. Clin Infect Dis 1998;27:1554.

50. Raad I, Hachem R, Hanna H, et al. Treatment of vancomycin-resistant enterococcal infections in the immunocompromised host: quinupristin-dalfopristin in combination with minocycline. Antimicrob Agents Chemother 2001;45:3202.

51. Stevens MP, Edmond MB. Endocarditis due to vancomycin-resistant enterococci: case report and review of the literature. Clin Infect Dis 2005;41:1134.

52. Arias CA, Torres HA, Singh KV, et al. Failure of daptomycin monotherapy for endocarditis caused by an *Enterococcus faecium* strain with vancomycin-resistant and vancomycin-susceptible subpopulations and evidence of in vivo loss of the vanA gene cluster. Clin Infect Dis 2007;45:1343.

53. Jenkins I. Linezolid- and vancomycin-resistant *Enterococcus faecium* endocarditis: successful treatment with tigecycline and daptomycin. J Hosp Med 2007; 2:343.

Why *Candida* Sepsis Should Matter to ICU Physicians

Yoanna Skrobik, MD, FRCP(c)[a,b,*], Michel Laverdiere, MD, FRCP(c)[c]

KEYWORDS

- Candidemia • Invasive candidiasis • Sepsis • Critical care • Intensive care

KEY POINTS

- Severe *candida* infections are prevalent in the critically ill.
- Prompt treatment with source control and timely antifungal initiation improves mortality.
- Because diagnosis is challenging in many clinical settings, stratification by risk factors improves its accuracy.
- Understanding local *candida* infection prevalence and resistance patterns is useful in clinical decision-making.

INTRODUCTION

Candidemia and/or invasive candidiasis (IC) infection significantly contribute to mortality and morbidity in the critically ill.[1,2] IC by definition refers to infection in deep-seated tissue or other normally sterile sites, excluding urine, documented by histopathology and/or microbiological culture. *Candida* bloodstream infection (ie, candidemia) is the most common form of documented IC; this pathologic condition is also almost exclusively the one reported in current epidemiology studies. Infection rates have increased dramatically (100- to 1000-fold) over the last 2 decades[3,4] in most environments, with increments within intensive care units (ICUs) as well as outside the ICU environment. Outpatient acquisition of *Candida* bloodstream infections is now reported[5]; it is likely to represent health care–associated infection because of its frequent association with central vein long-term use of indwelling catheters (peripherally inserted central catheter line, hemodialysis). True variations in candidemia/IC incidences and profiles between centers, regions, and countries have not been

Disclosures: The authors have nothing to disclose.
[a] Department of Medicine, Université de Montréal, 5415 Boulevard De l'Assomption, Montréal, Québec H1T 2M4, Canada; [b] Respiratory Critical Care Group, Respiratory Health Network of the FRQS, Montréal, Québec, Canada; [c] Department of Medicine, Hopital Maisonneuve Rosemont, Université de Montréal, 5415 Boulevard De l'Assomption, Montréal, Québec, H1T 2M4, Canada
* Corresponding author. Université de Montréal, 5415 Boulevard De l'Assomption, Montréal, Québec H1T 2M4, Canada
E-mail address: yoanna.skrobik@umontreal.ca

Crit Care Clin 29 (2013) 853–864
http://dx.doi.org/10.1016/j.ccc.2013.06.007

garnered from epidemiologically rigorous simultaneously collected data. The impact of Candida sepsis on the sickest of the sick seems considerable, however. Data collected in multiple sites in a single Canadian geographic region suggest septic shock is purportedly attributable to Candida in more than 7% of cases (**Table 1**), and in neutropenic patients in greater than 20% of cases (Kumar A, personal communication, 2012). Candida is the fourth leading cause of hematogenous infections in North American hospital in the 1990s,[4] and 33% of Candida episodes are identified in ICUs.[5] Among critically ill patients with nosocomial infections surveyed in a Western European 1-day point prevalence study including 1417 ICUs, 17% of samples yielded positive fungal cultures. In November 2004, a Canadian ICU point prevalence study aimed to identify all colonized or infected patients. Greater than 60% were colonized or infected with Candida, although patients with positive blood cultures for fungus within 4 days of the point prevalence sampling constituted less than 1% of the study population, making infection and colonization challenging to differentiate.

In addition to the worsening and worrisome prevalence of Candida among the critically ill, the risk of death is exceptionally high among patients with septic shock attributed to Candida infection. Delayed treatment of candidemia is an important determinant of patient outcome and mortality (**Fig. 1**).[6,7] Timely source control and antifungal treatment are associated with improved clinical outcomes.[8] Inappropriate antimicrobial therapy is associated with higher mortality and worse morbidity.[9] Prompt treatment of IC should therefore constitute a priority for critical care physicians.

RISK FACTORS

Patients are at greater risk for Candida infection if they have been exposed to broad-spectrum antibiotics; have diabetes, central lines, extensive (particularly

Table 1
Septic shock pathogens in the Cooperative Antimicrobial Therapy of Septic Shock (CATSS) Database (1996–2008)

Isolates	All Septic Shock (n = 5858) (%)	Neutropenic Septic Shock (n = 297) (%)
Pseudomonas	7.2	13.5
Enterobacter	3.3	3.0
Acinetobacter	1.2	0.7
Serratia	1.2	0.0
Citrobacter	0.8	0.3
Potentially resistant gram-negative bacilli	13.7	17.5
C albicans	4.5	13.5
C glabrata	1.0	1.3
C tropicalis	0.2	1.0
C parapsilosis	0.2	0.7
C krusei	0.1	1.0
C neoformans	0.1	0.0
Other yeast	0.4	1.0
Aspergillus/mucor	0.7	3.4
Blastomyces	0.3	0.0
Fungal pathogens	7.6	21.9

Courtesy of Dr Anand Kumar, MD, Winnipeg, Manitoba, Canada.

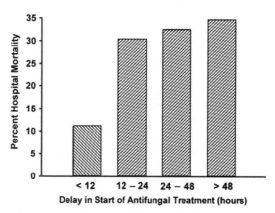

Fig. 1. Hospital mortality of patients with candidemia in relation to delay in initiating anti-fungal therapy after the index positive blood culture. Mortality risk climbs with increasing delays. (*Adapted from* Morrel M, Fraser VJ, Kollef MH. Delaying the empiric treatment of *Candida* bloodstream infection until positive blood culture results are obtained: a potential risk factor for hospital mortality. Antimicrob Agents Chemother 2005;49:3640–5; with permission.)

intra-abdominal) surgery, or burns; receive parenteral nutrition; are immunocompromised (whether in the context of chemotherapy, neutropenia, transplantation, or other); have renal failure; and/or are dialyzed. Prematurity and advanced age also considered risk factors.[10] As if these were insufficient to describe critically ill patients, prolonged ICU stay confers further risk.[11]

DIAGNOSIS

Diagnosis of candidemia or IC is notoriously challenging. The manifestations of IC are nonspecific. An abnormal culture may correspond to *Candida* infection or to colonization. Recovery of *Candida* species (spp) from a single specimen of normally sterile body fluid (except urine) in the critically ill establishes a diagnosis of IC or candidemia if recovered from blood cultures.[12] The detection of antigens, such as mannan and β-D-glucan, metabolites (arabinitol et enolase), or antibodies (anti-mannan) as well as fungal DNA amplification by polymerase chain reaction have been variable or disappointing in clinicians' and scientists' quests to diagnose severe *Candida* infections in a troponin-equivalent. Until now, these assays have generally showed variable diagnostic utility and are not ubiquitously available. The detection of β-D-glucan and polymerase chain reaction hold the greatest promise.[13]

Negative cultures of *Candida* in any site preclude the diagnosis of a *Candida* infection. How many *Candida*- positive sites are required to raise concern about the presence of candidemia/IC is unclear and may depend on patient population. The presence of *Candida* in cultures in up to 4 sites were poorly predictive and were associated with an only 18% probability of deep invasive infection or candidemia[14] in one study; however, the number of culture positive sites with *Candida* is associated with infection rate, as a percentage greater than 50% of sites is associated with a higher probability of invasive infection.[4] Prophylaxis does not improve outcomes nor mortality of IC in highly colonized patients.[15] Additional clinical challenges lie in the diagnostic value and the interpretation of the presence of *Candida* in sputum or urine. The presence of *Candida* in these specimens may be a marker of colonization or deep seated infection. In the case of candiduria it may reflect *Candida* bloodstream infection, or cystitis, whereas in the respiratory tract, it is frequently a marker of airway colonization and rarely documents deep pulmonary infections. Patients with *Candida* in their sputum cultures, however, have a worse prognosis in trials addressing ventilator associated pneumonia.[16] Unfortunately, feasibility of a randomized controlled trial testing the administration of antifungals to patients with suspected pulmonary *Candida* infection (CANTREAT[17]) was not demonstrated, and the question of how to best manage these patients (who are at low risk for a very morbid disease and may have worse prognosis, if only sputum cultures are positive for *Candida*) remains unanswered.

Predictive rules for the diagnosis of candidemia and IC in critical care patients have been modeled in 3 publications. In greater than 1100 patients in 3 countries, a score was created whereby surgery, total parenteral nutrition, and multiple colonization (meaning sites where *Candida* growth could be demonstrated, from wounds, drains, and catheters, or in body fluids) conferred one point, and severe sepsis conferred 2 points.[18] Patients with a score of less than 3 were unlikely to have *Candida*. Serum levels of (1–3)-β-D-glucan (a cell wall panfungal constituent) greater than 75 pg/mL predicted both candidiasis and response to treatment. In the second study, female sex, exposure to antibiotics for 48 hours or more, and upper gastrointestinal source of peritonitis, as well as perioperative cardiovascular failure, predicted peritoneal candidiasis in a surgical population of more than 220 ICU patients.[19] The combination of ICU stay, abdominal surgery, antibiotic exposure, dialysis, and central lines predicted *Candida* peritonitis in the third large multicenter study, including more than 2800 patients (odds ratio 4.3).[20]

INFECTION CONTROL

The 2 following principles govern controlling *Candida* infection: source control and use of antifungals antibiotics.

In source control, it is essential to consider central venous catheters as a potential source of *Candida* sepsis. The internal lumen of the infected central venous catheter from an ICU patient with candidiasis, obtained by scanning electronic microscopy, is shown in **Fig. 2**; *Candida albicans* hyphae and coagulase-negative staphylococci are seen embedded in the biofilm.

The failure to remove a colonized catheter is strongly associated with mortality in several studies in the critically ill[21,22] and any delay in efforts to do away with a central line is unjustified. On occasions when venous access catheters removal is impossible or ill advised, such as in patients with profound thrombocytopenia, administering antifungal agents via the catheter lumen daily can be considered a temporary measure.

The origin of *Candida* can frequently be endogenous from the colonized gastrointestinal tract; 50% of healthy individuals are colonized with *Candida* species,[4] which explains in part why surgical patients with gastrointestinal perforation or intervention involving disruption of the gastrointestinal tract are at high risk for *Candida* peritonitis and *Candida* sepsis. Gastric, jejunal, and colonic perforations contaminate the peritoneal cavity with *Candida* 64%, 50%, and 40% to 50% of the time, respectively.[23] This peritoneal contamination is associated with ICU patient mortality; only appendicular perforations confer a lower risk of such contamination (4%). However, nosocomial perforations seem to be associated with mortality attributable to *Candida* sepsis, whereas intestinal perforations originating in the community do not.[24] Surgical patients with candidiasis seem to have a better prognosis,[25] perhaps because of the higher prevalence of neutropenia, corticosteroid use, and high colonization indices noted in the comparative medical population. Patient and health care workers' skin

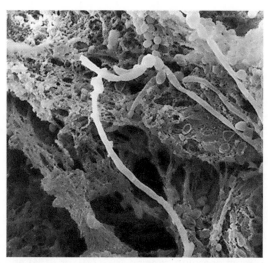

Fig. 2. Electron microscope image of the internal lumen of an infected central venous catheter from an ICU patient with candidiasis; *Candida albicans* hyphae and coagulase-negative staphylococci are seen embedded in the biofilm.

and hand colonization as a source of infection have been described, and epidemiologic linked transmission has also been reported.[4]

THERAPY

The use of antifungal antibiotics in the therapeutic management of IC infections in critically ill patients is based on 3 different strategies of interventions: prophylactic, preemptive, and targeted or definitive treatment.

Although azole-based antifungal prophylaxis reduces the event rate of invasive fungal infections,[26] it has not been shown to be useful in the critically ill.[27]

Preemptive therapy is probably the most commonly used strategy in the ICU setting. However, the preemptive treatment strategy in the nonneutropenic ICU patient has not been studied adequately. Prospectively most patients do not have a diagnosis, have a high index of suspicion based on the risk factors described earlier and warrant catheter removal and early antifungal therapy. Preemptive use of fluconazole may reduce proven candidiasis in surgical critically ill patients.[28] *Candida* infections occurred more frequently in the historical control cohort (7% vs 3.8%; $P = .03$) and microbiologically ICU-acquired proven infections decreased from 2.2% to 0% in the prospective interventional group. However, in the absence of reliable surrogate markers, and in the context of the current dearth of efficacy data, preemptive therapy in nonneutropenic patients cannot be advocated at this time in all patients. Despite the data from patients with *Candida*-colonized sputum cited earlier, preemptive antifungal therapy in hemodynamically stable ICU patients does not confer an overall mortality benefit when all patients (ie, those with subsequently proven *Candida* infection and patients without it [2/3 of the cohort]) are considered in a pooled outcomes analysis.[29] Management in the context of shock is less clear; the high probability of having *Candida* as a cause for shock (see **Table 1**) probably warrants early prescription and rapid administration of antifungals; when these are given to patients with candidemia within 2 hours of shock onset, the survival rates exceed 80%.[30] Practice surveys however suggest that most patients with candidemia with or without shock receive antifungals on average 35 hours[30] after the positive blood culture has been drawn in North America.

Targeted therapy refers to the use of antifungal antibiotics in patient with proven *Candida* infection; choice of agent is tempered by 3 considerations: efficacy, cost, and risk.

Efficacy against *Candida* infection should partly be guided by local patterns of resistance in *Candida* species, as *Candida* sp distributions and sensitivities vary by geographic region,[31] over time,[32] and in association with factors such as exposure to broad spectrum antibiotics.[33] Even though *C albicans* is the most common pathogen causing IC, the frequency with which other species, such as *Candida glabrata* or *Candida parapsilosis*, which are more likely to be resistant or less sensitive to certain antifungal antibiotics, should be considered. Of the 5 most common *Candida* species (*albicans, glabrata, parapsilosis, krusei*, and *tropicalis*) collected from candidemic patients with 779 positive blood cultures from ICUs in 79 medical centers around the world, none were susceptible to all 6 tested therapeutic agents (Anidulafungin, Caspofungin, Micafungin, Fluconazole, Posaconazole, and Voriconazole). *C albicans* was the most common species (393/779, or 51%) and was least likely to be resistant overall (0.3% to echinocandins, 0 to azoles). Echinocandins were less associated with resistant *C glabrata* (2.2%) than were azoles (4.4%–5.9%). No *C tropicalis* were resistant to echinocandins, and resistance to azoles ranged from 1.2% to 4.9%. Finally, both *C krusei* and *C parapsilosis* isolates were sensitive to all antifungals save one (Caspofungin and Fluconazole at 6.3% and 6.8%, respectively).[34]

Although the overall probability of resistance remains low, the narrow physiologic reserve inherent to most critically ill admissions suggests prudence and a comprehensive spectrum. The caveat about an IC caused by a less susceptible *Candida* species must be kept in mind, particularly in patients at higher risk for non-*albicans* species, such as those afflicted with hematologic malignancies, solid organ transplant recipients, or patients previously exposed to azoles.[33,35] Echinocandins are fungicidal and azoles are static. Pivotal studies on *Candida* bloodstream infection treatment suggest faster (albeit not statistically significant) fungal bloodstream clearance and more rapid symptom resolution with echinocandins, as well as higher overall success and survival rates compared with polyenes and azoles.[36] Adverse events and toxicities were also lesser with echinocandins. Newer triazoles, such as voriconazole, show enhanced activity against *Candida* species resistant to fluconazole. However, CYP2C19 genetic polymorphisms can have substantial impact on its pharmacokinetics. Asians inherit a larger proportion of CYP2C19 poor metabolizer gene (15%–20%) in relation to Caucasians (2%–3%).[37,38] Depending on phenotype, subtherapeutic or toxic blood levels of voriconazole have been documented with similar doses[39]; serum level monitoring has now been implemented to temper this drug characteristic in some bone marrow transplant centers.[40] Drug interactions,[41] a common problem in the ICU, are particularly frequent with azole antifungals. Initial treatment with an echinocandin (anidulafungin, caspofungin, micafungin) while awaiting species identification and susceptibility seems warranted in documented IC. How long antifungals should be administered in the critically ill has not been weighed with methodologically sound outcome studies; current Canadian recommendations suggest in neutropenic patients at least 48 hours after resolution of all infectious symptoms and resolution of the absolute neutrophil count to greater than 0.5×10^9/L. At least 14 days of antifungal therapy beyond clearance of organisms from bloodstream must also be completed. In nonneutropenic patients, at least 14 days after clearance of the *Candida* from the bloodstream and resolution of all signs and symptoms of infection is recommended.[11]

Cost needs to be considered in the selection of antifungal antibiotics. Fluconazole and amphotericin B are less expensive than the more recently marketed triazoles and echinocandins. Pharmacoeconomic analysis of the risk inherent to the surveillance and management of amphotericin B renal toxicity imposes the consideration of an alternative to polyene antifungals.[42] Despite their lesser intrinsic toxicities when compared with the Amphotericin B parent compound, the use of lipid preparations of amphotericin B remains risky because of significant nephrotoxicity and hepatotoxicity,[29] and proof of any benefit is limited in the critically ill population.

DRUG-DRUG INTERACTIONS

Multiple drugs, among them the opiate fentanyl (FEN) and the sedative benzodiazepine midazolam (MDZ), are commonly administered in the critical care setting[43] and are extensively metabolized by the same CYP450 isoenzymes, namely, CYP3A4/5.[44,45] Co-administration of FEN and MDZ, or of either, with other drugs such as fluconazole metabolized by the CYP3A4/5 isoenzyme[46] increases serum drug levels by competitive inhibition; in addition, the metabolism and excretion of these drugs decrease with age.[47] FEN and MDZ levels are increased when these drugs are administered simultaneously[48,49]; both increase independently with the co-administration of fluconazole or voriconazole in noncritically ill recipients.

The pharmacokinetics and pharmacodynamics of MDZ are predictable in healthy adults.[50] Metabolic clearance in healthy populations is preserved over a relatively narrow range.[51,52] Critical illness influences the pharmacokinetics and pharmacodynamics of midazolam. Plasma levels, half-life, and terminal half-life varied within a considerably broader range than that reported in healthy or noncritically ill patients,[53] with very broad intrasubject and intersubject variability. In addition, terminal half-life, which is determined after drug infusion cessation, is prolonged in all patients. These characteristics are also true of the pediatric critical care population[54] and thought to be attributable, among others, to covariates such as renal failure, hepatic failure, and concomitant administration of CYP3A inhibitors such as older and recent antifungal azoles. These issues take on particular importance given the growing awareness of the morbidity and mortality associated with deep sedation,[55] which is understood, in the context of multiple drug administration, to be more attributable to drug-drug interactions than to the administration of sedative doses.[56]

The limited clinical descriptions of drug interactions involving azole family drugs in the ICU, and their impact in day-to-day clinical practice, are nevertheless compelling. One example of potentially significant interactions is depicted in **Fig. 3** (prototypical individual patient; unpublished data). Mathematical modeling to project expected FEN levels based on administered doses and infusion rates failed to predict the measured FEN levels when fluconazole was being co-administered (such as the individual whose values in hours 0–50 are shown in **Fig. 3**). The higher FEN levels correlated with deep sedation. The effect was no longer present with similar FEN doses once fluconazole was discontinued (>100 hours, **Fig. 3**). How constant this effect is across cohorts and with different CYP 450 3A4 inhibitors is not known.

Computerized cytochromic interaction alerting software exists to identify potential drug interactions in vulnerable populations receiving multiple medications. It has been shown to improve detection and adjustment of medication based on identified interactions in geriatric patients.[57] In 100 elderly patients receiving 5 or more medications, a total of 238 cytochrome P450 drug-drug interactions were identified, of which more than 70% involved CYP3A4. Medication adjustments and follow-up were deemed to be required in more than 50% of the patients based on the information

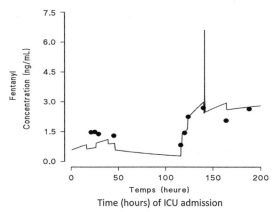

Fig. 3. Mathematical modeling to project expected FEN levels based on administered doses and infusion rates. The graph represents concentrations predicted by the ADAPT-V model (*lines*) and the observed plasma levels (*dots*); the peak represents a high predicted concentration corresponding to a bolus. Measured FEN plasma levels were significantly higher than predicted during hours 0 to 60, while fluconazole was being co-administered. These higher FEN levels correlated with deep sedation (Richmond Agitation and Sedation Scale [RASS] levels of −3 and −4). The effect was no longer present (ie, the levels are about the same as predicted or a little less) when FEN doses continued to be administered once fluconazole was discontinued (>100 hours, as depicted in the figure). The increase in measured/predicted levels at about 110 hours is due to an increase in dose of FEN. (*From* Michaud V, Skrobik Y, Tarasevych V, et al. Population pharmacokinetics of fentanyl during continuous infusion in patients admitted to the intensive care unit. American Society for Clinical Pharmacology and Therapeutics Meeting. Atlanta, March, 2010; with permission.)

provided by the software. Similar smart alert or detection systems have not been tested to date in critically ill adults or correlated with clinical outcomes.

SUMMARY

Candidemia and IC are significant and morbid clinical issues in the critically ill. Although much remains to be understood about determinants of disease progression and *Candida* species profiling and sensitivities, heightened awareness and education among critical care caregivers may help reduce the significant burden associated with these infections, particularly in patients with septic shock in whom rapid administration of echinocandins appears warranted.

REFERENCES

1. Leroy O, Gangneux JP, Montravers P, et al. Epidemiology, management, and risk factors for death of invasive Candida infections in critical care: a multicenter, prospective, observational study in France (2005-2006). Crit Care Med 2009; 37(5):1612–8.
2. Ostrosky-Zeichner L, Pappas PG. Invasive candidiasis in the intensive care unit. Crit Care Med 2006;34(3):857–63.
3. Marchetti O, Bille J, Fluckiger U, et al. Epidemiology of candidemia in Swiss tertiary care hospitals: secular trends, 1991-2000. Clin Infect Dis 2004;38(3): 311–20.

4. Eggimann P, Garbino J, Pittet D. Epidemiology of Candida species infections in critically ill non-immunosuppressed patients. Lancet Infect Dis 2003;3(11): 685–702.

5. Labbe AC, Pepin J, Patino C, et al. A single-centre 10-year experience with Candida bloodstream infections. Can J Infect Dis Med Microbiol 2009;20(2): 45–50.

6. Garey KW, Rege M, Pai MP, et al. Time to initiation of fluconazole therapy impacts mortality in patients with candidemia: a multi-institutional study. Clin Infect Dis 2006;43(1):25–31.

7. Morrell M, Fraser VJ, Kollef MH. Delaying the empiric treatment of candida bloodstream infection until positive blood culture results are obtained: a potential risk factor for hospital mortality. Antimicrob Agents Chemother 2005;49(9): 3640–5.

8. Kollef M, Micek S, Hampton N, et al. Septic shock attributed to Candida infection: importance of empiric therapy and source control. Clin Infect Dis 2012; 54(12):1739–46.

9. Kumar A, Ellis P, Arabi Y, et al. Initiation of inappropriate antimicrobial therapy results in a fivefold reduction of survival in human septic shock. Chest 2009; 136(5):1237–48.

10. Ostrosky-Zeichner L. New approaches to the risk of Candida in the intensive care unit. Curr Opin Infect Dis 2003;16(6):533–7.

11. Bow EJ, Evans G, Fuller J, et al. Canadian clinical practice guidelines for invasive candidiasis in adults. Can J Infect Dis Med Microbiol 2010;21(4):e122–50.

12. De Pauw B, Walsh TJ, Donnelly JP, et al. Revised definitions of invasive fungal disease from the European Organization for Research and Treatment of Cancer/ Invasive Fungal Infections Cooperative Group and the National Institute of Allergy and Infectious Diseases Mycoses Study Group (EORTC/MSG) Consensus Group. Clin Infect Dis 2008;46(12):1813–21.

13. Nguyen MH, Wissel MC, Shields RK, et al. Performance of Candida real-time polymerase chain reaction, beta-D-glucan assay, and blood cultures in the diagnosis of invasive candidiasis. Clin Infect Dis 2012;54(9):1240–8.

14. Pelz RK, Lipsett PA, Swoboda SM, et al. The diagnostic value of fungal surveillance cultures in critically ill patients. Surg Infect (Larchmt) 2000;1(4):273–81.

15. Eggimann P, Garbino J, Pittet D. Management of Candida species infections in critically ill patients. Lancet Infect Dis 2003;3(12):772–85.

16. Delisle MS, Williamson DR, Albert M, et al. Impact of Candida species on clinical outcomes in patients with suspected ventilator-associated pneumonia. Can Respir J 2011;18(3):131–6.

17. Available at: http://www.zapthevap.com/index.php?option=com_content& task=view&id=89&Itemid=62.

18. Leon C, Ruiz-Santana S, Saavedra P, et al. Usefulness of the "Candida score" for discriminating between Candida colonization and invasive candidiasis in non-neutropenic critically ill patients: a prospective multicenter study. Crit Care Med 2009;37(5):1624–33.

19. Dupont H, Bourichon A, Paugam-Burtz C, et al. Can yeast isolation in peritoneal fluid be predicted in intensive care unit patients with peritonitis? Crit Care Med 2003;31(3):752–7.

20. Ostrosky-Zeichner L, Sable C, Sobel J, et al. Multicenter retrospective development and validation of a clinical prediction rule for nosocomial invasive candidiasis in the intensive care setting. Eur J Clin Microbiol Infect Dis 2007;26(4): 271–6.

21. Garnacho-Montero J, Diaz-Martin A, Garcia-Cabrera E, et al. Impact on hospital mortality of catheter removal and adequate antifungal therapy in Candida spp. bloodstream infections. J Antimicrob Chemother 2013;68(1): 206–13.

22. Labelle AJ, Micek ST, Roubinian N, et al. Treatment-related risk factors for hospital mortality in Candida bloodstream infections. Crit Care Med 2008;36(11): 2967–72.

23. Dupont H, Paugam-Burtz C, Muller-Serieys C, et al. Predictive factors of mortality due to polymicrobial peritonitis with Candida isolation in peritoneal fluid in critically ill patients. Arch Surg 2002;137(12):1341–6 [discussion: 1347].

24. Montravers P, Dupont H, Gauzit R, et al. Candida as a risk factor for mortality in peritonitis. Crit Care Med 2006;34(3):646–52.

25. Charles PE, Doise JM, Quenot JP, et al. Candidemia in critically ill patients: difference of outcome between medical and surgical patients. Intensive Care Med 2003;29(12):2162–9.

26. Playford EG, Lipman J, Sorrell TC. Prophylaxis, empirical and preemptive treatment of invasive candidiasis. Curr Opin Crit Care 2010;16(5):470–4.

27. Schuster MG, Edwards JE, Sobel JD, et al. Empirical fluconazole versus placebo for intensive care unit patients: a randomized trial. Ann Intern Med 2008;149:83–90.

28. Piarroux R, Grenouillet F, Balvay P, et al. Assessment of preemptive treatment to prevent severe candidiasis in critically ill surgical patients. Crit Care Med 2004; 32(12):2443–9.

29. Azoulay E, Dupont H, Tabah A, et al. Systemic antifungal therapy in critically ill patients without invasive fungal infection*. Crit Care Med 2012;40(3): 813–22.

30. Group, A.K.a.t.C.D.R., The High Mortality of Candida Septic Shock is Explained by Excessive Delays in Initiation of Antifungal Therapy. ICAAC 2007, K-2174, 2007.

31. Kotwal A, Biswas D, Sharma JP, et al. An observational study on the epidemiological and mycological profile of Candidemia in ICU patients. Med Sci Monit 2011;17(11):CR663–8.

32. Cleveland AA, Farley MM, Harrison LH, et al. Changes in incidence and antifungal drug resistance in candidemia: results from population-based laboratory surveillance in Atlanta and Baltimore, 2008-2011. Clin Infect Dis 2012;55(10): 1352–61.

33. Garnacho-Montero J, Diaz-Martin A, Garcia-Cabrera E, et al. Risk factors for fluconazole-resistant candidemia. Antimicrob Agents Chemother 2010;54(8): 3149–54.

34. Pfaller MA, Messer SA, Moet GJ, et al. Candida bloodstream infections: comparison of species distribution and resistance to echinocandin and azole antifungal agents in Intensive Care Unit (ICU) and non-ICU settings in the SENTRY Antimicrobial Surveillance Program (2008-2009). Int J Antimicrob Agents 2011;38(1): 65–9.

35. Diekema DJ, Messer SA, Brueggemann A, et al. Epidemiology of candidemia: 3-year results from the emerging infections and the epidemiology of Iowa organisms study. J Clin Microbiol 2002;40:1298–302.

36. Kett DH, Shorr AF, Reboli AC, et al. Anidulafungin compared with fluconazole in severely ill patients with candidemia and other forms of invasive candidiasis: support for the 2009 IDSA treatment guidelines for candidiasis. Crit Care 2011;15(5):R253.

37. Chen L, Qin S, Xie J, et al. Genetic polymorphism analysis of CYP2C19 in Chinese Han populations from different geographic areas of mainland China. Pharmacogenomics 2008;9(6):691–702.
38. Kimura M, Ieiri I, Mamiya K, et al. Genetic polymorphism of cytochrome P450s, CYP2C19, and CYP2C9 in a Japanese population. Ther Drug Monit 1998;20(3):243–7.
39. Scholz I, Oberwittler H, Riedel KD, et al. Pharmacokinetics, metabolism and bioavailability of the triazole antifungal agent voriconazole in relation to CYP2C19 genotype. Br J Clin Pharmacol 2009;68(6):906–15.
40. Trifilio SM, Yarnold PR, Scheetz MH, et al. Serial plasma voriconazole concentrations after allogeneic hematopoietic stem cell transplantation. Antimicrob Agents Chemother 2009;53(5):1793–6.
41. Mikus G, Scholz IM, Weiss J. Pharmacogenomics of the triazole antifungal agent voriconazole. Pharmacogenomics 2011;12(6):861–72.
42. Abele-Horn M, Kopp A, Sternberg U, et al. A randomized study comparing fluconazole with amphotericin B/5-flucytosine for the treatment of systemic Candida infections in intensive care patients. Infection 1996;24(6):426–32.
43. Mehta S, Burry L, Fischer S, et al. Canadian survey of the use of sedatives, analgesics, and neuromuscular blocking agents in critically ill patients. Crit Care Med 2006;34(2):374–80.
44. Feierman DE, Lasker JM. Metabolism of fentanyl, a synthetic opioid analgesic, by human liver microsomes. Role of CYP3A4. Drug Metab Dispos 1996;24(9):932–9.
45. Gorski JC, Hall SD, Jones DR, et al. Regioselective biotransformation of midazolam by members of the human cytochrome P450 3A (CYP3A) subfamily. Biochem Pharmacol 1994;47(9):1643–53.
46. Saari TI, Laine K, Neuvonen M, et al. Effect of voriconazole and fluconazole on the pharmacokinetics of intravenous fentanyl. Eur J Clin Pharmacol 2008;64(1):25–30.
47. Greenblatt DJ, Abernethy DR, Locniskar A, et al. Effect of age, gender, and obesity on midazolam kinetics. Anesthesiology 1984;61(1):27–35.
48. Hamaoka N, Oda Y, Hase I, et al. Propofol decreases the clearance of midazolam by inhibiting CYP3A4: an in vivo and in vitro study. Clin Pharmacol Ther 1999;66(2):110–7.
49. McKillop D, Wild MJ, Butters CJ, et al. Effects of propofol on human hepatic microsomal cytochrome P450 activities. Xenobiotica 1998;28(9):845–53.
50. Albrecht S, Ihmsen H, Hering W, et al. The effect of age on the pharmacokinetics and pharmacodynamics of midazolam. Clin Pharmacol Ther 1999;65(6):630–9.
51. Malacrida R, Fritz ME, Suter PM, et al. Pharmacokinetics of midazolam administered by continuous intravenous infusion to intensive care unit patients. Crit Care Med 1992;20:1123–6.
52. Dresser GK. Coordinate induction of both cytochrome P4503A and MDR1 by St John's wort in healthy subjects. Clin Pharmacol Ther 2003;73:41–50.
53. Ovakim D, Bosma KJ, Young GB. Effect of critical illness on the pharmacokinetics and dose-response relationship of midazolam. Crit Care Med 2012;16(Suppl 1):330.
54. de Wildt SN, de Hoog M, Vinks AA, et al. Population pharmacokinetics and metabolism of midazolam in pediatric intensive care patients. Crit Care Med 2003;31(7):1952–8.
55. Shehabi Y, Bellomo R, Reade MC, et al. Early intensive care sedation predicts long-term mortality in ventilated critically ill patients. Am J Respir Crit Care Med 2012;186(8):724–31.

56. Skrobik Y, Leger C, Cossette M, et al. Factors predisposing to coma and delirium: fentanyl and midazolam exposure, CYP3A5, ABCB1 and ABCG2 genetic polymorphisms, and inflammatory factors. Crit Care Med 2013;41(4): 999–1008.

57. Zakrzewski-Jakubiak H, Doan J, Lamoureux P, et al. Detection and prevention of drug-drug interactions in the hospitalized elderly: utility of new cytochrome p450-based software. Am J Geriatr Pharmacother 2011;9(6):461–70.

Management of Severe Malaria in the Intensive Care Unit

Matthew P. Cheng, MD[a], Cedric P. Yansouni, MD, FRCPC[b],*

KEYWORDS

- Severe malaria • Sepsis • Adjunctive therapy • Antimalarials • Fluid management
- Respiratory failure • Acidosis

KEY POINTS

- Early recognition and diagnosis of severe malaria is vital.
- Intravenous artesunate should be used as first-line antimalarial treatment.
- The threshold for using antibiotic therapy should be low, particularly in children, in hypotensive patients, and in critically ill patients originating from endemic areas.
- Patients with severe malaria without hypotension or signs of significant volume depletion should generally receive fluids conservatively, in contrast with the recommendation for bacterial sepsis.
- There is currently insufficient evidence to recommend any specific adjunctive therapy.

BACKGROUND

Severe malaria is a medical emergency requiring early intervention to prevent death. Malaria remains one of the top 3 infectious killers in the world, alongside human immunodeficiency virus (HIV)/acquired immunodeficiency syndrome (AIDS) and tuberculosis, with global mortality estimates of around 1 million deaths per year.[1,2] Although most deaths occur in low-resource settings with high transmission intensity, malaria also accounts for most life-threatening illness in travelers returning from the tropics.[3]

Disclosures: C.P. Yansouni is supported by Grand Challenges Canada and the Research Institute of the McGill University Health Centre. The authors declare no conflicts of interest.
Contributors: M.P. Cheng performed literature searches and drafted several sections. C.P. Yansouni conceived the article and was responsible for the overall content.
[a] Department of Medicine, University of British Columbia, 2775 Laurel Street, Vancouver, BC V5Z 1M9, Canada; [b] Division of Infectious Diseases, Department of Medical Microbiology, J.D. MacLean Centre for Tropical Diseases, McGill University Health Centre, 1650 Cedar Avenue, Room L10.509, Montreal H3G 1A4, Canada
* Corresponding author.
E-mail address: cedric.yansouni@mcgill.ca

Crit Care Clin 29 (2013) 865–885
http://dx.doi.org/10.1016/j.ccc.2013.06.008
0749-0704/13/$ – see front matter © 2013 Elsevier Inc. All rights reserved.

criticalcare.theclinics.com

This article highlights key aspects of the management of severe malaria syndromes, with a focus on *Plasmodium falciparum*, because it accounts for most of the deaths. Individual case management of imported malaria is emphasized, because clinicians in nonendemic settings may be less accustomed to treating severe malaria than their counterparts in high-transmission areas. However, because most data for the management of severe disease are from malaria-endemic regions, differences in management strategies between endemic and nonendemic areas and between children and adults are highlighted.

LIFE CYCLE

Malaria results from infection by *Plasmodium* parasites, of which 5 species are known to cause disease in humans: *P falciparum*, *Plasmodium vivax*, *Plasmodium ovale*, *Plasmodium malariae* and *Plasmodium knowlesi*. Humans are the only reservoir for pathogenic species except *P knowlesi*. The principle means of transmission of *Plasmodium* parasites is via the bite of female *Anopheles* mosquitoes. The parasite's life cycle involves distinct life stages that differ with respect to pathogenic effect and susceptibility to drugs. After ingesting parasitized blood from an infected person, sporozoites develop within mosquito salivary glands. Sporozoites are subsequently transmitted to another host at the next blood meal, at which point they enter hepatocytes within approximately 30 minutes. On parasite maturation, infected hepatocytes rupture and release thousands of merozoites into the bloodstream. These organisms then infect erythrocytes and enter the intraerythrocytic lifecycle, which is responsible for disease manifestations. A minority of intraerythrocytic parasites develop by sexual reproduction into gametocytes, to be ingested eventually by another mosquito.

EPIDEMIOLOGY

Global mortality estimates for malaria range from 709,000 (95% confidence interval [CI], 554,000 to 892,000) deaths per year[1] to 1,133,000 (95% CI, 848,000 to 1,591,000) deaths in 2010.[2] Africa bears the highest burden of malaria, with 70 million reported cases in 2009, and estimates reaching 176 million (95% CI, 117 million to 241 million).[4] The incidence is thought to be decreasing in Africa, except in west and central Africa where transmission rates are the highest, with infections almost exclusively from *P falciparum*.[5,6] Most countries in southeast Asia remain endemic for the disease. It is estimated that 70% of the population is at risk for malaria, representing around 450 million people. Most cases are attributable to infection with *P falciparum*, although *P vivax* predominates in some localities.[1] *P knowlesi* is a recently emerging pathogen in this region. In the last decade, the incidence of malaria has significantly decreased in most countries in the Americas, and most now have low malaria transmission intensity. Countries in the Americas with the highest incidence of infection with *P falciparum* include Haiti, Guyana, and Suriname.[1]

Imported malaria is increasingly reported in low-incidence countries of Europe and North America. The number of imported malaria cases varies by country, with France reporting approximately 8000 cases per year,[7] the United Kingdom 1500 to 2000 cases per year,[8] the United States 1691 cases in 2010,[9] and Canada 350 to 1000 cases per year,[10] although underreporting is estimated at 30% to 50%.[11] *P falciparum* malaria accounted for 77% of potentially life-threatening tropical diseases among 82,825 ill Western travelers reported to GeoSentinel (a worldwide network of surveillance for travel-related illness) over a 15-year period.[3] Severe disease is reported in approximately 4% to 10% of imported cases.[7,9,10]

Predictors of severe disease include advanced age, originating from a nonendemic country, travel to Africa, absence of chemoprophylaxis, and delayed diagnosis.[12,13] **Fig. 1** shows how clinical presentations of severe falciparum malaria differ by age and by local epidemiology.

DIAGNOSIS
Severe Malaria Definitions

Box 1 shows who should be managed as having severe malaria. More detailed criteria are outlined in current World Health Organization (WHO) guidelines, and this is helpful for the standardization of clinical research.[14]

Diagnosis of Malaria

Clinical signs and basic laboratory data are notoriously nonspecific for the diagnosis of malaria, and microbiologic tests for malaria should always be ordered when any exposure history exists within the preceding year, or occasionally longer.[15] In settings in which malaria is rare, early consultation with a microbiologist or infectiologist may help expedite testing and appropriate management. Microbiologic diagnosis relies on detection of asexual parasites in the blood or sequestered in tissues. Blood smear microscopy has been the reference standard for more than a century, but is time consuming and is limited by the need for considerable expertise. Although high parasitemia is expected with severe malaria, microscopy may be negative on the first assessment because of parasite sequestration in tissues, particularly in patients who have been ill for several days. When there is clinical suspicion for malaria, testing must be repeated for up to 48 hours, which is the duration of the intraerythrocytic lifecycle of *P falciparum*. An interval of 8 to 12 hours between blood films is reasonable.

Rapid diagnostic tests (RDTs) for malaria were developed to address the shortcomings of microscopy. RDTs for detection of *P falciparum* parasites in blood have been extensively field validated[16,17] are recommended by WHO.[14] They are based on the detection of either the Histidine-Rich Protein II (HRP2) antigen or of *P falciparum*–specific parasite lactate dehydrogenase (Pf pLDH). Although HRP2-based RDTs tend to have higher sensitivity,[18] the advantages of using Pf pLDH instead of HRP2/pan pLDH include that (1) Pf pLDH rapidly becomes undetectable after successful treatment, whereas HRP2 positivity can represent cured infection from several weeks

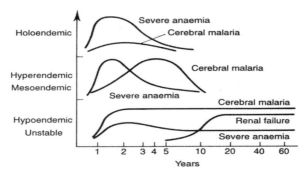

Fig. 1. The clinical presentations of severe falciparum malaria by age and transmission intensity. Nonimmune travelers are expected to behave like inhabitants of a zone of unstable transmission. (*From* White NJ. Malaria. In: Cook GC, Zumla AI, editors. Manson's tropical diseases. 22nd edition. Philadelphia: Saunders Ltd; 2009. p. 1205; with permission.)

Box 1
Criteria for severe falciparum malaria

Either

    History of recent possible exposure and no other related disorder

Or

    Asexual forms of *P falciparum* on blood smear

And

    One or more of the following 11 features:

        Impaired consciousness or coma

        Severe normocytic anemia

        Renal failure

        Pulmonary edema

        Hypoglycemia

        Circulatory collapse, shock

        Spontaneous bleeding/disseminated intravascular coagulation

        Repeated generalized convulsions

        Acidemia/acidosis

        Hemoglobinuria

        Parasitemia of greater than or equal to 2% in nonimmune individuals, greater than or equal to 5% in semi-immune individuals

Adapted from WHO. Guidelines for the treatment of malaria. 2nd edition. Geneva (Switzerland): World Health Organization; 2010. p. 1–194; with permission.

---

earlier; and (2) Pf pLDH does not yield false-negative results in hyperparasitemic individuals.[19,20] However, current RDTs cannot assess the degree of parasitemia, and this parameter is of paramount importance for the diagnosis, prognosis, and assessment of response to treatment of patients with severe malaria.

The limit of detection of both microscopy and RDTs is approximately 50 parasites/μL, roughly equivalent to a parasitemia of 0.001% and a total body burden of 1×10^8 parasites. The sensitivity of RDTs is less than that of expert microscopy at parasite densities less than 100 to 500 parasites/μL (about 0.002%–0.01%), depending on the type of RDT used.[21] PCR is more sensitive than expert microscopy but is not widely available at present.

Diagnosis of Cerebral Malaria in Endemic Settings

Distinguishing people with cerebral malaria from those with coma from other causes is difficult, particularly in areas where most people are semi-immune and in whom asymptomatic parasitemia is common. In endemic settings standard definitions of cerebral malaria (any sign of cerebral dysfunction with asexual *P falciparum* parasitemia and no other evident cause for coma[14,22]) lack specificity compared with postmortem findings, with one prospective series documenting a false-positive diagnosis in 23% of presumed cases (7 of 31 clinically diagnosed deceased patients had no findings of cerebral malaria at autopsy).[23] Several studies have established a characteristic malarial retinopathy as the best single discriminator between coma of malarial and nonmalarial origin, when applied to patients meeting standard definitions of cerebral malaria.[23,24] However, the necessary skill and equipment are barriers to implementation.

Current Innovations in Diagnostics

Recent publications report that quantitative assessment of HRP2 is highly correlated with malarial retinopathy in patients with coma[25] and is a strong predictor of severe illness and mortality irrespective of coma.[26] These data suggest the possibility in the near future of diagnosing cerebral malaria as well as discriminating severe from nonsevere disease with a single RDT quantitatively measuring HRP2.

INITIAL MANAGEMENT OF SUSPECTED SEVERE MALARIA

Death from severe malaria often occurs within hours of admission. Severe malaria suspects should receive the highest available level of care with appropriate therapy instituted as soon as possible. Delayed treatment is associated with high mortality despite subsequent high-level care.[12] In addition to detecting malaria parasites and assessing the degree of parasitemia, the initial diagnostic assessment of patients should include assessing clinical signs of neurologic dysfunction or convulsions, any end-organ dysfunction, hypoglycemia, acidosis and hyperlactemia, and anemia. Body weight should be measured or estimated early to optimize dosing of drugs and fluid. Blood should be sent for crossmatch and bacterial culture. Patients with neurologic dysfunction should have a lumbar puncture to rule out bacterial meningitis, but this should not delay antimalarial or antibacterial treatment. Blood glucose should be monitored frequently in all patients, because severe hypoglycemia can result from malaria infection as well as from quinine derivatives. If blood glucose measurement is delayed, empiric intravenous glucose should be administered in all patients with altered consciousness. Invasive monitoring of intravascular volume status should be considered early to help titrate fluids, and over-resuscitation should be avoided. If delayed laboratory confirmation of malaria is expected (>1 hour), empiric antimalarial treatment should be started immediately when clinical suspicion is high (**Box 2**). Care should be taken when prescribing quinine derivatives to patients who have taken other antimalarials before presentation, because cardiac toxicity may arise (see **Box 2**). If artesunate is subsequently required, no known interactions with other antimalarials preclude its use. Empiric antimicrobials should always be considered, particularly when hypotension is present or in patients from malaria-endemic areas in whom parasitemia may be asymptomatic and therefore not responsible for the presenting symptoms.

ANTIMALARIAL MANAGEMENT

Adequate doses of effective antimalarial drugs should be given parenterally as soon as possible in all patients with severe malaria. Two classes of parenteral agents are available for the treatment of severe malaria: the artemisinin derivatives (artesunate and artemether) and the cinchona alkaloids (quinine and quinidine). Injectable antibacterial agents with antimalarial activity should not be used alone without one of the classes mentioned earlier, because their spectrum and speed of action are inadequate (**Fig. 2** and **3**). Dosing regimens and precautions are detailed in **Box 2**, and drug availability by region is given in **Table 1**.

Artemisinin Derivatives

Artemisinins have been used medicinally as antipyretic agents in China for at least 2000 years, but only began development as potential antimalarial agents during the

---

Box 2
Antimalarial regimens for severe malaria

Intravenous artesunate is the treatment of choice in all cases of severe malaria, including pregnant women:

> Artesunate intravenous (IV): 2.4 mg/kg at 0, 12, and 24 hours, then daily

> Quinine IV: loading dose 20 mg salt/kg over 4 hours, followed by 10 mg salt/kg 8 hours after starting initial dose, over 2 to 4 hours, then 10 mg salt/kg every 8 hours over 2 to 4 hours

> Other parenteral options include arthemeter intramuscular (IM), quinine IM, and quinidine IV

> Oral agents: see text

Notes:

- All drugs should be ordered as urgent
- In endemic areas, artesunate should never be administered without a second agent because of concerns about generating transmissible artesunate-resistant parasites
- Cardiac monitoring and reduced doses of IV quinine should be used in patients who received quinoline-related agents in the hours preceding treatment, including oral quinine, quinidine, mefloquine, chloroquine, halofantrine, piperaquine, and halofantrine
- Quinine infusion should be held if either (1) QT interval (QTc) is increased 25% more than baseline, (2) QTc exceeds 600 milliseconds, or (3) if hypotension occurs

---

Vietnam War in the 1970s.[27] The first large-scale clinical trials comparing early artemisinin derivatives with quinine were performed in the 1990s.[28] In vitro and in vivo, artesunate has the broadest and most rapid parasite-killing activity of any agent known.[27] In addition, artesunate has a preferable side effect profile to that of quinine and is effective against the sexual forms of *P falciparum*, which serves to reduce parasite transmission. Several randomized clinical trials have established that artemisinins are the most effective antimalarial agents and reduce mortality from severe malaria in both adults and children, compared with parenteral quinine.

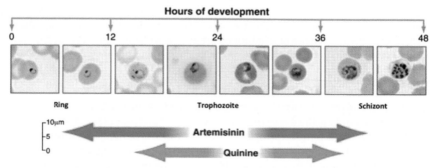

Fig. 2. The intraerythrocytic life cycle of *P falciparum* and the spectrum of action of parenteral antimalarial agents. Parasitized red blood cells circulate for the first third of the 48-hour cycle and then sequester in the microcirculation. Artemisinins inhibit development of a broader age range of the parasites than other antimalarial drugs. The effect on the young rings prevents the formation of mature parasites able to localise in the microcirculation. Antibacterial agents such as doxycycline and clindamycin inhibit development of a narrower age range of the parasites than quinine. (*From* White NJ. Qinghaosu (artemisinin): the price of success. Science 2008;320:330; with permission.)

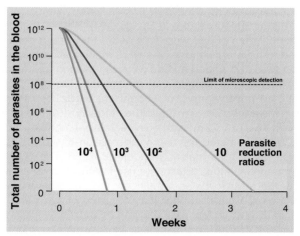

Fig. 3. Speed of parasite clearance with antimalarial drugs in vivo. The starting point shows infections of 10^{12} parasites (roughly equivalent to 2% parasitemia in an adult). Weak antimalarials, such as many antibacterials with antimalarial action, reduce the body burden of parasites by a factor of about 10 per asexual cycle (ie, a parasite reduction ratio [PRR] of 10) and thus need weeks to clear an infection. Most antimalarials (eg, quinine and chloroquine) have PRR values of 100 to 1000 per cycle. The artemisinins are the most potent antimalarial drugs, with PRR values around 10,000 per cycle, and thus take only 3 to 4 cycles (6–8 days) to eradicate the infection. (*From* White NJ. Qinghaosu (artemisinin): the price of success. Science 2008;320:332; with permission.)

Table 1
Distributor contact information and manufacturer of artesunate supply in various regions of the world. Outside North America, commercial distributors source artesunate from Guilin Pharmaceutical (Shanghai) Co, Ltd, which is WHO prequalified but not Good Manufacturing Practices (GMP) certified. In North America, no US Food and Drug Administration or Public Health Agency of Canada–approved product is available for commercial distribution because of lack of GMP certification. In these countries, GMP-certified artesunate is available through special access programs

Region	Who to Contact	Product Manufacturer
Malaria-endemic countries	Individual national malaria control programs	Guilin Pharmaceutical (Shanghai) Co, Ltd
Europe	Artesunate distributed by: ACE Pharmaceuticals BV PO Box 1262 NL-3890 BB Zeewolde, The Netherlands Customer service +31-36-5474092 http://www.ace-pharm.nl	Guilin Pharmaceutical (Shanghai) Co, Ltd
United States	CDC Malaria Hotline: +1-770-488-7788 (Monday to Friday, 8:00 AM to 4:30 PM, eastern time) or After hours, call +1-770-488-7100 and request CDC Malaria Branch clinician	US Army Medical Materiel Development Activity
Canada	Canadian Malaria Network 24 h/d Numbers by city: http://www.phac-aspc.gc.ca/tmp-pmv/quinine/index-eng.php	US Army Medical Materiel Development Activity

Abbreviation: CDC, US Centers for Disease Control and Prevention.

The largest such trial in adults is the SEAQUAMAT trial,[29] a multicentre, open-label, randomized trial that included centers in Bangladesh, Burma, India, and Indonesia. Patients more than 2 years of age were included if they had a positive RDT results and were deemed to have a diagnosis of severe malaria according to the admitting physician. Certain sites also added oral doxycycline to each treatment arm once the patients were well enough to tolerate oral medication. The trial was stopped after the enrollment of 1461 patients, most of whom were adults, because of a significant mortality benefit in the artesunate arm (absolute mortality, 107/730 [15%] with artesunate compared with 164/731 [22%] with quinine; relative mortality reduction, 34.7%; $P = .0002$). The WHO promoted the use of artemisinin-based therapies to first-line treatment of severe falciparum malaria in adults in 2006. The AQUAMAT trial was designed to evaluate intravenous artesunate use in African children with severe malaria. Similar to SEAQUAMAT, it was a multicentre, open-label trial with 11 centers in 9 African countries. Children younger than 15 years of age were included if they had a positive rapid diagnostic test for *P falciparum* and if they fulfilled criteria for severe malaria. As in SEAQUAMAT, a substantial, although smaller, mortality benefit was noted (absolute mortality, 230/2712 [8.5%] with artesunate compared with 297/2713 [10.9%] with quinine; relative mortality reduction, 22.5%; $P = .0002$). No serious adverse drug effects were reported.[30] These two trials formed the basis of a global paradigm shift in the treatment of severe malaria, toward the use of parenteral artesunate instead of parenteral quinine.

Previous studies had already established that another artemisinin derivative, arthemeter, is at least as effective as quinine in terms of mortality, but had fewer adverse effects.[28,31] The presumed superiority of intravenous artesunate compared with intramuscular arthemeter is derived from pharmacokinetic and pharmacodynamic data,[32,33] confirmed by a striking mortality difference in clinical trials versus quinine. At present, artesunate is universally effective for infections acquired around the world. However, fears of resistance have emerged following the description of decreased speed of parasite killing in vivo in some areas of southeast Asia.[34]

Toxicity concerns with artesunate have emerged amid sporadic delayed hemolytic reactions occurring up to 32 days after treatment, particularly in Europe.[35,36] Such reactions have not previously been reported from North American patients, leading to speculation that distinct drug supplies might account for this difference.[36] However, the first known North American instance of postartesunate delayed hemolysis has recently been identified in Canada, and may alter this hypothesis (Stan Houston, personal communication, 2013). Other hematologic toxicities, such as severe neutropenia, have been reported.[37]

Quinine and Quinidine

Quinine has been the standard treatment of severe malaria for centuries, and remains highly effective in all areas of the world. In addition to its inferior outcomes compared with artesunate, its use is limited by frequent and potentially fatal toxicity, which can include infusional hypotension, cardiac arrhythmia, and hypoglycemia via the stimulation of pancreatic islet cells. Hypoglycemia with quinine is especially frequent in pregnant patients. Quinidine is as effective as quinine, but is considered more toxic and should only be used when neither artemisinins nor parenteral quinine are available. For both drugs, the capacity for electrocardiographic monitoring and serial assessment of blood pressure and glycemia is required.[14,38]

Oral Agents

Oral agent can be substituted for parenteral drugs after greater than or equal to 24 hours of treatment when patients are able to tolerate oral medications. Acceptable oral regimens include the full recommended course of effective oral artemisinin combination therapies (ACT), artesunate (plus doxycycline or clindamycin), quinine (plus doxycycline or clindamycin), and atovaquone-proguanil. Chloroquine may be used for falciparum malaria from areas with known chloroquine-susceptible parasites. Mefloquine should be avoided in patients with severe malaria, especially if cerebral dysfunction is present, because of an increased risk of neuropsychiatric sequelae.[14,39]

SUPPORTIVE CARE AND SPECIFIC COMPLICATIONS

Several aspects of end-organ dysfunction from severe malaria differ from that with bacterial sepsis. Salient examples are discussed later. The relative frequency and severity of specific complication vary by age[40] and local malaria transmission intensity (see **Fig. 1**).

Fluid Management

Uncertainty surrounds optimal fluid management strategies in severe malaria, in which microvascular obstruction decreases circulatory volume and tissue perfusion.[41] Studies of children with severe malaria showing lack of significant intravascular volume depletion[42,43] have supported standard recommendations to avoid aggressive fluid administration in this setting.[44,45]

The Fluid Expansion as Supportive Therapy (FEAST) trial found an increased 48-hour mortality among 2097 severely ill African children randomized to receiving a fluid bolus of 20 to 40 mL/kg, compared with 1044 children who received maintenance fluids only.[46] Mortality at 48 hours was 10.5% in the bolus group compared with 7.3% in the no-bolus group (Relative Risk [RR] 1.45; 95% CI, 1.13–1.86). Most of the children had confirmed malaria (57%), and patients were included if they had severe febrile illness complicated by impaired consciousness and/or respiratory distress together with clinically defined impaired perfusion (median age, 24 months). Only 29 of 3170 children enrolled were severely hypotensive, and all of these were given fluid boluses. Although the trial is a major achievement in the presence of severe logistical challenges, interpretation of these results is complicated by lack of information on the causes of excess deaths, and by the lack of evidence of different outcomes in the subgroup without malaria. It is possible that the limited capacity in the study setting for monitoring and managing reversible complications of fluid administration (such as pulmonary and cerebral edema) were responsible for the observed results, rather than particularities in the pathophysiology of severe malaria.

More recently, Taylor and colleagues[47] reported on a series of 28 adults with severe malaria in whom transpulmonary thermodilution was used to assess global end diastolic volume (a measure of intravascular volume), extravascular lung water (a measure of pulmonary edema), and pulmonary vascular permeability. Unlike previous studies in children, all patients were hypovolemic on arrival and received a median of 3.4 L (range 1.0–7.3 L) of fluid resuscitation in the first 6 hours of admission. By 72 hours, a total of 15/28 patients (54%) developed clinical pulmonary edema with increased pulmonary vascular permeability, 7 of whom died despite mechanical ventilation. Although there was no correlation between the amount of fluid received and the development of acute lung injury (ALI), those patients who eventually developed pulmonary vascular leakage could not be identified by any parameter at the time of admission, suggesting a need for caution with fluid administration.

In summary, available information supports current guidelines and the widespread clinical practice that patients with severe malaria who do not have hypotension or signs of significant volume depletion should generally receive fluids conservatively.[8,14]

This is in contrast with the management of shock from bacterial sepsis, in which early fluid administration is advocated and is shown to decrease mortality, at least in high-income settings.[48,49]

Hypotension

Hypotensive shock in severe malaria is unusual and is associated with high mortality in all age groups.[50,51] In addition to nonmalarial causes of distributive shock, such as concomitant bacterial sepsis, hypovolemic shock from splenic rupture or other causes should be specifically excluded. In this setting, cautious administration of fluid boluses is recommended. The optimal timing for the introduction of inotropic agents is unknown and has not been evaluated in clinical trials. When inotropes are required, the greatest published experience in severe malaria supports the safety of dopamine.[50,52] Norepinephrine and dobutamine have also been used safely. Epinephrine can induce profound lactic acidosis in patients with malaria,[52] although the clinical implications of this are not clear. Many authorities advocate avoidance of epinephrine in this setting.[53,54]

Empiric Antimicrobials

Malaria is a predisposing factor to bacterial infections during and following illness.[55] This predisposition seems to be more significant in endemic areas than for imported malaria in returning travelers. Moreover, people from areas of high malaria transmission frequently have some degree of asymptomatic parasitemia unrelated to presenting febrile illnesses, suggesting the importance of ruling out bacterial infections in critically ill patients.[26,56,57] Among adults with severe imported *P falciparum* malaria, significant concomitant bacterial infections are reported in 24% to 30% of cases.[58–60] Published rates of concomitant bacteremia were 4.5% among 400 consecutive cases of severe malaria in French ICUs (10 on admission and 8 nosocomial),[58] 3.3% in Portugal (2/59 cases, both nosocomial),[61] and 0% in Sweden (0/30 cases).[60] Among adults in malaria-endemic settings, the rate of concomitant bacteremia was 13% in India (39/301[62] – 31/39 were nosocomial from ventilator-associated pneumonia [VAP]), and 0.2% (1/500) in a Vietnamese series.[47] Empiric use of antimicrobials may confound these data.

Concurrent bacteremia on hospital admission among children with severe malaria in endemic areas is more frequent than in adults, with multiple series reporting rates of 4% to 21%,[63–68] and up to 42% in outbreak settings.[69] In African studies, bacteremia greatly increases mortality, although this was not the case among adults in France.[58] Nontyphoidal *Salmonella* sp and other Enterobacteriaceae predominate in most series of African patients,[64,69–71] although *Streptococcus pneumoniae* and *Haemophilus influenzae* are also frequently isolated.[68] The flora associated with nosocomial infections reflects local epidemiology.

Nosocomial infections are an important complication of severe malaria, and VAP accounts for most of them. VAP was reported in 12% (48/400) of patients in France,[58] 39% (31/79) of patients with acute respiratory distress syndrome (ARDS) in India,[62] and 24% (20/83) of children in Senegal.[72]

In summary, there should be a low threshold for administering antimicrobials in severe malaria, particularly in any hypotensive patient; in children; in critically ill patients native to areas with a high burden of malaria, such as recently arrived refugees and immigrants; and in patients at risk for secondary nosocomial infections. Empiric therapy for community-acquired infections should optimally include an agent active against potentially resistant Salmonella species. Empiric nosocomial coverage should be guided by local susceptibility patterns.

Cerebral Malaria

Central nervous system dysfunction is the most frequent manifestation of severe falciparum malaria. The main presentations of cerebral malaria are decreased level of consciousness and/or convulsions. The pathogenesis of coma is not well defined but is generally understood to involve parasitized erythrocytes adhering to microvascular endothelial cells, leading to microvascular obstruction.[73] In turn, tissue hypoxia, acidosis, and local inflammation result.[74] Increased intracranial pressure may be seen, most commonly in children, and is thought to result from increased cerebral blood volume with or without interstitial edema.[75] Opening pressures correlate closely with brain swelling on computed tomography (CT) imaging, but neither of these predicts depth of coma or survival.[75]

The use of corticosteroids as adjunctive agents, presumably to reduce host inflammation and intracranial pressure, has been evaluated in 3 randomized, placebo-controlled trials in Asia (2 in adults[76,77] and 1 in Indonesian children).[78] Neither trial could show clinical benefit from dexamethasone, and the largest trial yielded more frequent complications in the treatment group, including prolonged coma, pneumonia, and gastrointestinal bleeding. However, no data exist on corticosteroid use in African children, in whom increased intracranial pressure is most marked. Several clinical trials have similarly evaluated the use of mannitol in both children and adults, all either failing to show clinical benefit or showing harm.[75,79,80]

Convulsions should be managed with standard anticonvulsant regimens after oxygenation and airway management are achieved. The use of prophylactic anticonvulsants drugs has been studied in 3 randomized trials comparing phenobarbital with placebo or no treatment. A Cochrane meta-analysis on the data found that, although the use of anticonvulsants was associated with fewer convulsions (RR, 0.30; 95% CI, 0.19–0.45), it also resulted in an increased risk of overall mortality (RR, 2.0; 95% CI, 1.20–3.33), arguing against using prophylactic phenobarbital in the treatment of cerebral malaria.[81]

In addition, aspiration pneumonia is an important complication of cerebral malaria. Mechanical ventilation is frequently used for airway protection in patients with decreased levels of consciousness. A recent study of adults with cerebral malaria in a low-resource setting where mechanical ventilation is not available found that aspiration pneumonia occurred in 33% of patients in whom enteral feeding was started on admission.[82] Half of patients with aspiration died. In contrast, whether prophylactic airway protection reduces morbidity and mortality in malaria remains unproved.[72]

Respiratory Failure

Respiratory distress in malaria may arise from severe anemia, severe metabolic acidosis, pneumonia, or ALI/ARDS, and occurs in 25% of adults and 40% of children with severe malaria from *P falciparum*.[47,83] ALI/ARDS may complicate infection with *P falciparum*, *P vivax*, and *P knowlesi*. ARDS is seen in 5% to 25% of adults with severe *P falciparum* malaria,[47] compared 0.1% in US soldiers with uncomplicated malaria.[84] ARDS is rare among young children with malaria. The prognostic impact of malaria-related ALI/ARDS depends on the availability and quality of intensive care with mechanical ventilation. In the largest published series of severe malaria in a high-income setting, ARDS was not an independent prognosticator.[58]

The timing of malaria-related respiratory dysfunction is distinct from that of other complications in that onset is often during the clinical recovery phase, after parasitemia has begun to decrease. For example, 18 of 301 (6%) patients with severe malaria in India had ALI or ARDS on ICU admission. An additional 33/301 (11%) developed

ARDS within 48 hours, and a further 36/301 (12%) developed ARDS later than 48 hours into therapy.[62] As mentioned previously, there are currently no available biomarkers for the early diagnosis of noncardiogenic pulmonary complications, and this argues for a conservative fluid strategy. Ventilation strategies in severe malaria can generally follow guidelines for non–malaria-related ARDS,[48] with the exception that permissive hypercapnia is discouraged in patients with cerebral malaria, because this may exacerbate increased intracranial pressure. Other aspects of pulmonary complications of malaria have been extensively reviewed by Taylor and colleagues.[47]

Acidosis

Metabolic acidosis increases with the severity of malaria infection and is strongly associated with death in all age groups.[40] The principal acid involved is unidentified, but increased production of lactate and ketoacids, as well as impaired renal bicarbonate handling, are important contributors.[85,86] A key driver of lactic acidosis seems to be tissue anaerobic glycolysis following microvascular obstruction by parasites. This theory is supported by studies in children using isotope techniques showing that lactate production was the main cause of hyperlactemia, rather than decreased clearance.[86] Moreover, visualization of parasite sequestration in vivo supports a correlation of microvascular obstruction with hyperlactemia.[87] In addition, in severe malaria, lactate/pyruvate ratios frequently exceed 30, reflecting tissue hypoxia, compared with typical values of less than 15 for bacterial sepsis.[88] Short-term peritoneal dialysis decreased mortality from acidosis with malaria-associated acute kidney injury by 50% in a Vietnamese referral hospital,[89] but was significantly clinically inferior to hemofiltration in a later randomized comparison in the same center.[86] In this setting, hemofiltration rapidly cleared acidemia in patients with malaria with combined renal failure and lactic acidosis. It is not known whether the early use of hemofiltration in patients with acidosis and early kidney injury (ie, before the development of overt renal failure) is clinically beneficial.

Anemia and Blood Transfusion

Profound anemia from massive hemolysis and reticuloendothelial clearance is most frequent in children but may complicate malaria at any age. Anemia decreases tissue oxygenation and contributes to acidosis, organ dysfunction, and death. Transfusion of whole blood or packed red blood cells is warranted clinically but existing data do not allow recommendations on the optimal hemoglobin cutoffs at which transfusion should be given. Benefits should outweigh the risk of acquiring blood-borne infections in areas of uncertain blood supply safety.

When parasitemia is extremely high (eg, >10%), exchange blood transfusion (EBT) is sometimes used in addition to antimalarial drugs to decrease the number of parasitized erythrocytes, reduce microcirculatory obstruction, and improve tissue oxygenation. Although EBT can rapidly decrease parasite biomass with minimal adverse events,[90] few data on outcomes support its use. A meta-analysis of 8 studies comparing the addition of EBT with antimalarials alone did not find that mortality was reduced (odds ratio, 1.2; 95% CI, 0.7–2.1).[91] A retrospective cohort of 146 Austrian cases found no increase in survival when EBT was used in addition to standard therapy.[92] Overall, the role of EBT as an adjunctive measure in hyperparasitemic patients has a strong rationale but weak supporting evidence. Interpretation of available data is complicated by problems with the comparability of various published EBT protocols, and because EBT recipients in unblinded studies generally have higher parasitemia and more severe disease than those without EBT. A sufficiently powered randomized controlled trial is necessary to determine whether exchange transfusion is beneficial.

OTHER ADJUNCTIVE THERAPIES

Numerous other adjunctive measures have been studied to improve outcomes in severe malaria, with limited success thus far. Interventions with data from human trials are summarized in **Table 2**. Several immunomodulators, including and anti–tumor necrosis factor (TNF) monoclonal antibodies, have been evaluated in the setting of severe malaria. Pentoxifylline was among the first agents studied, and was thought to act by reducing cytokine secretion and inhibiting erythrocyte rosette formation.[93] Patients receiving pentoxifylline had lower TNF serum levels and had significantly shorter coma duration, with a trend toward lower overall mortality.[94,95] However, recent data from a small nonrandomized controlled trial showed an unexpected trend toward increased mortality.[96] A double-blind, placebo-controlled trial of B-C7, an anti-TNF monoclonal antibody, similarly yielded an increased risk of neurologic sequelae without an improvement in overall survival in patients with cerebral malaria.[97]

A key feature of the pathogenesis of severe falciparum malaria is the expression of adhesion proteins on the surface of erythrocytes, which leads them to sequester in the microcirculation and eventually cause microvascular obstruction in end organs. Uninfected erythrocytes are able to pass through channels of 2 μm in diameter, whereas *P falciparum*–infected erythrocytes are limited to vessels of at least 6 μm.[98] The mechanism by which this occurs is thought to be the expression of the parasite-derived protein PfEMP-1, which binds to receptors on endothelial surfaces, including ICAM-1 and CD36. Infected red blood cells also form rosettes with uninfected erythrocytes, and this phenotype is associated with severe malaria.[99] In vitro data reveal that heparin can disrupt rosettes, suggesting a novel therapeutic approach in the treatment of severe malaria. However, no clinical studies to date have shown a benefit to the use of heparin as an adjunctive measure in the treatment of severe malaria.[100]

Desferrioxamine and *N*-acetylcysteine have been studied for their antioxidant properties. As a potent iron chelator, desferrioxamine was thought to potentially remove a key nutrient for the growth of *P falciparum* while simultaneously reducing the damages caused by free radical stress.[101] Although initial data suggested a decrease in coma resolution time coupled with increased parasite clearance, subsequent trials have yielded a trend toward increased mortality.[102] *N*-acetylcysteine was evaluated for its antioxidant effect and its inhibition of TNF release. However, the results of a randomized, double-blind, placebo-controlled trial showed no effect in patients with severe malaria.[103]

Other adjunctive therapies are currently being studied, including the use of erythropoietin, activated charcoal, arginine, inhaled nitric oxide, and levamisole. There are currently insufficient data to recommend the use of any adjunctive measures in the treatment of severe falciparum malaria.

FATAL OUTCOMES

The mortality caused by untreated severe malaria is extremely high, and outcomes in treated patients depend on age, setting, antimalarial agents used, and presenting clinical syndromes. In adults with imported severe malaria, reported in-hospital mortality varies from 10% to 25%.[58,59,61] The largest published series reported an ICU mortality of 10.5% (42/400 cases), and identified advanced age, altered consciousness, and hyperparasitemia as independent risk factors for death.[58] This series predated the widespread use of artesunate, and current adult mortality in high-income settings may be lower. In malaria-endemic settings, overall adult mortality from treated severe malaria generally varies around 15% to 25%.[29,62] Substantially higher mortalities occur with specific complications, such as renal failure[62,86] and respiratory failure.[47]

Table 2
Completed, ongoing, or planned trials of adjunctive therapy for severe malaria in humans

Intervention	Pathophysiologic Target	Net Effect	Comments
EBT	Parasite load	Unclear, Need RCT	Reasonable to try: reduces parasite clearance, but does not seem to reduce mortality
Pentoxifylline	TNF production Rosetting RBC deformability	Unclear	Early trials suggested an improvement in coma resolution time, but recent data suggest a trend toward increased mortality
Intravenous immunoglobulin	Cytoadherence of RBCs	No benefit	No difference in parasite clearance, defervescence, and coma resolution time
Curdlan sulfate	Cytoadherence of RBCs	No benefit	No difference in mortality
Desferrioxamine	Antioxidant Iron chelator	No benefit	No difference in mortality
N-acetylcysteine	Antioxidant RBC deformability TNF release	No benefit	RCT showed no difference in mortality, lactate clearance, or coma resolution time
Heparin	Microcirculatory flow Rosetting	No benefit	RCT showed no difference in parasite clearance, defervescence, or LOS
Dexamethasone	Intracranial pressure Systemic inflammation	Harmful	May prolong coma and increase risk of pneumonia and GI bleeding
Anti-TNF monoclonal antibody	TNF	Harmful	Increased risk of neurologic sequelae
Albumin	Hypovolemia	Harmful	Fluid bolus increased mortality in severely ill African children
Mannitol	Intracranial pressure Microcirculatory flow Free radical damage	Harmful	Prolongs coma resolution time
Phenobarbital	Anticonvulsant	Harmful	Reduces convulsions but likely increases mortality
Erythropoietin	Neuroprotection	Beneficial? Ongoing	May reduce risk of neurologic sequelae
Rosiglitazone	Phagocytosis of infected RBCs Systemic inflammation	Beneficial? Planned	Increased parasite clearance
Activated charcoal	Neuroprotection	Ongoing	—
Arginine	Endothelial function Oxygen delivery	Ongoing	—
Inhaled nitric oxide	Endothelial function	Ongoing	—
Levamisole	Cytoadherence of RBCs	Ongoing	—

Ongoing trials can be found at http://www.controlled-trials.com.
Abbreviations: GI, gastrointestinal; LOS, length of stay; RBC, red blood cell; RCT, randomized controlled trial; TNF, tumor necrosis factor.
Data from Refs.[46,75–81,90–97,100–103,105–117]

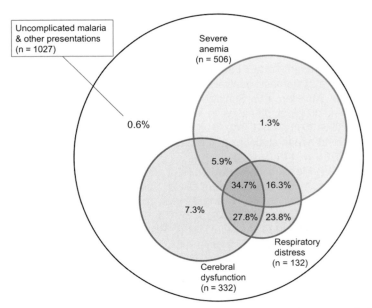

Fig. 4. Distribution and mortality of major clinical presentations of severe malaria among children in an area with high transmission intensity. Percentages are in-hospital mortality for each subgroup. Outcomes are in children treated with quinine. (*Data from* Marsh K, Forster D, Waruiru K, et al. Indicators of life-threatening malaria in African children. N Engl J Med 1995;332:1399–404.)

The 5-point Coma Acidosis Malaria (CAM) score reliably identifies adults with malaria who can safely be treated on general medical wards.[104]

Most pediatric data are from African children. As in adults, mortality varies by clinical syndrome (**Fig. 4**).[83] Overall mortality from severe malaria among children in 2 large recent clinical trials was 8.0% to 8.5%, which is generally lower than rates seen in adults from similar settings.[30,46] Moreover, in the SEAQUAMAT trial in Asia, the overall mortality in children 2 years of age or older with severe malaria treated with artesunate was approximately 5%, compared with overall mortalities in adults treated with artesunate of more than 3 times that, at 16%.[29] The reasons for this observed difference are not completely understood.

SUMMARY

Early recognition and diagnosis of severe malaria is vital. Intravenous artesunate should be used as first-line antimalarial treatment. The threshold for using antibiotic therapy should be low, particularly in children, in hypotensive patients, and in critically ill patients originating from endemic areas. Patients with severe malaria without hypotension or signs of significant volume depletion should generally receive fluids conservatively, in contrast with the recommendation for bacterial sepsis. Current data are insufficient to recommend any specific adjunct adjunctive therapy.

ACKNOWLEDGMENTS

We thank Drs Makeda Semret and Michael Libman (Montreal, Canada) and Professor Emmanuel Bottieau (Antwerp, Belgium) for critical review and insight on earlier versions of this article.

REFERENCES

1. WHO. World malaria report 2010. Geneva (Switzerland): World Health Organization; 2010. p. 238.
2. Murray CJ, Rosenfeld LC, Lim SS, et al. Global malaria mortality between 1980 and 2010: a systematic analysis. Lancet 2012;379:413–31.
3. Jensenius M, Han PV, Schlagenhauf P, et al. Acute and potentially life-threatening tropical diseases in western travelers–a GeoSentinel multicenter study, 1996–2011. Am J Trop Med Hyg 2013;88:397–404.
4. WHO. World health statistics 2011. Geneva (Switzerland): World Health Organization; 2011. p. 171.
5. O'Meara WP, Mangeni JN, Steketee R, et al. Changes in the burden of malaria in sub-Saharan Africa. Lancet Infect Dis 2010;10:545–55.
6. Feachem RG, Phillips AA, Hwang J, et al. Shrinking the malaria map: progress and prospects. Lancet 2010;376:1566–78.
7. Legros F, Bouchaud O, Ancelle T, et al. Risk factors for imported fatal *Plasmodium falciparum* malaria, France, 1996–2003. Emerg Infect Dis 2007;13:883–8.
8. Lalloo DG, Shingadia D, Pasvol G, et al. UK malaria treatment guidelines. J Infect 2007;54:111–21.
9. Mali S, Kachur SP, Arguin PM. Malaria surveillance–United States, 2010. MMWR Surveill Summ 2012;61:1–17.
10. CATMAT. Canadian recommendations for the prevention and treatment of malaria among international travellers–2009. Can Commun Dis Rep 2009; 35(Suppl 1):1–82.
11. Watkins K, McCarthy AE, Molnar-Szakacs H, et al. A survey of the accuracy of malaria reporting by the laboratories in Ontario and British Columbia. Can Commun Dis Rep 2003;29:121–5.
12. Seringe E, Thellier M, Fontanet A, et al. Severe imported *Plasmodium falciparum* malaria, France, 1996–2003. Emerg Infect Dis 2011;17:807–13.
13. Phillips A, Bassett P, Zeki S, et al. Risk factors for severe disease in adults with falciparum malaria. Clin Infect Dis 2009;48:871–8.
14. WHO. Guidelines for the treatment of malaria. 2nd edition. Geneva (Switzerland): World Health Organization; 2010. p. 1–194.
15. Taylor SM, Molyneux ME, Simel DL, et al. Does this patient have malaria? J Am Med Assoc 2010;304:2048–56.
16. D'Acremont V, Lengeler C, Mshinda H, et al. Time to move from presumptive malaria treatment to laboratory-confirmed diagnosis and treatment in African children with fever. PLoS Med 2009;6:e252.
17. D'Acremont V, Malila A, Swai N, et al. Withholding antimalarials in febrile children who have a negative result for a rapid diagnostic test. Clin Infect Dis 2010;51: 506–11.
18. Abba K, Deeks JJ, Olliaro P, et al. Rapid diagnostic tests for diagnosing uncomplicated *P. falciparum* malaria in endemic countries. Cochrane Database Syst Rev 2011;(7):CD008122. http://dx.doi.org/10.1002/14651858.CD008122.pub2.
19. Gillet P, Mori M, Van Esbroeck M, et al. Assessment of the prozone effect in malaria rapid diagnostic tests. Malar J 2009;8:271.
20. Gillet P, Scheirlinck A, Stokx J, et al. Prozone in malaria rapid diagnostics tests: how many cases are missed? Malar J 2011;10:166.
21. Maltha J, Gillet P, Jacobs J. Malaria rapid diagnostic tests in travel medicine. Clin Microbiol Infect 2013;19:408–15. http://dx.doi.org/10.1111/1469-0691. 12152.

22. Birbeck GL, Beare N, Lewallen S, et al. Identification of malaria retinopathy improves the specificity of the clinical diagnosis of cerebral malaria: findings from a prospective cohort study. Am J Trop Med Hyg 2010;82:231–4.
23. Taylor TE, Fu WJ, Carr RA, et al. Differentiating the pathologies of cerebral malaria by postmortem parasite counts. Nat Med 2004;10:143–5.
24. Beare N, Taylor T, Harding S, et al. Malarial retinopathy: a newly established diagnostic sign in severe malaria. Am J Trop Med Hyg 2006;75:790–7.
25. Seydel KB, Fox LL, Glover SJ, et al. Plasma concentrations of parasite histidine-rich protein 2 distinguish between retinopathy-positive and retinopathy-negative cerebral malaria in Malawian children. J Infect Dis 2012;206:309–18.
26. Hendriksen IC, Mwanga-Amumpaire J, von Seidlein L, et al. Diagnosing severe falciparum malaria in parasitaemic African children: a prospective evaluation of plasma PfHRP2 measurement. PLoS Med 2012;9:e1001297.
27. White NJ. Qinghaosu (artemisinin): the price of success. Science 2008;320:330–4.
28. Artemether-Quinine Meta-analysis Study Group. A meta-analysis using individual patient data of trials comparing artemether with quinine in the treatment of severe falciparum malaria. Trans R Soc Trop Med Hyg 2001;95:637–50.
29. Dondorp A, Nosten F, Stepniewska K, et al. Artesunate versus quinine for treatment of severe falciparum malaria: a randomised trial. Lancet 2005;366:717–25.
30. Dondorp AM, Fanello CI, Hendriksen IC, et al. Artesunate versus quinine in the treatment of severe falciparum malaria in African children (AQUAMAT): an open-label, randomised trial. Lancet 2010;376:1647–57.
31. Tran TH, Day NP, Nguyen HP, et al. A controlled trial of artemether or quinine in Vietnamese adults with severe falciparum malaria. N Engl J Med 1996;335:76–83.
32. Hien TT, Davis TM, Chuong LV, et al. Comparative pharmacokinetics of intramuscular artesunate and artemether in patients with severe falciparum malaria. Antimicrobial Agents Chemother 2004;48:4234–9.
33. Gomes M, Ribeiro I, Warsame M, et al. Rectal artemisinins for malaria: a review of efficacy and safety from individual patient data in clinical studies. BMC Infect Dis 2008;8:39.
34. Dondorp AM, Nosten F, Yi P, et al. Artemisinin resistance in *Plasmodium falciparum* malaria. N Engl J Med 2009;361:455–67.
35. Zoller T, Junghanss T, Kapaun A, et al. Intravenous artesunate for severe malaria in travelers, Europe. Emerg Infect Dis 2011;17:771–7.
36. CDC. Published reports of delayed hemolytic anemia after treatment with artesunate for severe malaria — worldwide, 2010–2012. MMWR Morb Mortal Wkly Rep 2013;62:5–8.
37. Bethell D, Se Y, Lon C, et al. Dose-dependent risk of neutropenia after 7-day courses of artesunate monotherapy in Cambodian patients with acute *Plasmodium falciparum* malaria. Clin Infect Dis 2010;51:e105–14.
38. White NJ. Cardiotoxicity of antimalarial drugs. Lancet Infect Dis 2007;7:549–58.
39. Nguyen TH, Day NP, Ly VC, et al. Post-malaria neurological syndrome. Lancet 1996;348:917–21.
40. Dondorp AM, Lee SJ, Faiz MA, et al. The relationship between age and the manifestations of and mortality associated with severe malaria. Clin Infect Dis 2008;47:151–7.
41. Dondorp AM, Pongponratn E, White NJ. Reduced microcirculatory flow in severe falciparum malaria: pathophysiology and electron-microscopic pathology. Acta Trop 2004;89:309–17.

42. Planche T, Onanga M, Schwenk A, et al. Assessment of volume depletion in children with malaria. PLoS Med 2004;1:e18.
43. Macallan DC, Abaye DA, Dottin S, et al. Blood volume and red cell mass in children with moderate and severe malaria measured by chromium-53 dilution and gas chromatography/mass spectrometric analysis. Rapid Commun Mass Spectrom 2009;23:2467–75.
44. Planche T. Malaria and fluids–balancing acts. Trends Parasitol 2005;21:562–7.
45. Planche T. Not yet time to use mortality as an outcome in trials of intravenous fluid therapy in severe malaria. Trends Parasitol 2007;23:138–9.
46. Maitland K, Kiguli S, Opoka RO, et al. Mortality after fluid bolus in African children with severe infection. N Engl J Med 2011;364:2483–95.
47. Taylor WR, Hanson J, Turner GD, et al. Respiratory manifestations of malaria. Chest 2012;142:492–505.
48. Dellinger RP, Levy MM, Carlet JM, et al. Surviving Sepsis Campaign: international guidelines for management of severe sepsis and septic shock: 2008. Crit Care Med 2008;36:296–327.
49. Rivers E, Nguyen B, Havstad S, et al. Early goal-directed therapy in the treatment of severe sepsis and septic shock. N Engl J Med 2001;345:1368–77.
50. Bruneel F, Gachot B, Timsit JF, et al. Shock complicating severe falciparum malaria in European adults. Intensive Care Med 1997;23:698–701.
51. Maitland K, Pamba A, Newton CR, et al. Response to volume resuscitation in children with severe malaria. Pediatr Crit Care Med 2003;4:426–31.
52. Day NPJ, Phu NH, Bethell DP, et al. The effects of dopamine and adrenaline infusions on acid-base balance and systemic haemodynamics in severe infection. Lancet 1996;348:219–23.
53. Day N, Dondorp AM. The management of patients with severe malaria. Am J Trop Med Hyg 2007;77:29–35.
54. Krishna S. Adjunctive management of malaria. Curr Opin Infect Dis 2012;25:484–8.
55. Scott JA, Berkley JA, Mwangi I, et al. Relation between falciparum malaria and bacteraemia in Kenyan children: a population-based, case-control study and a longitudinal study. Lancet 2011;378:1316–23.
56. Hendriksen IC, White LJ, Veenemans J, et al. Defining falciparum-malaria-attributable severe febrile illness in moderate-to-high transmission settings on the basis of plasma PfHRP2 concentration. J Infect Dis 2013;207:351–61.
57. Koram KA, Molyneux ME. When is "malaria" malaria? The different burdens of malaria infection, malaria disease, and malaria-like illnesses. Am J Trop Med Hyg 2007;77:1–5.
58. Bruneel F, Tubach F, Corne P, et al. Severe imported falciparum malaria: a cohort study in 400 critically ill adults. PLoS One 2010;5:e13236.
59. Gonzalez A, Nicolas JM, Munoz J, et al. Severe imported malaria in adults: retrospective study of 20 cases. Am J Trop Med Hyg 2009;81:595–9.
60. Sandlund J, Naucler P, Dashti S, et al. Bacterial coinfections in travelers with malaria: rationale for antibiotic therapy. J Clin Microbiol 2013;51:15–21.
61. Santos LC, Abreu CF, Xerinda SM, et al. Severe imported malaria in an intensive care unit: a review of 59 cases. Malar J 2012;11:96.
62. Krishnan A, Karnad DR. Severe falciparum malaria: an important cause of multiple organ failure in Indian intensive care unit patients. Crit Care Med 2003;31:2278–84.
63. Nadjm B, Amos B, Mtove G, et al. WHO guidelines for antimicrobial treatment in children admitted to hospital in an area of intense Plasmodium falciparum transmission: prospective study. BMJ 2010;340:c1350.

64. Bronzan RN, Taylor TE, Mwenechanya J, et al. Bacteremia in Malawian children with severe malaria: prevalence, etiology, HIV coinfection, and outcome. J Infect Dis 2007;195:895–904.
65. Berkley JA, Maitland K, Mwangi I, et al. Use of clinical syndromes to target antibiotic prescribing in seriously ill children in malaria endemic area: observational study. BMJ 2005;330:995.
66. Nielsen MV, Sarpong N, Krumkamp R, et al. Incidence and characteristics of bacteremia among children in rural Ghana. PLoS One 2012;7:e44063.
67. Ukaga CN, Orji CN, Orogwu S, et al. Concomitant bacteria in the blood of malaria patients in Owerri, southeastern Nigeria. Tanzan Health Res Bull 2006;8:186–8.
68. Berkley JA, Bejon P, Mwangi T, et al. HIV infection, malnutrition, and invasive bacterial infection among children with severe malaria. Clin Infect Dis 2009; 49:336–43.
69. Yansouni CP, Bottieau E, Chappuis F, et al. Rapid diagnostic tests for a coordinated approach to fever syndromes in low-resource settings. Clin Infect Dis 2012;55:610–1 [author reply: 611–2].
70. Were T, Davenport GC, Hittner JB, et al. Bacteremia in Kenyan children presenting with malaria. J Clin Microbiol 2011;49:671–6.
71. Bassat Q, Guinovart C, Sigauque B, et al. Severe malaria and concomitant bacteraemia in children admitted to a rural Mozambican hospital. Trop Med Int Health 2009;14:1011–9.
72. Gerardin P, Rogier C, Ka AS, et al. Outcome of life-threatening malaria in African children requiring endotracheal intubation. Malar J 2007;6:51.
73. Ponsford MJ, Medana IM, Prapansilp P, et al. Sequestration and microvascular congestion are associated with coma in human cerebral malaria. J Infect Dis 2012;205:663–71.
74. Mishra SK, Newton CR. Diagnosis and management of the neurological complications of falciparum malaria. Nat Rev Neurol 2009;5:189–98.
75. Mohanty S, Mishra SK, Patnaik R, et al. Brain swelling and mannitol therapy in adult cerebral malaria: a randomized trial. Clin Infect Dis 2011;53:349–55.
76. Warrell DA, Looareesuwan S, Warrell MJ, et al. Dexamethasone proves deleterious in cerebral malaria. A double-blind trial in 100 comatose patients. N Engl J Med 1982;306:313–9.
77. Hoffman SL, Rustama D, Punjabi NH, et al. High-dose dexamethasone in quinine-treated patients with cerebral malaria: a double-blind, placebo-controlled trial. J Infect Dis 1988;158:325–31.
78. Rampengan TH. Cerebral malaria in children. Comparative study between heparin, dexamethasone and placebo. Paediatr Indones 1991;31:59–66.
79. Namutangula B, Ndeezi G, Byarugaba JS, et al. Mannitol as adjunct therapy for childhood cerebral malaria in Uganda: a randomized clinical trial. Malar J 2007; 6:138.
80. Okoromah CA, Afolabi BB. Mannitol and other osmotic diuretics as adjuncts for treating cerebral malaria. Cochrane Database Syst Rev 2004;(4):CD004615. http://dx.doi.org/10.1002/14651858.CD004615.pub2.
81. Meremikwu M, Marson AG. Routine anticonvulsants for treating cerebral malaria. Cochrane Database Syst Rev 2002;(2):CD002152. http://dx.doi.org/10.1002/14651858.CD002152.
82. Maude RJ, Hoque G, Hasan MU, et al. Timing of enteral feeding in cerebral malaria in resource-poor settings: a randomized trial. PLoS One 2011;6:e27273.
83. Marsh K, Forster D, Waruiru K, et al. Indicators of life-threatening malaria in African children. N Engl J Med 1995;332:1399–404.

84. Sheehy TW, Reba RC. Complications of falciparum malaria and their treatment. Ann Intern Med 1967;66:807–9.

85. Dondorp AM, Chau TT, Phu NH, et al. Unidentified acids of strong prognostic significance in severe malaria. Crit Care Med 2004;32:1683–8.

86. Phu NH, Hien TT, Mai NT, et al. Hemofiltration and peritoneal dialysis in infection-associated acute renal failure in Vietnam. N Engl J Med 2002;347:895–902.

87. Dondorp AM. Clinical significance of sequestration in adults with severe malaria. Transfus Clin Biol 2008;15:56–7.

88. Day NP, Phu NH, Mai NT, et al. The pathophysiologic and prognostic significance of acidosis in severe adult malaria. Crit Care Med 2000;28:1833–40.

89. Trang TT, Phu NH, Vinh H, et al. Acute renal failure in patients with severe falciparum malaria. Clin Infect Dis 1992;15:874–80.

90. van Genderen PJ, Hesselink DA, Bezemer JM, et al. Efficacy and safety of exchange transfusion as an adjunct therapy for severe *Plasmodium falciparum* malaria in nonimmune travelers: a 10-year single-center experience with a standardized treatment protocol. Transfusion 2010;50:787–94.

91. Riddle MS, Jackson JL, Sanders JW, et al. Exchange transfusion as an adjunct therapy in severe *Plasmodium falciparum* malaria: a meta-analysis. Clin Infect Dis 2002;34:1192–8.

92. Auer-Hackenberg L, Staudinger T, Bojic A, et al. Automated red blood cell exchange as an adjunctive treatment for severe *Plasmodium falciparum* malaria at the Vienna General Hospital in Austria: a retrospective cohort study. Malar J 2012;11:158.

93. Lehman LG, Vu-Quoc B, Carlson J, et al. *Plasmodium falciparum*: inhibition of erythrocyte rosette formation and detachment of rosettes by pentoxifylline. Trans R Soc Trop Med Hyg 1997;91:74–5.

94. Di Perri G, Di Perri IG, Monteiro GB, et al. Pentoxifylline as a supportive agent in the treatment of cerebral malaria in children. J Infect Dis 1995;171:1317–22.

95. Das BK, Mishra S, Padhi PK, et al. Pentoxifylline adjunct improves prognosis of human cerebral malaria in adults. Trop Med Int Health 2003;8:680–4.

96. Lell B, Kohler C, Wamola B, et al. Pentoxifylline as an adjunct therapy in children with cerebral malaria. Malar J 2010;9:368.

97. van Hensbroek MB, Palmer A, Onyiorah E, et al. The effect of a monoclonal antibody to tumor necrosis factor on survival from childhood cerebral malaria. J Infect Dis 1996;174:1091–7.

98. Taylor-Robinson A. In-vitro model offers insight into the pathophysiology of severe malaria. Lancet 2004;363:1661–3.

99. Juillerat A, Lewit-Bentley A, Guillotte M, et al. Structure of a *Plasmodium falciparum* PfEMP1 rosetting domain reveals a role for the N-terminal segment in heparin-mediated rosette inhibition. Proc Natl Acad Sci U S A 2011;108:5243–8.

100. Hemmer CJ, Kern P, Holst FG, et al. Neither heparin nor acetylsalicylic acid influence the clinical course in human *Plasmodium falciparum* malaria: a prospective randomized study. Am J Trop Med Hyg 1991;45:608–12.

101. Gordeuk V, Thuma P, Brittenham G, et al. Effect of iron chelation therapy on recovery from deep coma in children with cerebral malaria. N Engl J Med 1992;327:1473–7.

102. Thuma PE, Mabeza GF, Biemba G, et al. Effect of iron chelation therapy on mortality in Zambian children with cerebral malaria. Trans R Soc Trop Med Hyg 1998;92:214–8.

103. Charunwatthana P, Abul Faiz M, Ruangveerayut R, et al. N-acetylcysteine as adjunctive treatment in severe malaria: a randomized, double-blinded placebo-controlled clinical trial. Crit Care Med 2009;37:516–22.

104. Hanson J, Lee SJ, Mohanty S, et al. A simple score to predict the outcome of severe malaria in adults. Clin Infect Dis 2010;50:679–85.

105. Hemmer CJ, Hort G, Chiwakata CB, et al. Supportive pentoxifylline in falciparum malaria: no effect on tumor necrosis factor alpha levels or clinical outcome: a prospective, randomized, placebo-controlled study. Am J Trop Med Hyg 1997;56:397–403.

106. Taylor TE, Molyneux ME, Wirima JJ, et al. Intravenous immunoglobulin in the treatment of paediatric cerebral malaria. Clin Exp Immunol 1992;90:357–62.

107. Havlik I, Looareesuwan S, Vannaphan S, et al. Curdlan sulphate in human severe/cerebral *Plasmodium falciparum* malaria. Trans R Soc Trop Med Hyg 2005;99:333–40.

108. Higgins SJ, Kain KC, Liles WC. Immunopathogenesis of falciparum malaria: implications for adjunctive therapy in the management of severe and cerebral malaria. Expert Rev Anti Infect Ther 2011;9:803–19.

109. Casals-Pascual C, Idro R, Picot S, et al. Can erythropoietin be used to prevent brain damage in cerebral malaria? Trends Parasitol 2009;25:30–6.

110. Casals-Pascual C, Idro R, Gicheru N, et al. High levels of erythropoietin are associated with protection against neurological sequelae in African children with cerebral malaria. Proc Natl Acad Sci U S A 2008;105:2634–9.

111. Boggild AK, Krudsood S, Patel SN, et al. Use of peroxisome proliferator-activated receptor gamma agonists as adjunctive treatment for *Plasmodium falciparum* malaria: a randomized, double-blind, placebo-controlled trial. Clin Infect Dis 2009;49:841–9.

112. Serghides L, Patel SN, Ayi K, et al. Rosiglitazone modulates the innate immune response to *Plasmodium falciparum* infection and improves outcome in experimental cerebral malaria. J Infect Dis 2009;199:1536–45.

113. de Souza JB, Okomo U, Alexander ND, et al. Oral activated charcoal prevents experimental cerebral malaria in mice and in a randomized controlled clinical trial in man did not interfere with the pharmacokinetics of parenteral artesunate. PLoS One 2010;5:e9867.

114. Yeo TW, Lampah DA, Gitawati R, et al. Recovery of endothelial function in severe falciparum malaria: relationship with improvement in plasma L-arginine and blood lactate concentrations. J Infect Dis 2008;198:602–8.

115. Hawkes M, Opoka RO, Namasopo S, et al. Nitric oxide for the adjunctive treatment of severe malaria: hypothesis and rationale. Med Hypotheses 2011;77:437–44.

116. Hawkes M, Opoka RO, Namasopo S, et al. Inhaled nitric oxide for the adjunctive therapy of severe malaria: protocol for a randomized controlled trial. Trials 2011;12:176.

117. Dondorp AM, Silamut K, Charunwatthana P, et al. Levamisole inhibits sequestration of infected red blood cells in patients with falciparum malaria. J Infect Dis 2007;196:460–6.

Prevention, Diagnosis, and Management of Surgical Site Infections

Relevant Considerations for Critical Care Medicine

Charles de Mestral, MD, PhD[a],*, Avery B. Nathens, MD, PhD, MPH[b,c]

KEYWORDS

- Surgical site infection • Wound infection • Postoperative infection
- Critical care medicine • Intensive care

KEY POINTS

- Prevention of surgical site infection (SSI) begins and ends in the operating room.
- SSI presentation varies based on the type of surgery and whether the infection involves superficial incisional, deep incisional, or organ/space sites. A high level of suspicion is required for patients with an implanted foreign body or after bariatric surgery.
- Ruling out a rapidly progressive group A streptococcal or clostridial infection and obtaining source control are critical early steps in SSI management.
- In the setting of a nonhealing wound or failure to improve, source control should be reassessed.

DEFINITION OF SURGICAL SITE INFECTION

As the name implies, a surgical site infection (SSI) is an infection directly resulting from a surgical intervention. While interventions in the operating room environment are susceptible to SSI, it is important to consider a broader context. For example, an empyema that occurs after chest tube insertion would be considered an SSI.

The Centers for Disease Control and Prevention (CDC) further characterizes SSIs as superficial incisional, deep incisional, or organ/space. An incisional SSI is limited to the skin and subcutaneous fatty tissue (superficial incisional) or the deeper soft tissues,

Disclosures: The authors have no relevant financial interests to disclose.

[a] Division of General Surgery, Sunnybrook Health Sciences Center, Sunnybrook Research Institute, University of Toronto, 2075 Bayview Avenue, K3W-28H, Toronto, ON M4N 3M5, Canada; [b] Division of General Surgery and Critical Care, Sunnybrook Health Sciences Center, Sunnybrook Research Institute, University of Toronto, 2075 Bayview Avenue, D578, Toronto, ON M4N 3M5, Canada; [c] Li Ka Shing Knowledge Institute, St. Michael's Hospital, University of Toronto, 209 Victoria Street, Toronto, ON M5B 1T8, Canada
* Corresponding author.
E-mail address: charles.demestral@mail.utoronto.ca

such as muscle and fascia (deep incisional). An organ/space SSI affects an organ or organ space that was manipulated during surgical intervention (**Fig 1**).[1,2]

Most SSIs occur within 30 days of the surgical intervention. Depending on the surgery, almost half of these infections may present after discharge.[1,3] A longer window of 1 year from surgical intervention is generally used when defining an SSI in the case of an implanted device (eg, vascular graft, hernia mesh, orthopedic hardware). Thus, in addition to the SSI anatomic classification, the time frame since surgical intervention is a critical consideration, both in the context of SSI surveillance and in the evaluation and management of sepsis in patients who have undergone surgery.

EPIDEMIOLOGY

SSIs are estimated to complicate 2% to 5% of all operative procedures.[4–6] Among hospitalized patients, SSIs account for 14% to 31% of all health care–associated infections and lead to prolonged length of stay and increased costs.[5–7] Patients with an SSI are also 60% more likely to be admitted to the intensive care unit (ICU).[8] Furthermore, many of the risk factors for SSIs are present in patients typically requiring postoperative ICU care.

RISK FACTORS

The importance of various risk factors for SSI differs based on the procedure performed. The risk factors (**Box 1**) can be classified into 3 broad categories relating to

- Patient characteristics
- The disease process requiring surgical intervention
- Characteristics of the surgical procedure

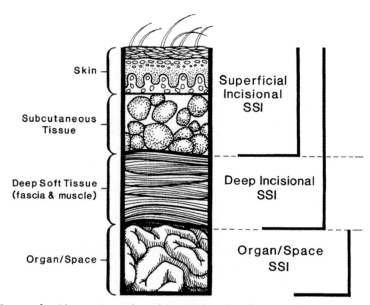

Fig. 1. Centers for Disease Controls and Prevention classification of surgical site infection. (*From* Horan TC, Gaynes RP, Martone WJ, et al. CDC definitions of nosocomial surgical site infections, 1992: a modification of CDC definitions of surgical wound infections. Infect Control Hosp Epidemiol 1992;13(10):606–8; with permission.)

Box 1
Risk factors for surgical site infection

Patient characteristics

- Older age
- Obesity
- Diabetes
- Smoking
- Hyperglycemia
- Malnutrition
- Immunosuppressive therapy: radiotherapy, chemotherapy, steroids

Disease process

- Contaminated wounds: a higher degree of wound contamination increases the risk of SSI. The wound classification system developed by the National Academy of Science in the 1960s is widely used and remains applicable to all surgical procedures. The 4 categories include:

  1. Clean: a procedure without break of sterile technique in which no inflammation is encountered and the gastrointestinal, respiratory, and genitourinary tracts are not entered or transected (eg, inguinal hernia repair, breast lumpectomy, femoropopliteal bypass).

  2. Clean-contaminated: a procedure involving controlled entry into gastrointestinal, respiratory, or genitourinary tract without important contamination (eg, Roux-en-Y gastric bypass, elective right hemicolectomy for colorectal cancer).

  3. Contaminated: a procedure during which a major break in sterile technique or gross spillage from the gastrointestinal tract occurs or the incision is through inflamed tissues.

  4. Dirty/infected: incision is through purulent infected tissues or devitalized tissues, or in the setting of perforated viscus.

- American Society of Anesthesiologists (ASA) physical status classification of 3 or greater: the ASA physical status classification reflects the patient's preoperative condition and underlying illness:

  1. Levels 1 and 2 are healthy patients and patients with mild systemic disease.

  2. Levels 3 and greater are patients with severe systemic disease (level 3), patients with severe systemic disease that is a constant threat to life (level 4), and moribund patients not expected to survived without an operation (level 5).

Surgical procedure

- Prolonged duration of operative intervention: increased risk is associated with duration of operation longer than the 75th percentile in hours for the given procedure.

- Minimally invasive surgical approach: compared with open surgery, minimally invasive approaches (eg, laparoscopic) are generally associated with a lower incidence of SSI.

- Surgical technique: excessive tissue manipulation and ischemia, poor hemostasis, and not approximating subcutaneous tissues.

A recent systematic review of the evidence for each risk factor presented in **Box 1** can be freely accessed online in the National Institute for Health and Clinical Excellence's guideline on SSI prevention.[3]

PATHOGENS

Organisms that cause SSIs are acquired at surgery and involve either microbes endogenous to the surgical site (complete track of dissection) or, less commonly, exogenous microbes from contaminated surgical equipment or personnel. In clean procedures, such as most cardiac, orthopedic, neurologic, breast, and hernia surgeries, skin flora are the most frequent pathogens, including the gram-positive cocci: *Staphylococcus aureus* or coagulase-negative *Staphylococcus* spp.[9]

Enteric organisms are frequently isolated from SSIs, complicating clean-contaminated procedures involving the gastrointestinal tract, whereas SSIs after procedures involving the upper aerodigestive tract (eg, oropharynx, trachea) are often caused by streptococcal species.[1] Contaminated and dirty procedures are more frequently polymicrobial, involving gram-negative bacteria (*Escherichia coli*, *Pseudomonas* spp, *Enterobacter* spp) and anaerobes in cases of fecal contamination.[9]

An increasing number of SSIs involve antibiotic-resistant organism species that should be considered in management.[1] A recent CDC survey involving 463 American hospitals identified high proportions of antibiotic resistance among culture positive SSIs with *S aureus* (49% methicillin-resistant), *E coli* (23% fluoroquinolone-resistant), *Enterococcus* spp (20% vancomycin-resistant), and *Pseudomonas aeruginosa* (16% fluoroquinolone-resistant and 12% carbapenem-resistant).[9] An increased risk of colonization with methicillin-resistant *S aureus* (MRSA) among hospitalized surgical patients has been reported in association with age older than 70 years, nursing home residency, recent hospitalization, recent antibiotic exposure, and chronic skin diseases or ulcers.[10,11]

PREVENTION

Methods of SSI prevention begin and end in the operating room. Antimicrobial prophylaxis should be administered within 30 minutes before incision and redosed if the procedure is prolonged (>3–4 hours). Postoperative antimicrobials have not been shown to be of benefit. Antisepsis preparation of the patient's skin using 70% alcohol with chlorhexidine (where possible), sterile operative technique, and maintenance of perioperative normothermia have all been shown to be beneficial.[3]

Even in cases of intraoperative contamination (eg, inadvertent spillage of gastrointestinal contents), there is no benefit from prolongue antimicrobial therapy (>24 hours).[12,13] This principle is distinct from treatment of surgical infections, for which a course of antimicrobial therapy in addition to source control is mandatory.

The few preventive strategies in the postoperative period that are relevant to care in the ICU include appropriate wound management and postoperative glycemic control.

Appropriate Wound Management

When a surgical incision is primarily closed (skin closed at the end of surgery), CDC recommendations state that the incision should remain covered by a sterile dressing for 24 to 48 hours.[1] In wounds initially left open for later closure (delayed primary closure) or secondary closure, daily packing with moist gauze covered by a dressing is standard. The packing technique and dressing supplies should be sterile.[1] Beyond this standard of care, evidence is insufficient to support routine use of other wound care measures, such as postoperative incision cleansing, topical antimicrobials, or specific products incorporated into dressings.[3]

Postoperative Glycemic Control

Theoretical support for perioperative glycemic control to reduce rates of SSIs can be based on data showing an association between hyperglycemia and SSI for a variety of procedures.[14–16] However, the issue of glycemic control in the ICU remains contentious, with variable efficacy observed with respect to a range of outcomes across different patient populations and targeted glycemic ranges.[17,18] What seems evident is that hypoglycemia should be avoided, because it has been associated with increased mortality in critically ill patients.[19] When considering solely the effect on SSI, postoperative glycemic control is most consistently beneficial in patients with diabetes undergoing cardiac surgery.[20,21] However, for most critically ill patients, moderate glucose control within 140 and 180 mg/dL (7.8 and 10.0 mmol/L) is most appropriate.[22,23]

DIAGNOSIS

SSI as a source of sepsis should be considered in any postoperative patient. The manifestations depend on the site, the type of SSI, and, to a lesser extent, the causal pathogens. A superficial incisional SSI typically presents with erythema, localized swelling, heat, and/or pain. Purulent discharge is frequently seen with S aureus infections. Patients with deep incisional SSIs may have tenderness outside the area of local erythema, and more often have signs of sepsis (eg, fever, leukocytosis, tachycardia, tachypnea). They might also present with incisional dehiscence. Organ/space SSIs reflect a deep contained abscess or uncontained pus that presents with sepsis and local symptoms. After gastrointestinal surgery, the initial manifestations might be a prolonged ileus or failure to tolerate enteral nutrition. Most organ space SSIs (eg, empyema, intra-abdominal abscess) present beyond day 4 to 5. Earlier computed tomography (CT) imaging is not likely to be informative, because early postoperative changes will not be easily differentiated from infection. Two rapidly progressive SSIs require urgent intervention. Infections from group A streptococcal species and clostridial species (most frequently Clostridium perfringens) are rare, but may be catastrophic. Group A streptococcal infections most frequently present within 24 to 48 hours of the surgical procedure, with rapidly progressive cellulitis and significant pain, often with systemic manifestations of sepsis. Clostridial infections present similarly to group A streptococcal infections but may also be associated with subcutaneous gas, often manifesting as crepitus.

MANAGEMENT
Initial Management

Opening the skin of an infected incision is therapeutic through evacuation of pus and allows examination of deeper fascia and muscle to differentiate superficial from deep incisional infections. Cellulitis without purulent drainage or evidence of an underlying abscess might be managed with antimicrobials alone. However, failure to resolve within 24 to 48 hours mandates either opening the incision or further evaluation.

Antimicrobials

In healthy patients, a superficial incisional SSI without a cellulitic component can be treated by opening the incision and changing the dressing without use of antimicrobials.[3] When significant cellulitis accompanies a superficial SSI, antimicrobials with a spectrum appropriate to the most likely pathogens should be administered.

Antimicrobial therapy alone is insufficient for deep incisional or organ space infections. The choice of antimicrobial will depend on the site of infection, the nature of the procedure, and knowledge of local resistance patterns. Discontinuation of antimicrobial therapy is appropriate once clinical signs and symptoms of infection have resolved.[13] If source control is not possible or a prosthesis (eg, implant or hardware) is present, then longer courses might be indicated.

Source Control

Source control represents any intervention designed to drain, debride, or divert the source or foci of infection. Source control might be obtained through debridement in the case of deep incisional or necrotizing infections. Diversion (eg, a defunctioning ileostomy) might be necessary in the case of a leaking intestinal anastomosis. Most frequently, organ space infections may be managed through abscess drainage, either percutaneous or operative. Rarely, antimicrobial therapy is sufficient for small (<2.5 cm) abscesses.

Promoting Healing Through Secondary Intention

Wounds opened in the context of an SSI are usually left to heal through secondary intention. Daily dressing changes allow for gentle mechanical debridement of the wound. Once the wound base is clean and granulation has begun, the frequency of dressing changes can decrease and negative pressure wound therapy can also be considered to remove excess wound edema and promote wound contraction.[24] Involvement of a wound care specialist is recommended for complex wounds.[3]

Treatment Failure

In the setting of a nonhealing wound, or a patient failing to improve, source control should be reassessed and antimicrobial type and dosage reviewed. Prolonged antimicrobial therapy is often not the appropriate solution. Furthermore, immune status should be optimized (eg, improve nutrition, stop steroids) and local wound care management reassessed.

SPECIAL CONSIDERATIONS
Implanted Foreign Body

A few important considerations merit mentioning regarding SSIs in the setting of an implanted foreign body, such as a vascular graft, an abdominal wall mesh, or a joint prosthesis. Given the relatively low microbial burden required to cause an SSI in the context of a foreign body and the nature of the organisms (eg, coagulase-negative *Staphylococcus*, *Enterococci*), infections tend to occur late (months and occasionally years after surgery)[25] and are often associated with limited clinical manifestations.[3] Thus, a high level of suspicion is required. Management remains challenging, with antimicrobials usually trialed before explantation, depending on the severity and site of infection.[25,26]

Obese Patients Post-Bariatric Surgery

Obese patients who undergo bariatric surgery have several of the previously mentioned risk factors for SSI. This patient population presents a diagnostic challenge, because physical examination is limited and intra-abdominal infection might only manifest as tachycardia without fever or peritonitis.[27] A low threshold for CT scan or exploratory laparoscopy/laparotomy is necessary.

SUMMARY

SSI complicates 2% to 5% of all surgical procedures. Many of the risk factors for the development of an SSI (eg, old age, major comorbidity, emergency surgery) are present in patients typically requiring postoperative admission to the ICU. Methods of SSI prevention begin and end in the operating room. Presentation varies based on the type of surgery and whether the infection involves superficial incisional, deep incisional, or organ/space sites. A high level of suspicion is required for patients with an implanted foreign body or after bariatric surgery. Ruling out a rapidly progressive group A streptococcal or clostridial infection and obtaining source control are critical early steps in management. In the setting of a nonhealing wound or failure to improve, source control should be reassessed.

REFERENCES

1. Mangram AJ, Horan TC, Pearson ML, et al. Centers for Disease Control and Prevention guideline for prevention of surgical site infection. Infect Control Hosp Epidemiol 1999;20:247–78.
2. Horan TC, Gaynes RP, Martone WJ, et al. CDC definitions of nosocomial surgical site infections, 1992: a modification of CDC definitions of surgical wound infections. Infect Control Hosp Epidemiol 1992;13(10):606–8.
3. National Institute for Health and Clinical Excellence. Clinical guideline: surgical site infection prevention and treatment. Available at: http://www.nice.org.uk/cg74. Accessed December 28, 2012.
4. Reilly J, Cairns S, Fleming S, et al. Results from the second Scottish national prevalence survey: the changing epidemiology of healthcare-associated infection in Scotland. J Hosp Infect 2012;82(3):170–4.
5. de Lissovoy G, Fraeman K, Hutchins V, et al. Surgical site infection: incidence and impact on hospital utilization and treatment costs. Am J Infect Control 2009;37:387–97.
6. Gravel D, Taylor G, Ofner M, et al. Point prevalence survey for healthcare-associated infections within Canadian adult acute-care hospitals. J Hosp Infect 2007;66(3):243–8.
7. Magill SS, Hellinger W, Cohen J, et al. Prevalence of health-care associated infections in acute care hospitals in Jacksonville, Florida. Infect Control Hosp Epidemiol 2012;33(3):283–91.
8. Kirkland KB, Briggs JP, Trivette SL, et al. The impact of surgical-site infections in the 1990s: attributable mortality, excess length of hospitalization, and extra costs. Infect Control Hosp Epidemiol 1999;20(11):725–30.
9. Hidron AI, Edwards JR, Patel J, et al. Antimicrobial-resistant pathogens associated with healthcare-associated infections: annual summary of data reported to the National Healthcare Safety Network at the Centers for Disease Control and Prevention, 2006-2007. Infect Control Hosp Epidemiol 2008;29(11):996–1011.
10. Pan A, Lee A, Cooper B, et al. Risk factors for previously unknown methicillin-resistant Staphylococcus aureus carriage on admission to 13 surgical wards in Europe. J Hosp Infect 2013;83(2):107–13.

11. Harbarth S, Sax H, Uckay I, et al. A predictive model for identifying surgical patients at risk of methicillin-resistant Staphylococcus aureus carriage on admission. J Am Coll Surg 2008;207(5):683–9.

12. Bratzler DW, Dellinger EP, Olsen KM, et al. Clinical practice guidelines for antimicrobial prophylaxis in surgery. Surg Infect (Larchmt) 2013;14(1):73–156.

13. Solomkin JS, Mazuski JE, Bradley JS, et al. Diagnosis and management of complicated intra-abdominal infection in adults and children: guidelines by the Surgical Infection Society and the Infectious Diseases Society of America. Surg Infect (Larchmt) 2010;11:79–109.

14. Richards JE, Kauffmann RM, Zuckerman SL, et al. Relationship of hyperglycemia and surgical-site infection in orthopaedic surgery. J Bone Joint Surg Am 2012; 94(13):1181–6.

15. Jackson RS, Amdur RL, White JC, et al. Hyperglycemia is associated with increased risk of morbidity and mortality after colectomy for cancer. J Am Coll Surg 2012;214(1):68–80.

16. Ata A, Lee J, Bestle SL, et al. Postoperative hyperglycemia and surgical site infection in general surgery patients. Arch Surg 2010;145(9):858–64.

17. Kavanagh BP, McCowen KC. Clinical practice. Glycemic control in the ICU. N Engl J Med 2010;363(26):2540–6.

18. Hirsch IB. Understanding low sugar from NICE-SUGAR. N Engl J Med 2012; 367(12):1150–2.

19. NICE-SUGAR Study Investigators, Finfer S, Liu B, et al. Hypoglycemia and risk of death in critically ill patients. N Engl J Med 2012;367(12):1108–18.

20. Lazar HL, Chipkin SR, Fitzgerald CA, et al. Tight glycemic control in diabetic coronary artery bypass graft patients improves perioperative outcomes and decreases recurrent ischemic events. Circulation 2004;109(12):1497–502.

21. Leibowitz G, Raizman E, Brezis M, et al. Effects of moderate intensity glycemic control after cardiac surgery. Ann Thorac Surg 2010;90(6):1825–32.

22. Moghissi ES, Korytkowski MT, DiNardo M, et al. American Association of Clinical Endocrinologists and American Diabetes Association consensus statement on inpatient glycemic control. Diabetes Care 2009;32:1119–31.

23. Lazar HL, McDonnell MM, Chipkin S, et al. Effects of aggressive versus moderate glycemic control on clinical outcomes in diabetic coronary artery bypass graft patients. Ann Surg 2011;254:458–64.

24. Venturi ML, Attinger CE, Mesbahi AN, et al. Mechanisms and clinical applications of the vacuum-assisted closure (VAC) device: a review. Am J Clin Dermatol 2005; 6:185–94.

25. Shuman EK, Urquhart A, Malani PN. Management and prevention of prosthetic joint infection. Infect Dis Clin North Am 2012;26:29–39.

26. Young MH, Upchurch GR, Malani PN. Vascular graft infections. Prosthetic joint infection. Infect Dis Clin North Am 2012;26:41–56.

27. Townsend CM, Beauchamp RD, Evers BM, et al. Sabiston textbook of surgery. 19th edition. Missouri: Elsevier; 2012.

Resistant Gram-Negative Infections

Henry Fraimow, MD[a],*, Raquel Nahra, MD[b]

KEYWORDS

- Enterobacteriaceae • *Pseudomonas aeruginosa* • *Acinetobacter* species
- Gram-negative bacilli • Septic shock • Antibiotic resistance

KEY POINTS

- Worldwide increased incidence of multidrug-resistant gram-negative bacilli (GNB) has been associated with worse outcomes.
- Strategies including combination therapy and extended antimicrobial infusion are increasingly being used in attempts to treat these infections.
- Source control remains an important part of managing septic shock as clinicians are faced with increasing incidence of multidrug-resistant GNB, a paucity of new agents, and ineffectiveness of older agents.

BACKGROUND

The global crisis in antimicrobial resistance continues to escalate. Infections caused by multidrug-resistant (MDR) gram-negative bacilli (GNB) are particularly challenging, with little immediate help forthcoming in the antimicrobial pipeline.[1–3] The crisis of MDR infections is especially vexing in the intensive care unit (ICU), where the highest rates of MDR GNB are found.[4] In the ICU, early effective antimicrobial therapy improves survival of patients with septic shock and other life-threatening infections, but selective pressures from intense antimicrobial exposure contribute to the emergence of MDR bacteria, including extensively drug-resistant (XDR) and even pan–drug-resistant (PDR) organisms.[5] MDR pathogens colonizing patients in ICUs can "leak" into the long-term patient population and even into the community setting, when former ICU patients cycle through the acute and chronic health care system.

Funding Sources: None.

Conflict of Interest: None.

[a] Department of Medicine, Cooper Medical School of Rowan University, 401 Haddon Avenue, Room 278, Camden, NJ 08103, USA; [b] Department of Medicine, Cooper Medical School of Rowan University, 401 Haddon Avenue, Room 261, Camden, NJ 08103, USA

* Corresponding author.

E-mail address: Fraimow-henry@cooperhealth.edu

Crit Care Clin 29 (2013) 895–921

http://dx.doi.org/10.1016/j.ccc.2013.06.010

criticalcare.theclinics.com

0749-0704/13/$ – see front matter © 2013 Elsevier Inc. All rights reserved.

This article reviews the major classes of resistant and MDR GNB and their current prevalence in ICUs worldwide. The authors discuss the older and new drugs of potential use in treating these infections, and current strategies to maximize their effectiveness, including rational combination therapy and dosing schemes optimizing the pharmacodynamics of these agents. Treatment options are presented for specific classes of resistant GNB encountered in the ICU, including extended β-lactamase (ESBL)-producing, AmpC-producing, and carbapenem-resistant Enterobacteriaceae (CRE), MDR and carbapenem-resistant *Acinetobacter baumannii* (ACCB), and MDR *Pseudomonas aeruginosa* (PA).

EPIDEMIOLOGY

Antimicrobial resistance is a major public health catastrophe. Following the introduction of each new antimicrobial, reports of resistance rapidly appear. In the late 1970s, reports described mechanisms of resistance of GNB to aminoglycoside and the newly introduced cefamandole.[6] More recently, the lag from introduction of new agents to reports of resistance has markedly decreased, with resistance often identified even before release of the drug. A wide variety of resistance mechanisms are described in GNB. Some mechanisms, such as ESBL production, are found in many species. Others are highly specific, such as overexpression of the MexAB-OprM efflux pump in PA.[7] GNB resistance mechanisms are reviewed elsewhere.[8,9] Important classes of resistance are summarized in **Table 1**.

The trend toward increased resistance among GNB is reported in numerous local, regional and international studies. Recent data from a few of these studies are shown in **Table 2**. In the United States, 10-year surveillance from the Tracking Resistance in the United States Today (TRUST) study describes the steady increase in resistant and MDR GNB isolated in 26 institutions.[10] For example, imipenem-resistant PA increased from 5% in 2003 to 15% in 2009. The prevalence of ESBL-producing *Escherichia coli* increased from 20.8% to 65 % over 7 years among intra-abdominal infection isolates in China.[11] This trend toward increased resistance has been especially significant in ICUs in both tertiary care centers and community hospitals worldwide.[12,13] ACCB are particularly problematic, with resistance rates of up to 60% to 70% in international studies.[11,14] Studies also demonstrate that colonization with MDR GNB is a risk for subsequent infections and bacteremia with same organism.[15] The US Centers for Disease Control and Prevention (CDC) is currently performing population-based surveillance of infection caused by CRE and MDR ACCB through the Multi-Site Resistant Gram-Negative Bacilli Surveillance Initiative (MuGSI), with data expected in 2013.[16] The goals of this project are to determine the extent of CRE and MDR ACCB infections in the United States, identify those most at risk for infection, and measure trends of disease over time.

DEFINITIONS AND DIAGNOSIS OF INFECTIONS CAUSED BY RESISTANT AND MDR GNB

Until recently there was little consensus on the definitions of MDR, XDR, and PDR.[17–22] To remedy the issue, an expert panel sponsored by CDC and the European Center for Disease Prevention and Control (ECDC) met in 2008 to establish interim standard definitions for MDR, XDR, and PDR for epidemiologically significant microorganisms, as well as to begin to establish consistency in categorization of "susceptible" and "nonsusceptible" for different organisms and antimicrobial classes.[23] These definitions were developed specifically for public health and epidemiology purposes and not for clinical management. An organism was designated as nonsusceptible to an antibiotic when it tested intermediate or resistant when using clinical breakpoints as interpretive criteria.

Table 1
Definitions of multidrug resistance and predominant mechanisms of resistance to traditional gram-negative antibiotics

	Common Resistance Phenotypes	Major Mechanisms of Resistance
Enterobacteriaceae	Third- ± fourth-generation cephalosporins	ESBL, AmpC β-lactamases
	Carbapenem resistance	Carbapenemases
	Fluoroquinolones	DNA gyrase and topoisomerase mutations
	Aminoglycosides	Aminoglycoside-modifying enzymes
Pseudomonas aeruginosa	Carbapenem resistance and other β-lactam resistance	Metallo-β-lactamases AmpC and other β-lactamases Multidrug efflux pumps Deletion of membrane porins
	Fluoroquinolones	DNA gyrase and topoisomerase mutations
	Aminoglycosides	Aminoglycoside-modifying enzymes
Acinetobacter spp	Cephalosporin and carbapenem resistance	Cephalosporinases Carbapenemases Multidrug efflux pumps Porin mutations Penicillin-binding protein changes
	Aminoglycoside resistance	Aminoglycoside-modifying enzymes
	Fluoroquinolone resistance	DNA gyrase and topoisomerase mutations
Resistance category definitions	MDR is defined as resistant to more than 1 agent in 3 or more antimicrobial categories XDR is defined as nonsusceptible to more than 1 agent in all but 2 categories PDR is defined as resistant to all categories Intrinsic resistance to specific antimicrobial agent would automatically eliminate that agent from being included in defining resistance	

Only acquired resistance was considered, thus intrinsic species-wide resistance to specific antimicrobial agents was not considered in defining classes of resistance. MDR is defined as nonsusceptible to more than 1 agent from 3 or more antimicrobial categories, XDR is defined as nonsusceptible to more than 1 agent in all but 2 categories, and PDR is defined as resistant to all categories. The antimicrobial categories and breakpoints for determining nonsusceptibility are individually defined for each clinically significant class of GNB (ie, Enterobacteriaceae, PA, and ACCB) (**Table 3**).

Epidemiologic definitions used for nonsusceptibility are not always concordant with outcome data from treating infections attributable to nonsusceptible organisms. For some drug-organism combinations, minimum inhibitory concentration (MIC) values are shown to be more predictive of clinical outcome than characterization as susceptible, intermediate, or resistant by MIC. For most GNB, the Clinical Laboratory and Standards Institute (CLSI) have recently reduced the MIC breakpoint for susceptibility to most cephalosporins and carbapenems to 1 μg/mL or less, based on clinical outcome data (see **Table 3**).[24] However, patients with GNB bloodstream infections nonsusceptible to a carbapenems with a MIC of 2 μg/mL or less were more likely to have a good outcome than those with a MIC of 4 μg/mL or greater.[25] Conversely, for

Table 2
Representative global surveillance data for resistant gram-negative bacilli

Study	Location	Site of Isolation	No. of Isolates (Gram-Negative)	Isolates	Surveillance Period
Tracking Resistance in the United States (TRUST) Surveillance	USA	Not specified	EN (35,847) PA (8882) AC (1621)	ESBL EC: 1% (2003) to 3.5% (2009) ESBL KP: 4% (2003) to 5.8% (2009) EN MDR[a]: 7.5% (1999) to 12.3% (2009) PA MDR[a]: 7.3% (1999) to 7.7% (2009) AC MDR[a]: 24.7% (1999) to 43.6%(2009)	1999–2009
Study for Monitoring Antimicrobial Resistance Trends (SMART) Surveillance Program	Canada/Rest of World	Urine Intra-abdominal infections	Canada: 936 Rest of world: 19,276	ESBL EC: 8%[b], 21%[c] ESBL *Klebsiella* spp: 6%[b], 33%[c]	2002–2010
SMART Surveillance (China)	China	Intra-abdominal infections	3420 EC ESBL+ 882 KP ESBL+ 193 PA 286 AC 154	ESBL EC 20.8% (2002) to 64.9% (2009) ESBL KP 24% (2002) to 31.9% (2009) PA 80% retained susceptibility to AG AC <30% susceptibility to all agents	2002–2009
MDR GNR reported to the National Healthcare Safety Network	USA	Sputum Blood Urine Surgical site	15,275 isolates PA 7092 AC 2068 KP 6115	KP 15% resistant to 3 antimicrobial classes and 7% resistant to 4 antimicrobial classes PA 10% resistant to 3 antimicrobial classes and 2% resistant to 4 antimicrobial classes ACCB 60% resistant to 3 antimicrobial classes and 34% resistant to 4 antimicrobial classes	2006–2008

CAN-ICU	Canada ICU	Sputum Blood Wound/tissue Urine	EC 536 KP 224 PA 419	FQ-resistant EC 21% MDR EC 0.2% MDR PA 12.6%	2005–2006
International Nosocomial Infection Control Consortium (INICC) Report	422 ICUs in 36 countries in Central and South America, South Asia, Oceania, Europe, North Africa, and the Middle East	Urine Sputum Blood Other	PA 589 tested for piperacillin susceptibility 517 tested for imipenem susceptibility KP 447 tested for ceftriaxone/ceftazidime susceptibility 508 tested for carbapenem susceptibility AC 667 tested for carbapenem susceptibility EC 171 tested for ceftriaxone/ceftazidime susceptibility 182 tested for imipenem/meropenem/ertapenem susceptibility 133 tested for fluoroquinolone susceptibility	Data below are reported as % of strains resistant PA Fluoroquinolone 42.1% Piperacillin/tazobactam 36% Amikacin 27.7% Imipenem or Meropenem 47.2% Cefepime100% KP Ceftriaxone/ceftazidime 76.3% Imipenem/meropenem/ertapenem 7.9% AC Imipenem/meropenem 55.3% EC Ceftriaxone/ceftazidime 66.7% Imipenem/meropenem/ertapenem 4.4% Fluoroquinolone 53.4%	2004–2009

Abbreviations: AC, *Acinetobacter* spp; EC, *E coli*; EN, Enterobacteriaceae; KP, *K pneumoniae*; PA, *P aeruginosa*.
a MDR (Defined as resistant to ≥3 antibiotic classes).
b Canada isolates.
c Rest of the world.
Data from Refs.[10–14,106]

Table 3
Breakpoints for susceptibility as approved by EUCAST, SCLIS, and FDA (in μg/mL)

	EUCAST Cefepime/ Imipenem/ Tobramycin			CLSI Cefepime/ Imipenem/ Tobramycin			FDA Cefepime/ Imipenem/ Tobramycin		
Enterobacteriaceae	≤1	≤2	≤2	≤2	≤1	≤4	≤8	≤4	≤4
Pseudomonas aeruginosa	≤8	≤4	≤4	≤8	≤2	≤4	≤8	≤4	≤4
Acinetobacter spp	—	≤2	≤4	≤8	≤4	≤4	≤8	≤4	≤4

Abbreviations: CLSI, Clinical and Laboratory Standards Institute; EUCAST, The European Committee on Antimicrobial Susceptibility Testing; FDA, US Food and Drug Administration.

levofloxacin, patients with GNB bacteremia in whom levofloxacin MIC was 1 μg/mL, well below the susceptibility cutoff, had poorer outcomes than those with MICs of 0.5 μg/mL or less.[26] The conclusion to be drawn from these data is that breakpoints for susceptibility need to be continually reassessed based on clinical outcomes for emerging resistances. However, there may still be reasons for using agents that test as nonsusceptible for the treatment of resistant organisms.

MANAGEMENT OF INFECTIONS CAUSED BY RESISTANT GNB

The cornerstone of treating of resistant gram-negative infections is administration of maximally effective antimicrobial therapy. Whether this can be accomplished depends on several key factors including host status, the type of resistance(s) encountered and available treatment options, the site(s) of infection, and whether source control of infection is achievable. Many resistant GNB infections are treatable with available gram-negative agents such as third- and fourth-generation cephalosporins, β-lactam/β-lactamase inhibitor (BL/BI) agents, carbapenems, or fluoroquinolones. However, some MDR infections are only treatable with more toxic agents including polymyxins and aminoglycosides.[27,28] Treatment of XDR and PDR organisms may require combinations of partially active or individually inactive agents. Optimizing pharmacodynamics of available agents by use of extended infusion times and novel delivery methods including aerosolization may also improve outcomes for marginally treatable infections.[29–31] PDR infections for which there are no available effective treatments are increasingly reported.[1,2] This discussion focuses on treatment of documented resistant GNB infections, but similar principles apply to empiric therapy for severe infections in individuals at high risk for resistant GNB, including colonized patients or patients in an outbreak setting.

ANTIMICROBIAL AGENTS FOR INFECTIONS CAUSED BY MDR GNB

There are often many options for treating resistant GNB with single-class antimicrobial resistance. Rarely, however, do resistant GNB demonstrate single-class resistance. Multidrug resistance is selected by sequential exposures to different antibiotics, by horizontal transfer of multiple resistance traits clustered on mobile genetic elements, or by selection for characteristics such as permeability changes or upregulation of efflux pumps that alter susceptibility to multiple drug classes.[8] Knowledge of local susceptibility patterns from current antibiograms, especially unit-specific antibiograms, may help guide initial therapy. Combination antibiograms demonstrating patterns of cross-resistance may be even more useful for this.[32] Standard broad-spectrum gram-negative agents including third- and fourth-generation cephalosporins, carbapenems, BL/BI agents, aminoglycosides, fluoroquinolones, and trimethoprim-sulfamethoxazole may be effective against some MDR GNB, especially ESBL-producing and AmpC-expressing strains. This section focuses on newer agents and some older agents with particular activity, used alone or in combination against resistant GNB (**Table 4**).

Recently Approved Agents: Doripenem and Tigecycline

There have been only 3 agents with broad-spectrum gram-negative activity approved by the US Food and Drug Administration since 2005. Ceftaroline, a novel fifth-generation cephalosporin, has enhanced gram-positive/methicillin-resistant *Staphylococcus aureus* activity, and offers little new for resistant GNB. Doripenem is a newer carbapenem with a spectrum similar to that of imipenem and meropenem. Some isolates, especially PA, with low-level resistance to imipenem and meropenem via permeability or efflux remain susceptible to doripenem.[33] Doripenem is hydrolyzed by *Klebsiella pneumoniae* carbapenemases (KPCs) and metallo-β-lactamases (MBLs), and is not significantly more active alone than other carbapenems for CRE or carbapenem-resistant (CR) ACCB.[9] Doripenem has good stability in solution, and is thus well suited for extended interval infusions.[33] Doripenem was more active in in vitro combinations than other carbapenems for some XDR and PDR strains, although the clinical significance of this is unknown.[34]

Another recently approved agent is tigecycline, a glycylcycline tetracycline analogue with broad-spectrum activity first introduced in the United States in 2005. Tigecycline has activity against most Enterobacteriaceae and ACCB. PA and also *Proteus*, *Morganella*, and *Providencia* spp are intrinsically resistant via efflux pumps, and acquired tigecycline resistance is reported in other GNB via enhanced expression of multidrug efflux systems.[27,35] Emergence of resistance on therapy can occur during treatment of CRE and ACCB.[27] Recent large surveys show no significant worsening resistance trends among Enterobacteriaceae including ICU strains, although increased resistance among ACCB is reported.[36] Tigecycline achieves low levels in serum and only 20% is excreted in urine, and is a poor monotherapy agent for MDR GNB bloodstream or urinary tract infections (UTIs) at standard doses.[37] Higher doses of 100 mg every 12 hours have been used for MDR bloodstream infections.[27,37]

Older Agents Active Against MDR, XDR, and PDR GNB

Fosfomycin is an older broad-spectrum antibiotic widely used outside of the United States that inhibits phosphoenolpyruvate, an early step in peptidoglycan synthesis.[38] Oral and parenteral formulations are available in some European and Asian countries, although only oral fosfomycin is available in the United States for treating cystitis. The oral prodrug has good oral bioavailability and achieves high urine levels, although serum levels are low.[38] Fosfomycin has broad activity against Enterobacteriaceae including most *E coli* and *Klebsiella* strains. Some PA are susceptible, although not ACCB. There is no cross-resistance with other agents, and fosfomycin remains active against many MDR CRE. The primary niche for fosfomycin is treatment of MDR GNB UTIs, but there are reports from Europe on the use of parenteral fosfomycin for systemic infections. Fosfomycin is used in combination therapy to prevent emergence of resistance.[39] There are only limited data on outcome or emergence of resistance in these settings.[39]

Of the older tetracyclines, minocycline maintains the best activity against ACCB.[40] Like tigecycline, minocycline is a poor substrate for most tetracycline-resistance efflux pumps in GNB. The intravenous formulation is widely available in Europe and Asia, and since 2009 has also been available in the United States. Minocycline may be active against sulbactam-resistant and carbapenem-resistant ACCB strains, and even some tigecycline-resistant strains, and has been used for the treatment of a variety of complicated ACCB infections, including ventilator-associated pneumonia (VAP), although experience remains limited.[41]

The β-lactamase inhibitor sulbactam binds to ACCB penicillin-binding protein PBP-2, and has specific potent inhibitory activity against many ACCB.[42] In most countries sulbactam is only available as a coformulation with ampicillin. Rates of ampicillin-sulbactam resistance are increasing among ACCB, especially CR ACCB.[27,43] Sulbactam has been studied in vitro combined with carbapenems, and this regimen has been used clinically for treatment of XDR and PDR ACCB.[43]

Aztreonam, a monobactam, is a substrate for most broad-spectrum β-lactamases including ESBL, AmpC, and KPC. However, aztreonam is uniquely resistant to hydrolysis by some MBLs including New Delhi MBL-1.[44] Aztreonam may have a role in infections caused by MBL-producing CRE, and some isolates are susceptible. However, most strains carry multiple β-lactamases in addition to the MBLs, so aztreonam needs to be combined with other agents. Combinations of aztreonam and other monobactams with novel β-lactamase inhibitors are being evaluated.

Rifampin is a potent, bactericidal broad-spectrum antimicrobial that inhibits DNA-dependent RNA polymerase. Primarily an antimycobacterial drug, rifampin is used in combination therapy for gram-positive infections but is increasingly used for MDR and XDR GNB. Rifampin has relatively poor activity against most GNB because of its poor outer membrane penetration, and resistance is easily selected in vivo when used as monotherapy. Rifampin combinations have been extensively studied in vitro, particularly rifampin plus polymyxins and/or carbapenems for CRE, MDR, ACCB, and PA.[45] These studies demonstrate potent synergy between rifampin and other agents.[45] Rifampin may delay the emergence of resistance to other agents in vitro, especially to polymyxins. Synergy may result in increased rifampin access to intracellular targets in the presence of cell membrane–damaging agents, even in some polymyxin-resistant isolates (**Fig. 1**).

Off of the Antibiotic Scrap Heap: the Resurrection of the Polymyxins

Polymyxins are cationic polypeptide antibiotics that bind to lipopolysaccharide (LPS) in gram-negative outer membranes and to cytoplasmic membranes, resulting in altered permeability and cell death. Polymyxins were introduced in the 1950s for the treatment of GNB, but owing to toxicity concerns virtually disappeared after the introduction of broad-spectrum β-lactams.[27,46] Polymyxins were "rediscovered" in the 1990s for the treatment of MDR GNB. Polymyxins have broad activity against many GNB including *E coli, Klebsiella, Enterobacter*, PA, and ACCB, although several important pathogens, notably *Proteus, Providencia*, and most *Serratia*, are intrinsically resistant. Because of the unique mechanism of action, there is no cross-resistance with other agents. Resistance to polymyxins is uncommon, but may occur by modification of LPS outer-membrane target components, including lipid A.[46–48] Colistin resistance is increasingly reported in ACCB.[48]

The available polymyxins are colistin (polymyxin E), which is more widely used in the United States, and polymyxin B. Colistin is administered as the inactive prodrug colistimethate sodium (CMS), which is converted in vivo to the active colistin sulfate; polymyxin B is administered as the active sulfate moiety. Polymyxins appear to have relatively poor distribution into lung tissue, pleural fluid, and cerebrospinal fluid (CSF). A recent multicenter study sponsored by the National Institutes of Health has led to new proposed guidelines for dosing CMS, including administration of a loading dose.[49] CMS is also administered by aerosol therapy for resistant respiratory tract infections.[31] Susceptibility testing for polymyxins remains problematic. Disc-diffusion testing is highly unreliable in comparison with Etests or other MIC methods. The limiting toxicity of colistin is nephrotoxicity.[46,47] Reported rates in recent series range from as low as 6% to as high as 32% to 55% in other studies in critically ill patients.[46] Definitions of nephrotoxicity and dosing regimens varied in these studies. Most nephrotoxicity is reversible.

Gram-Negative Agents on the Horizon

Despite the overall lack of new drug classes and paucity of new gram-negative agents in the antibiotic pipeline, there are several agents currently in phase 1 or phase 2 trials that may improve the treatment of resistant GNB.[50] These agents include several novel β-lactamase inhibitors with activity against KPC enzymes, although not against MBLs. One of these, avibactam (formerly NXL-104), is in trials in combination with several β-lactams. BLI-489, another novel inhibitor, is entering clinical trials. BAL30376 is a monobactam–clavulanic acid combination drug with specific activity against MBLs. New aminoglycosides such as plazomicin, which are stable to common gram-negative aminoglycoside-modifying enzymes, are also under study. Other agents with novel mechanisms of activity against GNB are in early phases of development.[27,50]

EVIDENCE FOR EFFECTIVENESS OF TREATMENT OF MDR, XDR, AND PDR GNB

Ample evidence exists from in vitro susceptibility data, pharmacokinetic and pharmacodynamic modeling, and clinical outcome data to make recommendations for the treatment of infections caused by ESBL and AmpC GNB (**Table 5**). The evidence for treatment of more resistant pathogens, including CRE, MDR and PDR PA, and ACCB is less robust. Combination therapy may be assessed in vitro by synergy testing in checkerboard and time-kill assays. Polymyxins are challenging to study in the laboratory because of binding of drug to surfaces and other poorly understood in vitro phenomena. Pharmacodynamic models are extensively used to optimize dosing regimens for organisms with borderline susceptibility. A few drug combinations have been tested in animal models. However, the pool of experimental data is small, the clinical correlates of in vitro testing are uncertain, and the limited number of strains studied may not adequately represent the diversity of MDR and XDR clinical isolates.

Human treatment data most often consist of case reports or uncontrolled case series, making comparison of different regimens difficult. There are a small number of well-conducted nonrandomized studies with case-control designs, and there have been several recent systematic reviews focusing on specific pathogens or the effectiveness of specific drugs.[39,51] Randomized clinical trials comparing monotherapy and combination regimens for MDR and XDR infections are currently enrolling subjects in Europe and the United States, although recruitment is challenging.[52,53]

OPTIMIZING THE USE OF AVAILABLE AGENTS TO TREAT MDR GNB
Extended Infusion of β-Lactams for MDR GNB

The most important pharmacodynamic parameter for killing by β-lactams is the time above the MIC of the target organism. This criterion is the theoretical basis for extended-infusion or continuous-infusion β-lactam strategies for treating GNB (**Fig. 2**).[29,54] Some agents (eg, imipenem) are not suitable for extended infusion owing to their poor stability in solution. Most experience with extended-interval dosing is with piperacillin-tazobactam, which is increasingly used in such a manner for both efficacy and economic considerations.[55] Experience is also increasing with doripenem and meropenem, and with cephalosporins including ceftazidime and cefepime. Initial

Table 4
Some new and older antimicrobials with activity against multidrug-resistant gram-negative bacilli

Antimicrobial Agent	Drug Class/Mechanism	Formulations	Standard and Maximal Dosing	MDR GNB Activity	Comments
Doripenem	Carbapenem	Intravenous	500 mg every 8 h Maximum: 1000 mg every 8 h	ESBL AmpC CS ACCB CS PA	Active against some imipenem- or meropenem-resistant PA Used in combination therapy for CR ACCB, CR PA, and CRE Extended-infusion time dosing
Tigecycline	Tetracycline	Intravenous	100 mg load then 50 mg every 12 h Maximum: 100 mg every 12 h	ESBL AmpC CRE MDR ACCB	Low serum and urine levels Breakthrough bacteremias while on therapy Used as monotherapy or combination therapy
Fosfomycin	Phosphoenolpyruvate inhibitor	Oral Parenteral (in some countries)	Oral (for UTI): 3 g every 48–72 h Intravenous: 2–4 g every 6 h	ESBL AmpC CRE PA	High urine levels Resistance develops while on therapy Only as combination therapy for systemic infections
Sulbactam	β-Lactam inhibitor with β-lactam activity	Intravenous (as ampicillin-sulbactam)	1 g every 4 h (3 g ampicillin-sulbactam every 4 h)	ACCB only	Used as monotherapy for susceptible ACCB. Used in combination therapy for sulbactam-resistant ACCB

				NDM-producing CRE	
Aztreonam	Monobactam	Intravenous	2 g every 8 h		Must be used in combination to overcome other resistances
Rifampin	RNA polymerase inhibitor	Oral Intravenous	Oral and intravenous: 600 mg every 24 h Maximum: 600 mg every 8 h	CRE MDR ACCB MDR PA	Only used in combination therapy Synergy with polymyxins Resistance emerges on therapy
Minocycline	Tetracycline	Intravenous Oral	Oral and Intravenous: 100 mg every 12 h	MDR ACCB	Used as monotherapy or combination therapy
Polymyxins (colistin, polymyxin B)	Cationic polypeptide Damages lipid membranes	Parenteral Aerosolized Intrathecal	See Table 6 for dosing information	CRE MDR ACCB MDR PA	Active against *E coli, Klebsiella, Enterobacter*, PA, ACCB Significant nephrotoxicity Synergy with many other agents, even against colistin-resistant strains

Abbreviations: CS, carbapenem-sensitive; NDM, New Delhi metallo-β-lactamase.

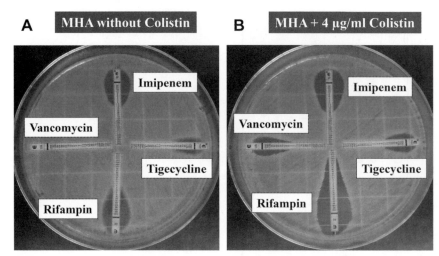

Fig. 1. Demonstration of synergy of other antibiotics with colistin for a carbapenem-resistant and colistin-resistant ACCB strain. Susceptibility to vancomycin, rifampin, tigecycline and imipenem was determined by Etest on plates without (A) or with (B) addition of 4 μg/ml of colistin. Susceptibility to vancomycin and rifampin was dramatically increased and susceptibility to tigecycline and imipenem was modestly increased in presence of colistin. (*Courtesy of* C. Knob.)

randomized controlled trials failed to demonstrate significant differences in outcome in comparison with standard administration.[30,54]

However, patients in these trials may not have been "sick" enough or infected with resistant enough GNB to show benefits of improved attainment of pharmacodynamics targets. In one study, superiority of extended piperacillin-tazobactam infusion was limited to only the sickest patients.[56] A recent systematic review and meta-analysis of predominantly nonrandomized trials showed benefit with extended or continuous infusion of pipericillin-tazobactam or carbapenems in patients with all sites of infection, and specifically those with pneumonia.[30] A recent small, randomized trial of continuous infusion of piperacillin-tazobactam, meropenem, and ticarcillin–clavulanic acid in 5 ICUs demonstrated both better drug levels and cure rates.[57] With limited options in critically ill patients with borderline or low-level resistant organisms, extended infusion is a rational strategy. Extended infusion of antibiotics demonstrating concentration-dependent killing, such as aminoglycosides, is not indicated. Colistin has been administered by continuous infusion, but pharmacokinetic and safety data do not currently support such dosing strategies.

Aerosolized Aminoglycosides and Polymyxins for Respiratory Infections

Aerosolized administration provides benefits of enhanced delivery to epithelial lining fluid (ELF) for drugs that have poor pulmonary penetration or significant toxicity with systemic dosing. Aerosolized therapy is used for preventing or treating respiratory infections in patients with cystic fibrosis and bronchiectasis, and has been studied for the treatment of VAP. Use in the ICU has increased with the increase in VAP caused by MDR GNB.[31] Most experience is with aminoglycosides and polymyxins, agents with potent in vitro gram-negative activity but with significant systemic toxicity and poor lung penetration.[31]

There are several recent studies of aerosolized aminoglycoside therapy for VAP, but only one small randomized study comparing aerosolized with intravenous therapy.[58]

Two larger retrospective observational studies compared benefits of aerosolized therapy added to intravenous therapy that included many MDR pathogens. Reported cure rates were 59% and 73%.[59,60] Gentamicin and tobramycin doses are 300 mg every 12 hours, and amikacin doses are 500 to 1000 mg every 12 hours. Treatment has been generally well tolerated.

There are multiple reports of treating VAP caused by resistant ACCB and PA with aerosolized colistin, with overall reported cure rates of 58% to 100%.[31] Use of concurrent systemic therapy and choice of systemic agents varied in these trials. One well-designed retrospective case-control study for VAP comparing intravenous plus aerosolized colistin with intravenous therapy alone demonstrated a trend toward better outcomes and lower mortality in the aerosol-treated group.[61] Respiratory symptoms are more frequently reported with aerosolized colistin than with aminoglycosides, and drug preparation in accordance with standard protocols is important to prevent toxicity.[31] The recommended dose of colistin is 150 mg every 12 hours.[31]

Definitive recommendations for the use of aerosolized aminoglycosides or polymyxins in addition to systemic drug, or in combination with other agents, are lacking. Aerosolized regimens should be considered in patients failing or relapsing after systemic treatment, and for MDR infections with limited treatment options. Systemic therapy is still necessary when treating concurrent bacteremia or other sites of infection outside the respiratory tract.

RECOMMENDATIONS FOR THE TREATMENT OF SPECIFIC CLASSES OF RESISTANT GNB
ESBL-Producing Enterobacteriaceae

There are numerous case series assessing treatment of ESBLs, but no randomized, comparative trials. Options also depend on the site and severity of infection, the specific ESBL enzyme, and additional associated resistances (see **Table 5**). For ESBL bacteremia, most expert opinion and a recent meta-analysis support using a carbapenem.[62–65] Carbapenems are highly active in vitro, stable to hydrolysis by ESBLs, and do not demonstrate an inoculum effect (decreased in vitro activity with large bacterial concentrations), and there is extensive clinical experience. Experience with the narrower-spectrum drug ertapenem for ESBL infections for bacteremia is less than for other carbapenems.[66] Piperacillin-tazobactam has been used for bloodstream and urinary tract ESBL infections, and in a recent meta-analysis was not inferior to carbapenems for bacteremia caused by susceptible isolates.[65,67]

Recommendations regarding cephalosporins for ESBL Enterobacteriaceae have changed following revision of the CLSI susceptibility breakpoints in 2010.[24] These new lower breakpoints eliminate the broad characterization of ESBL strains as pan-cephalosporin resistant, and support treatment with third- or fourth-generation cephalosporins when MICs are 1 µg/mL or less, regardless of the presence of ESBL enzymes. Some cephalosporins are more stable to hydrolysis by specific ESBL enzymes, and demonstrate good outcomes for treating ESBLs when MICs are in these lower ranges. In one study, 11 of 12 patients with ESBL-producing K pneumoniae and E coli infections with MICs to cefepime of 2 µg/mL or less had cure or improvement.[68] Good outcomes were also reported with ceftazidime for cefotaxime-resistant but ceftazidime-susceptible ESBL E coli bacteremia.[69] When using cefepime for bacteremia and pneumonia caused by susceptible ESBL strains, maximal doses may be necessary.[70]

There is limited information on the use of fluoroquinolones or aminoglycosides for serious ESBL infections. Fluoroquinolone resistance rates are high, and even if quinolone susceptible, the outcome of patients with bacteremia treated with fluoroquinolones is poorer than with a carbapenem.[71] Resistance can also be selected in vivo,

Table 5
Options for treatment of different classes of multidrug-resistant gram-negative bacilli

Resistance Class	Site of Infection	Preferred Option	Alternatives	Comments
ESBL	Bacteremia and pneumonia	Carbapenem	Third-/fourth-generation cephalosporin if MIC ≤1 Piperacillin-tazobactam	
	Urine and other low-severity, low-inoculum infections		Fluoroquinolone Aminoglycoside Trimethoprim-sulfamethoxazole Fosfomycin	
AmpC	Bacteremia and pneumonia	Carbapenem or cefepime	Piperacillin-tazobactam Fluoroquinolone	Resistance to third-generation cephalosporin develops on therapy
	Urine and other low-severity, low-inoculum infections		Third-generation cephalosporin Aminoglycoside Trimethoprim-sulfamethoxazole	
CRE	Bacteremia	Colistin[a]	Tigecycline Carbapenem (if MIC ≤4) Only in combination therapy: Rifampin Fosfomycin Aztreonam (for NDM strains)	If susceptible can use: Aminoglycoside Fluoroquinolone Trimethoprim-sulfamethoxazole Usually combination therapy Combination therapy usually includes 2–3 drugs
ACCB	All sites	Carbapenem	Sulbactam Colistin Tigecycline	Sulbactam may be equivalent to carbapenem

Organism	Infection	Therapy		Comments
CR ACCB and pan-resistant ACCB	Bacteremia	If Susceptible: Sulbactam Colistin[a] Tigecycline In combination only: Rifampin		Combination therapy commonly used
	Pneumonia	Systemic therapy plus aerosolized aminoglycoside or colistin		
MDR PA	Bacteremia	Colistin[a] Aminoglycosides If susceptible: Doripenem For combination therapy only: Rifampin Fosfomycin		Combination therapy if possible for bacteremia Susceptibilities vary: some isolates remain susceptible to ceftazidime, cefepime, piperacillin-tazobactam, or aztreonam
	Pneumonia	Systemic therapy plus aerosolized aminoglycoside or colistin		
	UTI only	Fosfomycin		
Stenotrophomonas maltophilia	Pneumonia and bacteremia	Trimethoprim-sulfamethoxazole	Ticarcillin–clavulanic acid Fluoroquinolone	Levofloxacin and moxifloxacin more active than ciprofloxacin

[a] Colistin or polymyxin B.

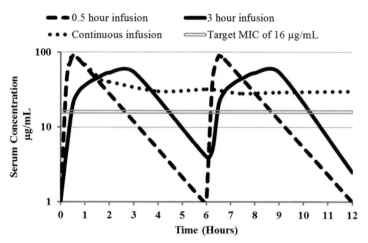

Fig. 2. Pharmacokinetics of standard-, prolonged-, and continuous-infusion β-lactam regimens. The graph shows the representative pharmacokinetics of a standard dose of β-lactam with a short half-life such as piperacillin-tazobactam when administered by 0.5-hour infusion (*dashed line*) or by a 3-hour infusion (*solid line*) every 6 hours. When treating an organism with a higher minimum inhibitory concentration (MIC) of 16 μg/mL, the time that drug concentration is above the MIC is increased using the prolonged infusion time. Administration of a standard bolus dose followed by continuous infusion of drug can theoretically provide even greater time above the MIC (*dotted line*).

especially in higher inoculum infections. Treatment failures with aminoglycosides have also been reported.[72] For nonbacteremic infections, especially those with low bacterial inoculum and lower potential for emergence of resistance, fluoroquinolones and aminoglycosides may be appropriate. Trimethoprim-sulfamethoxazole is also an option for susceptible isolates, especially UTIs.[64] Cephamycins, including cefoxitin, are not inactivated by ESBLs and are active in vitro, but because resistance can develop by other mechanisms, these are poor choices for serious infections.[64] Fosfomycin is active against most ESBL *E coli* and *Klebsiella* isolates, and is an option for UTIs.[38,39]

AmpC-Producing Enterobacteriaceae

Up to 20% of AmpC-producing *Enterobacter cloacae* may fail therapy with a third-generation cephalosporin during treatment of bacteremia, owing to emergence of resistance.[73,74] Use of these agents is not recommended for serious infections caused by AmpC-expressing GNB, especially bacteremia, pneumonia, and intra-abdominal infections.[74] Carbapenems and cefepime are not readily hydrolyzed by AmpC and are treatments of choice. Rare strains are resistant to carbapenems or cefepime because of altered permeability or expression of additional β-lactamases. Resistance is less likely to develop to piperacillin-tazobactam than to third-generation cephalosporins. Fluoroquinolones, aminoglycosides, and trimethoprim-sulfamethoxazole are acceptable options for susceptible strains.

Carbapenem-Resistant Enterobacteriaceae

Recommendations for the treatment of CRE are based on in vitro data and published experience from case reports, retrospective reviews, small case series, and recent systematic reviews.[75] Most data concern the treatment of KPC- or MBL-expressing CR *Klebsiella*. In recent studies, other variables that affect the outcome of CRE infections include site of infection and carbapenem MIC, as well as host factors such as age, underlying comorbidities, severity of illness, and being in an ICU.[75,76] Treatment options are limited by the high rates of resistance to other drug classes, including resistance to fluoroquinolone, aminoglycoside, and trimethoprim-sulfamethoxazole. Ninety percent to 100% of isolates may be fluoroquinolone resistant. Rates of pan-aminoglycoside resistance are variable especially for KPC strains, and aminoglycosides have been used alone or in combination.[77] CRE treatment regimens can be broadly characterized as monotherapy, generally with either a carbapenem, colistin, aminoglycoside, or tigecycline; or combinations that include colistin and/or a carbapenem.[75] Other components of combinations often include tigecycline or rifampin. Comparison of different regimens is difficult because of patient diversity and variable CRE susceptibility patterns. One recent review has attempted to compare the outcome of various regimens.[75] Although there are limitations to this analysis, there were some interesting observations. Ineffective therapy resulted in worse outcomes. Carbapenem-based combination regimens were among the most effective despite carbapenem nonsusceptibility, and carbapenem monotherapy was superior to no effective therapy. Effectiveness of carbapenems correlated with MIC, with some successes with monotherapy for strains having MICs as high as 8 μg/mL.[78] Despite reported susceptibility to tigecycline of most CRE, failure rates may be higher than for other monotherapy regimens, with reports of breakthrough bacteremia.[37,75] Higher tigecycline doses of 100 mg every 12 hours are recommended for bacteremic infections.[75]

Polymyxins are increasingly being used for the treatment of CRE, with more published data for colistin than for polymyxin B. Ninety percent to 100% of KPC-producing or MBL-producing *K pneumoniae* were reported as susceptible to polymyxins, but colistin-resistant strains are increasingly being described.[79]

Reported outcomes with colistin monotherapy vary greatly, in part likely because of nonstandardized colistin dosing. Routine use of more uniform, data-driven dosing regimens (**Table 6**), including an initial loading dose rapidly achieving levels above the MIC, may provide better comparative data on colistin effectiveness.[49]

Table 6 Colistin dosing	
Intravenous loading dose	T × 2 × body weight Not to exceed 300 mg First maintenance dose in 24 h
Intravenous maintenance dose	T × ((1.5 × creatinine clearance) + 30) Interval based on creatinine clearance <10 mL/min/1.73 m²: interval every 12 h 10–70 mL/min/1.73 m²: interval every 12–8 h >70 mL/min/1.73 m²: interval every 8 h Intermittent hemodialysis (HD): On non-HD days supplement with 30 mg of colistin On HD days infuse after HD 39 mg of colistin every 12 h Continuous hemofiltration: 192 mg every 8–12 h
Inhaled	150 mg every 12 h
Intrathecal	10–20 mg qd

T is defined as desired plasma colistin, which varies by MIC, organ, and severity of infection.

Data from Drusano GL, Lodise TP. Editorial commentary: saving lives with optimal antimicrobial chemotherapy. Clin Infect Dis 2013;56:245–7; and Petrosillo N, Ioannidou E, Falagas ME. Colistin monotherapy vs. combination therapy: evidence from microbiological, animal and clinical studies. Clin Microbiol Infect 2008;14:816–27.

Combination regimens, including some drugs that individually test as intermediate or resistant, are increasingly being used for CRE, especially XDR and PDR strains.[75] Regimens consist of at least 2 to 3 drugs from a menu including polymyxins, tigecycline, rifampin, carbapenems, and aminoglycosides. Assumptions of synergy are extrapolated from published experimental data rather than direct testing of clinical isolates, as few institutions have the ability to perform real-time in vitro synergy studies. In one in vitro study, polymyxin B plus rifampin was synergistic for 15 of 16 KPC *K pneumoniae*, including 2 polymyxin-resistant isolates.[80] Similar results were seen for 12 of 12 polymyxin-resistant KPC strains.[81] A double carbapenem regimen of ertapenem plus doripenem also showed activity in vitro.[82] There are numerous reports for other combinations as well.[75] Comparative outcome data for different regimens is lacking. Aerosolized aminoglycosides or colistin can be used for the treatment of CRE pneumonia, usually in combination with systemic therapy.[31]

MDR, XDR, and Pan-Resistant Acinetobacter baumannii

ACCB strains possess numerous intrinsic resistances, and readily assimilate and express new resistance mechanisms. MDR ACCB are important nosocomial pathogens, especially for VAP but also for traumatic wound infections, UTIs, and meningitis.[42] Previously considered a low-virulence, opportunistic pathogen, more recent studies demonstrate the morbidity attributable to ACCB infections, as well as the benefits of appropriate antibiotic therapy in improving survival in critically ill ICU patients with ACCB bacteremia.[42,43,83] Drugs used for the treatment of MDR ACCB alone or in combination include carbapenems, sulbactam (available as ampicillin-sulbactam), tigecycline, minocycline, aminoglycosides, rifampin, and polymyxins (see **Table 5**). Occasional isolates remain susceptible to fluoroquinolone or trimethoprim-sulfamethoxazole. Carbapenems are drugs of choice for ACCB, but rates of CR ACCB have increased over the past decade.[36,43,84,85] Carbapenem resistance is mediated by several classes of carbapenemases, most prominently the oxacillinase (OXA) and MBL enzymes; effects of carbapenemases are augmented by changes in outer membrane protein and multidrug efflux pumps. Unlike other GNB, ACCB may display differential susceptibilities for imipenem and meropenem.[43] Doripenem is not significantly more active than other carbapenems.[86] For ACCB with higher carbapenems MICs, higher doses and extended-interval dosing with meropenem (2 g every 8 hours) or doripenem (up to 1 g every 8 hours) may provide a pharmacodynamic advantage.[27] Sulbactam is active against many ACCB strains. In one study, outcomes for ACCB were better with ampicillin-sulbactam than with a carbapenem.[42] High total daily sulbactam doses of 6 g (18 g ampicillin-sulbactam) were used for bacteremia and meningitis. Sulbactam resistance is increasing.[43] A combination of a carbapenem and sulbactam was reported to be effective in 4 patients with sulbactam-resistant CR ACCB.[87]

Of other agents employed for CR ACCB, polymyxins maintain the highest susceptibility rates and are the most extensively studied.[27,36,43] Colistin monotherapy was equivalent to a carbapenem for the treatment of ACCB pneumonia, and a recent meta-analysis of 6 ACCB pneumonia studies suggested that colistin monotherapy was as effective as comparators, without evidence of higher toxicity.[51,88] For CR ACCB, colistin combined with carbapenems, rifampin, tetracyclines, macrolides, and even glycopeptides have been studied in vitro and in animal models for.[27,43,89–91] Colistin resistant strains may be hypersusceptible to non–gram-negative antibiotics, possibly because of enhanced outer membrane permeability (see **Fig. 2**).[90] There are only limited outcome data comparing colistin monotherapy with combination therapy. One retrospective study showed no benefit of colistin plus meropenem versus colistin alone for MDR infections.[17] Intravenous colistin has been combined with aerosolized colistin for treating MDR ACCB pneumonias.[31,61]

The tetracyclines tigecycline and minocycline are options for the treatment of CR ACCB infections, including colistin-resistant strains, although rates of tigecycline resistance are increasing.[36,40,43] Success rates for tigecycline monotherapy or combination therapy for nosocomial ACCB pneumonia are reported to be as high as 75%, although outcomes for bacteremia are worse.[43,92] Tigecycline doses of 100 mg every 12 hours have been used to optimize serum levels.[37,43] Susceptibility rates for minocycline are similar to those for tigecycline, and intravenous minocycline is now available in the United States. In vitro studies show synergy with minocycline and colistin and carbapenems, even against isolates resistant to some of these agents, although experience with minocycline for serious ACCB infections is limited.[41]

Treatment of nosocomial meningitis caused by ACCB, especially CR ACCB, is especially challenging. Sulbactam at maximal doses may not achieve adequate CSF levels. Colistin has been administered intrathecally, either alone or with systemic therapy, and appears to be well tolerated.[93]

MDR and XDR Pseudomonas aeruginosa

PA remains an important pathogen in the ICU. Like ACCB, PA expresses many antimicrobial resistances and demonstrates propensity to develop resistance while on therapy, although PA is a more virulent pathogen. PA is a major cause of health care–associated pneumonia and VAP, but is important in other settings, including neutropenic and burn patients, injection drug users, and patients with cystic fibrosis and chronic lung diseases. Although an MDR phenotype is less prevalent among PA than in ACCB, MDR PA infections, particularly respiratory infections and bacteremia, are extremely challenging and have high mortality.[94] Increasing rates of MDR PA are reported in surveys of ICUs internationally.[13,95]

PA express β-lactam resistance through expression of multiple β-lactamases including AmpC, MBLs, KPCs, and OXA enzymes, as well as by efflux pumps and changes in outer membrane permeability. Unlike in most CRE and CR ACCB, carbapenem resistance does not indicate broad resistance to all β-lactams or even resistance to all carbapenems, especially for resistance mediated primarily by permeability changes and not carbapenemases. For example, doripenem may be active against OprD outer membrane mutants with a low level of imipenem resistance, but imipenem and doripenem may be active against strains with efflux-mediated resistance to meropenem.[96] Susceptibility to cefepime, ceftazidime, or piperacillin-tazobactam may be preserved despite carbapenem resistance. However, PA strains susceptible to β-lactams such as piperacillin-tazobactam often have MICs near susceptibility breakpoints with a higher likelihood of emergence of resistance on therapy, thus use of maximal daily doses and extended-interval infusions may be appropriate.[56]

PA may remain susceptible to some aminoglycosides; tobramycin and amikacin are usually the most active. Aminoglycoside monotherapy is not recommended for most serious PA infections, especially pneumonia or bacteremia, but options for agents to combine with an aminoglycoside may be limited with concurrent β-lactam and quinolone resistance. Aerosolized aminoglycosides have been used for treatment of VAP caused by MDR PA.[31,59] Aerosolized therapy may be especially useful in cases where risks of toxicity of systemic aminoglycosides are high or where MICs are higher than levels achievable with systemic therapy.

Polymyxins remain active in vitro against most PA strains in recent surveys, although there are reports of resistance emerging on therapy.[97–99] Clinical experience with polymyxins for PA bacteremia is limited. Monotherapy has been effective in some patients but is inferior to β-lactam therapy.[98] Recent trials of aerosolized colistin have included VAP patients with MDR PA, with favorable reported outcomes.[31,61] Susceptible PA infections are commonly treated with combination therapy, most often with a β-lactam plus an aminoglycoside, although the benefits of this strategy remain controversial.[100] There are few clinical data available on combination therapy for MDR and XDR PA strains. There are in vitro data for colistin plus doripenem, or with rifampin for MDR and XDR PA.[34] Colistin-aminoglycoside combinations would be predicted to have high rates of nephrotoxicity. Parenteral fosfomycin remains an alternative for use in combination therapy for systemic MDR PA infections.[101]

MDR *Stenotrophomonas maltophilia*

Stenotrophomonas maltophilia (SM) is a low-virulence but highly resistant GNB that colonizes patients and occasionally causes respiratory infections in ICUs. SM is resistant to carbapenems and usually most other β-lactams, as well as aminoglycosides.[102] Trimethoprim-sulfamethoxazole is active against nearly all strains, and is the treatment of choice.[19,102] Ticarcillin-clavulanate may be effective, even for isolates resistant to all other β-lactams, and fluoroquinolones are also an alternative for susceptible isolates.[103] Unlike for most GNB, levofloxacin and moxifloxacin are more active than ciprofloxacin against SM in vitro. Tigecycline and minocycline also have excellent in vitro activity.[103]

ADJUVANT THERAPY FOR MDR INFECTIONS: SOURCE CONTROL AND INFECTION PREVENTION

With increasing drug resistance and few new antibiotics available, a crucial component of management of infections caused by MDR pathogens is source control. Source control is critical to the management of septic shock and severe sepsis.[104,105] Though not specifically studied for less severe MDR infections, prompt removal of infected venous catheters and devices, drainage of infected collections, and debridement of infected soft tissue are efficacious ways to decrease the bacterial burden and limit the development of even further resistance to the few useful drugs available. Surveillance and infection-prevention strategies are beyond the scope of this review but are also a critical component in identifying and limiting the spread of MDR infections in the ICU setting.

SUMMARY

MDR gram-negative infections are increasingly prevalent in ICUs worldwide, and therapeutic options are limited. Antibiotic choices vary with class of resistance. For the most resistant organisms such as CRE and MDR ACCB, treatment may include polymyxins and other older drugs, newer drugs such as tigecycline, and multidrug combinations. Current evidence for combinations is limited. Source control is also critical in the management of MDR infection.

REFERENCES

1. Boucher HW, Talbot GH, Bradley JS, et al. Bad bugs, no drugs: no ESKAPE! An update from the Infectious Diseases Society of America. Clin Infect Dis 2009; 48:1–12.
2. Livermore DM. Has the era of untreatable infections arrived? J Antimicrob Chemother 2009;64(Suppl 1):i29–36.
3. Spellberg B, Guidos R, Gilbert D, et al. The epidemic of antibiotic-resistant infections: a call to action for the medical community from the Infectious Diseases Society of America. Clin Infect Dis 2008;46:155–64.

4. Brusselaers N, Vogelaers D, Blot S. The rising problem of antimicrobial resistance in the intensive care unit. Ann Intensive Care 2011;1:47.

5. Kumar A, Roberts D, Wood KE, et al. Duration of hypotension before initiation of effective antimicrobial therapy is the critical determinant of survival in human septic shock. Crit Care Med 2006;34:1589–96.

6. Rosenthal SL, Freundlich LF, Quraishi MA. Sensitivity of gentamicin-resistant Enterobacteriaceae to cefamandole and cefoxitin. Chemotherapy 1979;25(3): 157–62.

7. Koch DC, Raunest M, Harder T, et al. Unilateral access regulation: ground state dynamics of the *Pseudomonas aeruginosa* outer membrane efflux duct OprM. Biochemistry 2013;52(1):178–87.

8. Fraimow HS, Tsigrelis C. Antimicrobial resistance in the intensive care unit: mechanisms, epidemiology, and management of specific resistant pathogens. Crit Care Clin 2011;27:163–205.

9. Kanj SS, Kanafani ZA. Current concepts in antimicrobial therapy against resistant gram-negative organisms: extended-spectrum beta-lactamase-producing Enterobacteriaceae, carbapenem-resistant Enterobacteriaceae, and multidrug-resistant *Pseudomonas aeruginosa*. Mayo Clin Proc 2011;86:250–9.

10. Pillar CM, Brown NP, Sahm DF, et al. Trends towards increased resistance among clinically important gram-negative pathogens in the US; results from 10 years of TRUST surveillance (1999-2009). Abstract C2-696, Interscience Conference on Antimicrobial Agents and Chemotherapy. Boston (MA): 2010. Available at: http://www.eurofins.com/media/1770121/C2-696.pdf. Accessed January 23, 2013.

11. Yang Q, Wang H, Chen M, et al. Surveillance of antimicrobial susceptibility of aerobic and facultative Gram-negative bacilli isolated from patients with intra-abdominal infections in China: the 2002-2009 Study for Monitoring Antimicrobial Resistance Trends (SMART). Int J Antimicrob Agents 2010;36:507–12.

12. Kallen AJ, Hidron AI, Patel J, et al. Multidrug resistance among gram-negative pathogens that caused healthcare-associated infections reported to the National Healthcare Safety Network, 2006-2008. Infect Control Hosp Epidemiol 2010;31:528–31.

13. Zhanel GG, DeCorby M, Laing N, et al. Antimicrobial-resistant pathogens in intensive care units in Canada: results of the Canadian National Intensive Care Unit (CAN-ICU) study, 2005-2006. Antimicrob Agents Chemother 2008; 52:1430–7.

14. Rosenthal VD, Bijie H, Maki DG, et al. International Nosocomial Infection Control Consortium (INICC) report, data summary of 36 countries, for 2004-2009. Am J Infect Control 2012;40:396–407.

15. Borer A, Saidel-Odes L, Eskira S, et al. Risk factors for developing clinical infection with carbapenem-resistant *Klebsiella pneumoniae* in hospitalized patients initially only colonized with carbapenem resistant *K. pneumoniae*. Am J Infect Control 2012;40:421–5.

16. Available at: http://www.cdc.gov/hai/eip/mugsi_techinfo.html. Accessed January 23, 2013.

17. Falagas ME, Koletsi PK, Bliziotis IA. The diversity of definitions of multidrug-resistant (MDR) and pandrug-resistant (PDR) *Acinetobacter baumannii* and *Pseudomonas aeruginosa*. J Med Microbiol 2006;55:1619–29.

18. Goossens H. Susceptibility of multi-drug-resistant *Pseudomonas aeruginosa* in intensive care units: results from the European MYSTIC study group. Clin Microbiol Infect 2003;9:980–3.

19. Falagas ME, Karageorgopoulos DE. Pandrug resistance (PDR), extensive drug resistance (XDR), and multidrug resistance (MDR) among gram-negative bacilli: need for international harmonization in terminology. Clin Infect Dis 2008;46:1121–2.

20. Apisarnthanarak A, Pinitchai U, Thongphubeth K, et al. A multifaceted intervention to reduce pandrug-resistant *Acinetobacter baumannii* colonization and infection in 3 intensive care units in a Thai tertiary care center: a 3-year study. Clin Infect Dis 2008;47:760–7.

21. Doi Y, Husain S, Potoski BA, et al. Extensively drug-resistant *Acinetobacter baumannii*. Emerg Infect Dis 2009;15:980–2.

22. Park YK, Peck KR, Cheong HS, et al. Extreme drug resistance in *Acinetobacter baumannii* infections in intensive care units, South Korea. Emerg Infect Dis 2009;15:1325–7.

23. Magiorakos AP, Srinivasan A, Carey RB, et al. Multidrug-resistant, extensively drug-resistant and pandrug-resistant bacteria: an international expert proposal for interim standard definitions for acquired resistance. Clin Microbiol Infect 2012;18(3):268–81.

24. Clinical and Laboratory Standards Institute. Performance standards for antimicrobial susceptibility testing: twentieth informational supplement CLSI document M100-S20. Wayne (PA): Clinical and Laboratory Standards Institute.

25. Esterly JS, Wagner J, McLaughlin MM, et al. Evaluation of clinical outcomes in patients with bloodstream infections due to Gram-negative bacteria according to carbapenem MIC stratification. Antimicrob Agents Chemother 2012;56(9):4885–90.

26. Defife R, Scheetz MH, Feinglass JM, et al. Effect of differences in MIC values on clinical outcomes in patients with bloodstream infections caused by gram-negative organisms treated with levofloxacin. Antimicrob Agents Chemother 2009;53(3):1074–9.

27. Kosmidis C, Poulakou G, Markogiannakis A. Treatment options for infections caused by carbapenem-resistant gram negative bacteria. Eur Infect Dis 2012;6:28–34.

28. Michalopoulos A, Falagas ME. Colistin and polymyxin B in critical care. Crit Care Clin 2008;24:377–91.

29. Drusano GL, Lodise TP. Editorial commentary: saving lives with optimal antimicrobial chemotherapy. Clin Infect Dis 2013;56:245–7.

30. Falagas ME, Tansarli GS, Ikawa K, et al. Clinical outcomes with extended or continuous versus short-term intravenous infusion of carbapenems and Piperacillin/Tazobactam: a systematic review and meta-analysis. Clin Infect Dis 2013;56:272–82.

31. Wood GC. Aerosolized antibiotics for treating hospital-acquired and ventilator-associated pneumonia. Expert Rev Anti Infect Ther 2011;9:993–1000.

32. Beardsley JR, Williamson JC, Johnson JW, et al. Using local microbiologic data to develop institution-specific guidelines for the treatment of hospital-acquired pneumonia. Chest 2006;130:787–93.

33. Mandell L. Doripenem: a new carbapenem in the treatment of nosocomial infection. Clin Infect Dis 2009;49(Suppl 1):S1–3.

34. Urban C, Mariano N, Rahal JJ. In vitro double and triple bactericidal activities of doripenem, polymyxin B, and rifampin against multidrug-resistant *Acinetobacter baumannii, Pseudomonas aeruginosa, Klebsiella pneumoniae*, and *Escherichia coli*. Antimicrob Agents Chemother 2010;54:2732–4.

35. Livermore DM. Tigecycline: what is it, and where should it be used? J Antimicrob Chemother 2005;56:611–4.

36. Wang YF, Dowzicky MJ. In vitro activity of tigecycline and comparators on *Acinetobacter* spp. isolates collected from patients with bacteremia and MIC change during the Tigecycline Evaluation and Surveillance Trial, 2004 to 2008. Diagn Microbiol Infect Dis 2010;68:73–9.

37. Burkhardt O, Rauch K, Kaever V, et al. Tigecycline possibly underdosed for the treatment of pneumonia: a pharmacokinetic viewpoint. Int J Antimicrob Agents 2009;34:101–2.

38. Raz R. Fosfomycin: an old–new antibiotic. Clin Microbiol Infect 2012;18:4–7.

39. Falagas ME, Kastoris AC, Kapaskelis AM, et al. Fosfomycin for the treatment of multidrug-resistant, including extended-spectrum beta-lactamase producing, Enterobacteriaceae infections: a systematic review. Lancet Infect Dis 2010;10: 43–50.

40. Arroyo LA, Mateos I, Gonzalez V, et al. In vitro activities of tigecycline, minocycline, and colistin-tigecycline combination against multi- and pandrug-resistant clinical isolates of *Acinetobacter baumannii* group. Antimicrob Agents Chemother 2009;53:1295–6.

41. Jankowski CA, Balada-Liasat J. A stewardship approach to combating multidrug-resistant *Acinetobacter* infections with minocycline. Infect Dis Clin Pract (Baltim Md) 2012;20:184–7.

42. Peleg AY, Seifert H, Paterson DL. *Acinetobacter baumannii*: emergence of a successful pathogen. Clin Microbiol Rev 2008;21:538–82.

43. Fishbain J, Peleg AY. Treatment of *Acinetobacter* infections. Clin Infect Dis 2010; 51:79–84.

44. Shakil S, Azhar EI, Tabrez S, et al. New Delhi metallo-beta-lactamase (NDM-1): an update. J Chemother 2011;23:263–5.

45. Drapeau CM, Grilli E, Petrosillo N. Rifampicin combined regimens for gram-negative infections: data from the literature. Int J Antimicrob Agents 2010;35: 39–44.

46. Yahav D, Farbman L, Leibovici L, et al. Colistin: new lessons on an old antibiotic. Clin Microbiol Infect 2012;18:18–29.

47. Nation RL, Li J. Colistin in the 21st century. Curr Opin Infect Dis 2009;22:535–43.

48. Cai Y, Chai D, Wang R, et al. Colistin resistance of *Acinetobacter baumannii*: clinical reports, mechanisms and antimicrobial strategies. J Antimicrob Chemother 2012;67:1607–15.

49. Garonzik SM, Li J, Thamlikitkul V, et al. Population pharmacokinetics of colistin methanesulfonate and formed colistin in critically ill patients from a multicenter study provide dosing suggestions for various categories of patients. Antimicrob Agents Chemother 2011;55:3284–94.

50. Freire-Moran L, Aronsson B, Manz C, et al. Critical shortage of new antibiotics in development against multidrug-resistant bacteria—time to react is now. Drug Resist Updat 2011;14:118–24.

51. Florescu DF, Qiu F, McCartan MA, et al. What is the efficacy and safety of colistin for the treatment of ventilator-associated pneumonia? A systematic review and meta-regression. Clin Infect Dis 2012;54:670–80.

52. Trial for the treatment of extensively drug-resistant gram-negative bacilli. Available at: http://clinicaltrials.gov/ct2/show/NCT01597973. Accessed January 24, 2013.

53. Multicenter open-label randomized controlled trial (RCT) to compare colistin alone versus colistin plus meropenem. Available at: http://clinicaltrials.gov/ct2/show/NCT01732250. Accessed January 24, 2013.

54. Abdul-Aziz MH, Dulhunty JM, Bellomo R, et al. Continuous beta-lactam infusion in critically ill patients: the clinical evidence. Ann Intensive Care 2012;2:37.

55. George JM, Colton BJ, Rodvold KA. National survey on continuous and extended infusions of antibiotics. Am J Health Syst Pharm 2012;69:1895–904.
56. Lodise TP Jr, Lomaestro B, Drusano GL. Piperacillin-tazobactam for *Pseudomonas aeruginosa* infection: clinical implications of an extended-infusion dosing strategy. Clin Infect Dis 2007;44:357–63.
57. Dulhunty JM, Roberts JA, Davis JS, et al. Continuous infusion of beta-lactam antibiotics in severe sepsis: a multicenter double-blind, randomized controlled trial. Clin Infect Dis 2013;56:236–44.
58. Hallal A, Cohn SM, Namias N, et al. Aerosolized tobramycin in the treatment of ventilator-associated pneumonia: a pilot study. Surg Infect (Larchmt) 2007;8: 73–82.
59. Czosnowski QA, Wood GC, Magnotti LJ, et al. Adjunctive aerosolized antibiotics for treatment of ventilator-associated pneumonia. Pharmacotherapy 2009;29: 1054–60.
60. Mohr AM, Sifri ZC, Horng HS, et al. Use of aerosolized aminoglycosides in the treatment of Gram-negative ventilator-associated pneumonia. Surg Infect (Larchmt) 2007;8:349–57.
61. Kofteridis DP, Alexopoulou C, Valachis A, et al. Aerosolized plus intravenous colistin versus intravenous colistin alone for the treatment of ventilator-associated pneumonia: a matched case-control study. Clin Infect Dis 2010;51: 1238–44.
62. Paterson DL, Ko WC, Von Gottberg A, et al. Antibiotic therapy for *Klebsiella pneumoniae* bacteremia: implications of production of extended-spectrum beta-lactamases. Clin Infect Dis 2004;39:31–7.
63. Peleg AY, Hooper DC. Hospital-acquired infections due to gram-negative bacteria. N Engl J Med 2010;362:1804–13.
64. Pitout JD. Infections with extended-spectrum beta-lactamase-producing Enterobacteriaceae: changing epidemiology and drug treatment choices. Drugs 2010;70:313–33.
65. Vardakas KZ, Tansarli GS, Rafailidis PI, et al. Carbapenems versus alternative antibiotics for the treatment of bacteraemia due to Enterobacteriaceae producing extended-spectrum beta-lactamases: a systematic review and meta-analysis. J Antimicrob Chemother 2012;67:2793–803.
66. Lye DC, Wijaya L, Chan J, et al. Ertapenem for treatment of extended-spectrum beta-lactamase-producing and multidrug-resistant gram-negative bacteraemia. Ann Acad Med Singapore 2008;37:831–4.
67. Gavin PJ, Suseno MT, Thomson RB Jr, et al. Clinical correlation of the CLSI susceptibility breakpoint for piperacillin- tazobactam against extended-spectrum-beta-lactamase-producing *Escherichia coli* and *Klebsiella* species. Antimicrob Agents Chemother 2006;50:2244–7.
68. Labombardi VJ, Rojtman A, Tran K. Use of cefepime for the treatment of infections caused by extended spectrum beta-lactamase-producing *Klebsiella pneumoniae* and *Escherichia coli*. Diagn Microbiol Infect Dis 2006;56:313–5.
69. Bin C, Hui W, Renyuan Z, et al. Outcome of cephalosporin treatment of bacteremia due to CTX-M-type extended-spectrum beta-lactamase-producing *Escherichia coli*. Diagn Microbiol Infect Dis 2006;56:351–7.
70. Lee NY, Lee CC, Huang WH, et al. Cefepime therapy for monomicrobial bacteremia caused by cefepime-susceptible extended-spectrum beta-lactamase-producing Enterobacteriaceae: MIC matters. Clin Infect Dis 2013;56:488–95.
71. Endimiani A, Luzzaro F, Perilli M, et al. Bacteremia due to *Klebsiella pneumoniae* isolates producing the TEM-52 extended-spectrum beta-lactamase: treatment

outcome of patients receiving imipenem or ciprofloxacin. Clin Infect Dis 2004; 38:243–51.

72. Kim YK, Pai H, Lee HJ, et al. Bloodstream infections by extended-spectrum beta-lactamase-producing *Escherichia coli* and *Klebsiella pneumoniae* in children: epidemiology and clinical outcome. Antimicrob Agents Chemother 2002;46:1481–91.

73. Chow JW, Fine MJ, Shlaes DM, et al. *Enterobacter* bacteremia: clinical features and emergence of antibiotic resistance during therapy. Ann Intern Med 1991; 115:585–90.

74. Jacoby GA. AmpC beta-lactamases. Clin Microbiol Rev 2009;22:161–82.

75. Tzouvelekis LS, Markogiannakis A, Psichogiou M, et al. Carbapenemases in *Klebsiella pneumoniae* and other Enterobacteriaceae: an evolving crisis of global dimensions. Clin Microbiol Rev 2012;25:682–707.

76. Ben-David D, Kordevani R, Keller N, et al. Outcome of carbapenem resistant *Klebsiella pneumoniae* bloodstream infections. Clin Microbiol Infect 2012;18: 54–60.

77. Souli M, Galani I, Antoniadou A, et al. An outbreak of infection due to beta-Lactamase *Klebsiella pneumoniae* carbapenemase 2-producing *K. pneumoniae* in a Greek University Hospital: molecular characterization, epidemiology, and outcomes. Clin Infect Dis 2010;50:364–73.

78. Daikos GL, Markogiannakis A. Carbapenemase-producing *Klebsiella pneumoniae*: (when) might we still consider treating with carbapenems? Clin Microbiol Infect 2011;17:1135–41.

79. Elemam A, Rahimian J, Mandell W. Infection with panresistant *Klebsiella pneumoniae*: a report of 2 cases and a brief review of the literature. Clin Infect Dis 2009;49:271–4.

80. Bratu S, Tolaney P, Karumudi U, et al. Carbapenemase-producing *Klebsiella pneumoniae* in Brooklyn, NY: molecular epidemiology and in vitro activity of polymyxin B and other agents. J Antimicrob Chemother 2005;56:128–32.

81. Elemam A, Rahimian J, Doymaz M. In vitro evaluation of antibiotic synergy for polymyxin B-resistant carbapenemase-producing *Klebsiella pneumoniae*. J Clin Microbiol 2010;48:3558–62.

82. Bulik CC, Nicolau DP. Double-carbapenem therapy for carbapenemase-producing *Klebsiella pneumoniae*. Antimicrob Agents Chemother 2011;55: 3002–4.

83. Lee YT, Kuo SC, Yang SP, et al. Impact of appropriate antimicrobial therapy on mortality associated with *Acinetobacter baumannii* bacteremia: relation to severity of infection. Clin Infect Dis 2012;55:209–15.

84. Gales AC, Jones RN, Sader HS. Contemporary activity of colistin and polymyxin B against a worldwide collection of Gram-negative pathogens: results from the SENTRY Antimicrobial Surveillance Program (2006-09). J Antimicrob Chemother 2011;66:2070–4.

85. Manchanda V, Sanchaita S, Singh N. Multidrug resistant *Acinetobacter*. J Glob Infect Dis 2010;2:291–304.

86. Paterson DL, Depestel DD. Doripenem. Clin Infect Dis 2009;49:291–8.

87. Lee NY, Wang CL, Chuang YC, et al. Combination carbapenem-sulbactam therapy for critically ill patients with multidrug-resistant *Acinetobacter baumannii* bacteremia: four case reports and an in vitro combination synergy study. Pharmacotherapy 2007;27:1506–11.

88. Garnacho-Montero J, Ortiz-Leyba C, Jimenez-Jimenez FJ, et al. Treatment of multidrug-resistant *Acinetobacter baumannii* ventilator-associated pneumonia

(VAP) with intravenous colistin: a comparison with imipenem-susceptible VAP. Clin Infect Dis 2003;36:1111–8.

89. Bassetti M, Repetto E, Righi E, et al. Colistin and rifampicin in the treatment of multidrug-resistant *Acinetobacter baumannii* infections. J Antimicrob Chemother 2008;61:417–20.

90. Gordon NC, Png K, Wareham DW. Potent synergy and sustained bactericidal activity of a vancomycin-colistin combination versus multidrug-resistant strains of *Acinetobacter baumannii*. Antimicrob Agents Chemother 2010;54:5316–22.

91. Petrosillo N, Ioannidou E, Falagas ME. Colistin monotherapy vs. combination therapy: evidence from microbiological, animal and clinical studies. Clin Microbiol Infect 2008;14:816–27.

92. Poulakou G, Kontopidou FV, Paramythiotou E, et al. Tigecycline in the treatment of infections from multi-drug resistant gram-negative pathogens. J Infect 2009; 58:273–84.

93. Cascio A, Conti A, Sinardi L, et al. Post-neurosurgical multidrug-resistant *Acinetobacter baumannii* meningitis successfully treated with intrathecal colistin. A new case and a systematic review of the literature. Int J Infect Dis 2010;14:e572–9.

94. Tam VH, Rogers CA, Chang KT, et al. Impact of multidrug-resistant *Pseudomonas aeruginosa* bacteremia on patient outcomes. Antimicrob Agents Chemother 2010;54:3717–22.

95. Croughs PD, Li B, Hoogkamp-Korstanje JA, et al. Thirteen years of antibiotic susceptibility surveillance of *Pseudomonas aeruginosa* from intensive care units and urology services in the Netherlands. Eur J Clin Microbiol Infect Dis 2012; 32(2):283–8.

96. Riera E, Cabot G, Mulet X, et al. *Pseudomonas aeruginosa* carbapenem resistance mechanisms in Spain: impact on the activity of imipenem, meropenem and doripenem. J Antimicrob Chemother 2011;66:2022–7.

97. Durakovic N, Radojcic V, Boban A, et al. Efficacy and safety of colistin in the treatment of infections caused by multidrug-resistant *Pseudomonas aeruginosa* in patients with hematologic malignancy: a matched pair analysis. Intern Med 2011;50:1009–13.

98. Kvitko CH, Rigatto MH, Moro AL, et al. Polymyxin B versus other antimicrobials for the treatment of *Pseudomonas aeruginosa* bacteraemia. J Antimicrob Chemother 2011;66:175–9.

99. Lee JY, Song JH, Ko KS. Identification of nonclonal *Pseudomonas aeruginosa* isolates with reduced colistin susceptibility in Korea. Microb Drug Resist 2011;17:299–304.

100. Chamot E, Boffi El Amari E, Rohner P, et al. Effectiveness of combination antimicrobial therapy for *Pseudomonas aeruginosa* bacteremia. Antimicrob Agents Chemother 2003;47:2756–64.

101. Apisarnthanarak A, Mundy LM. Use of high-dose 4-hour infusion of doripenem, in combination with fosfomycin, for treatment of carbapenem-resistant *Pseudomonas aeruginosa* pneumonia. Clin Infect Dis 2010;51:1352–4.

102. Nicodemo AC, Paez JI. Antimicrobial therapy for *Stenotrophomonas maltophilia* infections. Eur J Clin Microbiol Infect Dis 2007;26:229–37.

103. Insa R, Cercenado E, Goyanes MJ, et al. In vitro activity of tigecycline against clinical isolates of *Acinetobacter baumannii* and *Stenotrophomonas maltophilia*. J Antimicrob Chemother 2007;59:583–5.

104. Marshall JC, Maier RV, Jimenez M, et al. Source control in the management of severe sepsis and septic shock: an evidence-based review. Crit Care Med 2004;32:S513–26.

105. Sulaiman L, Hunter J, Farquharson F, et al. Mechanical thrombectomy of an infected deep venous thrombosis: a novel technique of source control in sepsis. Br J Anaesth 2011;106:65–8.

106. Rennie RP, Turnbull L, Johnson A. Surveillance of gram-negative intra-abdominal and urinary tract pathogens in Canada compared to the rest of the world: the SMART study Abstract C2-1789, Interscience Conference on Antimicrobial Agents and Chemotherapy. Chicago (IL): 2011.

Infective Endocarditis in the Intensive Care Unit

Yoav Keynan, MD[a,b,c],*, Rohit Singal, MD[d,e], Kanwal Kumar, MD[d], Rakesh C. Arora, MD, PhD[d,e,f,g], Ethan Rubinstein, MD[a,b]

KEYWORDS

- Endocarditis • Diagnosis • Infection site • ICU • Echocardiography

KEY POINTS

- Infective endocarditis (IE) is a disease with many facets and various expressions depending on the site of infection, microorganism, underlying heart lesion, immune status of the host, and remote effects such as emboli, organ dysfunction, and the general condition of the host.
- Diagnosis is the first crucial step, which depends on meticulous clinical examination, blood cultures, results, and echocardiographic findings.
- The management of the patient with endocarditis in the intensive care unit is complex and needs a multidisciplinary team, including the intensivist, a cardiologist, an experienced echocardiologist, an infectious diseases specialist, and a cardiac surgeon.
- The medical and surgical management of such patients is complex, and timely decisions are important.

The true incidence of endocarditis is difficult to estimate; various figures are based on diverse study designs, settings, and variable case definitions. In developed countries, the incidence is approximately 5 to 7.9 cases per 100,000 persons/y. An estimated 10,000 to 15,000 new cases of infective endocarditis (IE) are diagnosed in the United States each year.[1,2] These rates vary between geographic regions, and publications regarding the epidemiology are affected by referral bias, with a tendency for reporting from larger centers.[3,4] In addition to the range of incidence rates, the underlying conditions such as rheumatic heart disease, injection drug use, prosthetic devices, and

Disclosures: The authors have nothing to disclose.
[a] Department of Internal Medicine, University of Manitoba, Manitoba, Canada; [b] Department of Medical Microbiology, University of Manitoba, Manitoba, Canada; [c] Department of Community Health Sciences, University of Manitoba, Manitoba, Canada; [d] Department of Surgery, University of Manitoba, Manitoba, Canada; [e] Manitoba Cardiac Sciences Program, University of Manitoba, Manitoba, Canada; [f] Department of Anesthesia, University of Manitoba, Manitoba, Canada; [g] Department of Physiology, University of Manitoba, Manitoba, Canada
* Corresponding author. Department of Internal Medicine, Medical Microbiology and Community Health Sciences, University of Manitoba, Rm 507, 745 Bannatyne Avenue, Winnipeg, Manitoba R3E 0J9, Canada.
E-mail address: keynany@yahoo.com

Crit Care Clin 29 (2013) 923–951
http://dx.doi.org/10.1016/j.ccc.2013.06.011
0749-0704/13/$ – see front matter © 2013 Elsevier Inc. All rights reserved.
criticalcare.theclinics.com

immunosuppression have changed over time. The incidence seems to be increasing because of greater number of indwelling devices and prosthetic materials and higher levels of immune suppression.

IE is no longer commonly associated with rheumatic heart disease in developed countries, and it is more common in older adults.[5–7] In a study reporting 203 IE episodes among 193 patients,[5] the median age was 67 years, one-third were nosocomial and one-third involved a prosthetic valve. The other trend observed is the increase in *Staphylococcus aureus* (SA), which may also be related to prosthetic devices. SA is the most common pathogen associated with IE and has a predilection for individuals with intravascular devices, hemodialysis, and diabetes.[6–8] In a report of the results of the ICE-PCS (International Collaboration on Endocarditis-Prospective Cohort Study), patients in the United States were likely to be hemodialysis dependent, to have diabetes, to harbor an intravascular device and were more likely to be infected with methicillin-resistant SA (MRSA), and to receive vancomycin.[8] These underlying comorbidities resulted in an increased severity of illness manifested as higher mortality and higher incidence of embolic events and central nervous system (CNS) events, as well as higher rates of surgery.[6,7] A recent study noted a trend toward an increase in SA and a significant increase in the subgroup of patients without known underlying valvular disease.[9] A population-based study reported an incidence of 33.8 cases per million, highest among men aged 75 to 79 years, most of whom had no previously identified predisposing heart disease. Staphylococci were the most common causal agents, accounting for 36.2% of cases, and of those, SA accounted for more than a quarter, whereas coagulase-negative staphylococci (CONS) caused nearly 10%. Health care–associated IE accounted for 26.7% of cases. SA was the most important factor associated with in-hospital mortality for infections originating in the community as well as for nosocomially acquired cases.[10]

IE can be caused by many microorganisms; however, staphylococci and streptococci account for most cases (**Table 1**).

The higher incidence of SA compared with viridans group streptococci (VGS) is probably because this study was conducted in large tertiary-care centers, which may not reflect the epidemiology of uncomplicated IE in rural settings. This hypothesis is supported by a population-based survey using the Rochester Epidemiology Project of Olmsted County, Minnesota, in which VGS were the most common cause.[11] The same group reported a more recent accumulation of 150 patients with IE, with VGS accounting for 40% and SA for 26.7%.[12] SA epidemiology is changing, with increasing incidence and prevalence of MRSA. The emergence of community-associated MRSA

Table 1
Cause of IE in 2781 patients with definite endocarditis from 25 countries, ICE-PCS

Causative Organism	Overall Rate (%)	Native Valve (Excluding Drug Abusers) (%)	Prosthetic Valve (%)
SA	17–43 (31)	28	23
VGS	9–26 (17)	21	12
Enterococci	10–13 (11)	11	12
CONS	7–13 (11)	9	17
Streptococcus bovis and other streptococci	8–15	14	10

Data from Murdoch DR, Corey GR, Hoen B, et al. Clinical presentation, etiology, and outcome of infective endocarditis in the 21st century: the International Collaboration on Endocarditis-Prospective Cohort Study. Arch Intern Med 2009;169(5):466.

and its invasion into hospitals created a mixture of distinct SA pathogens that are capable of causing bacteremia and IE.

The rates of other causes vary greatly between geographic regions, with HACEK organisms being uncommon in North America and *Bartonella* and *Coxiella* reported mostly from centers in Europe.[13] In the Middle East, *Brucella* is an important cause of IE.[14,15] The role of CONS is being increasingly appreciated, in part because of multi-center studies providing an opportunity to study less frequent causative agents. In recent multicenter studies, it has become the third most common causative agent overall, with a growing appreciation as a pathogen in the context of native valve IE.[13,16] More cases of a more virulent CONS, *Staphylococcus lugdunensis,* have been reported in recent years, and this frequent colonizer of the groin, perineum, and long-term indwelling catheters has been shown to account for predominantly native valve endocarditis (NVE), responsible for up to 18% of CONS endocarditis cases.[17,18]

IE IN THE INTENSIVE CARE UNIT SETTING

It is difficult to estimate the proportion of patients with IE requiring admission to the intensive care unit (ICU). Many of those requiring surgery go through the ICU at some stage of their hospital admission. In addition, the associated cardiac and extrac-ardiac complications of IE may necessitate management in the ICU setting. Among the systemic complications are hemodynamic instability caused by sepsis, cardiogenic shock or a combination of the 2, embolization of infected materials, with resulting end-organ damage, sepsis, septic shock, and so forth. The causes for requiring ICU admission were reported in a study of 4106 patients admitted to 4 medical ICUs, of whom 33 had a complicated IE. More than half had IE diagnosed before ICU admission, whereas the remaining 15 were diagnosed while in the ICU. The most common reason for ICU admission was congestive heart failure (CHF), in almost two-thirds of cases; septic shock accounted for 21% cases and the third most common was neurologic deterioration in 15%. Seventy-nine percent required mechanical ventilation, 73% were on ionotropic support, and 39% suffered from renal failure, renal failure was the only independent risk factor for mortality in a multivariate analysis.[19] SA was the most common causative agent.

NEUROLOGIC COMPLICATIONS

Neurologic complications of IE are common among patients with IE admitted to ICU. The mechanisms that lead to these complications include embolic occlusion of cere-bral arteries; cerebral hemorrhage; infection of the brain parenchyma (septic purulent encephalitis) or meninges and mycotic aneurysms. Several of these complications may be present together in a given patient and can be accompanied by sepsis-related encephalopathy, leading to acute delirium and fluctuating level of conscious-ness; these factors may make the diagnosis of focal neurologic deficits even more difficult. Sonneville and colleagues[20] recently reported a series of 198 left-sided IE from 33 ICUs in France. Neurologic complications occurred in 55% of the patients. These complications included, in order of frequency, ischemic strokes, cerebral hem-orrhages, meningitis, brain abscesses, and mycotic aneurysms. The risk factors for these neurologic complications were SA as the cause of IE; mitral valve endocarditis; and embolic events elsewhere. Meningitis is not uncommon and may be caused by presence of bacteria in the cerebrospinal fluid (CSF) or represent an inflammatory reaction to a nearby parenchymal infection or ischemia; it occurs in 2% to 20% of patients with IE and up to 40% of those with neurologic complications. However, in most cases, the organisms are not recovered from the CSF because of absence, or transient presence only, with the notable exception of *Streptococcus pneumoniae*.

CNS embolization is frequent and may range from subclinical to catastrophic. The incidence of neurologic embolic events complicating IE varies between series and is probably higher among patients reported from referral centers, because they tend to be overrepresented in large multicenter studies. The importance of CNS emboli is shown by older studies of autopsies of patients succumbing to IE. In some, the presence of brain lesions is reported to occur in up to 90% of patients.[21] In most series that are based on clinical manifestations, CNS involvement during the course of IE occurs in 20% to 40% of cases. In a Finnish teaching hospital, one-quarter of cases were associated with neurologic complications, and SA was 2 to 3 times more likely to be associated with their presence.[22] A recent series from France reported lower occurrence of strokes (17%) among 264 IE cases caused by staphylococci or streptococci[23]; similar rates were observed among 513 episodes of complicated, left-sided native valve IE, from the United States.[24] In the ICE database,[13] which reported on 2781 patients from 58 hospitals in 25 countries, identical incidence of strokes was found. The use of computed tomography (CT) or magnetic resonance imaging (MRI) results in detection of some clinically silent embolic events. A study from France[25] identified cerebrovascular complications in 22.2% of patients with IE. CT led to identification of 17 (3.8%) additional unsuspected emboli (453 CT scans, 496 patients). Even more dramatic discrepancies were reported by Cooper and colleagues,[26] who studied 56 patients with definite left-sided IE. Clinical stroke was present in 25%. Forty patients underwent MRI, and the incidence rates of subclinical brain embolization and acute brain embolization were 48% and 80%, respectively. Patients with any stroke (clinical and subclinical) were more likely to have IE caused by SA (56% vs 13%). Some rarer pathogens such as *Streptococcus agalactiae* and fungi are associated with even higher rates of systemic and CNS embolization, attributed to the larger vegetation size that they cause. Although these pathogens lead to a higher proportion of embolic complications, because of their relative rarity, they account for a smaller absolute number.[27,28] The proportion of neurologic events is increased among individuals with IE requiring admission to the ICU as a result of selection of more severe cases with higher rates of comorbid conditions. The initiation of appropriate antimicrobial therapy leads to a precipitous decline in embolic complications evident as early as after the first week of therapy,[29] with further decreases in incidence in the ensuing weeks.

THE ROLE OF ECHOCARDIOGRAPHY IN DIAGNOSIS AND MANAGEMENT OF IE

Echocardiography is a cornerstone in the diagnosis of IE. Both the American Society of Echocardiography[30] and the European Association of Echocardiography[31] have provided guidelines for the appropriate use of transthoracic echocardiography (TTE) or transesophageal (TEE) echocardiography in patients with suspected IE. Echocardiography must be performed early in patients with suspected IE. Echocardiography is the preferred imaging modality to detect vegetations on cardiac valves and show lesions as small as 1 to 2 mm. In addition, two-dimensional imaging can show intracardiac abscesses and with the use of color Doppler, abnormal blood flow patterns (**Box 1**).

TTE OR TEE?

Both TTE and TEE have a role in the diagnosis of IE. Because of the noninvasive nature of TTE, it is the first-line technique, because it can provide useful information on the

> **Box 1**
> **Key echocardiographic findings of IE**
>
> Vegetations: an oscillating or sessile mass typically on the lower-pressure side of the valve apparatus
>
> Valvular disease: regurgitation, leaflet perforation, or destruction
>
> Abscess formation and valve annulus destruction
>
> Perivalvular lesions (pseudoaneurysms and fistulization)
>
> Dehiscence of prosthetic valves
>
> Ancillary findings
>
>   Alterations in left ventricular size and function
>
>   Increased right heart or pulmonary artery pressures
>
>   Presence of pericardial effusions
>
> *Data from* Habib G, Badano L, Tribouilloy C, et al. Recommendations for the practice of echocardiography in infective endocarditis. Eur J Echocardiogr 2010;11(2):204.

diagnosis and severity of the disease.[32] TTE generally has a lower sensitivity compared with TEE (46% vs 93%); however, both are highly specific (95% vs 96%).[33] A good-quality, negative TTE examination and a low clinical index of suspicion of IE should prompt clinicians to seek alternate diagnosis. However, an equivocal (ie, suboptimal examination) or a negative TTE examination in the setting of high pretest probability (ie, positive blood cultures, type of organism, presence of known IE risk factors, or new murmur) does not exclude the diagnosis of IE. TEE is required to show the cardiac lesion(s) consistent with IE and to further characterize the extent of perivalvular disease (ie, severity of regurgitation, valve leaflet perforation, aneurysm, and abscess formation). Furthermore, even with positive TTE, examining the extent of disease by the TEE may assist the surgical team in planning their operative management. An algorithm for suggested use of TTE/TEE is shown in **Fig. 1**. The use of TTE in patients admitted to the ICU may be even less sensitive because of the need of mechanical ventilation and suboptimal positioning of the patient for examination. In a multicenter review of echocardiographic examination in ICU patients,[34] TTE was diagnostic in only 33% and a subsequent TEE was required in 91% to confirm the diagnosis or fully to delineate the extent of disease. Others have reported sensitivity of TTE and TEE for endocarditis detection is 58% to 62% and 88% to 98%, respectively.[35,36]

The presence of prosthetic heart valve, particularly mechanical valves, can make the visualization more challenging, particularly with examination performed by the transthoracic technique. A study by Palraj and colleagues[37] reported the poor sensitivity (<50%) of TTE in the context of SA prosthetic endocarditis and has recommended the use of selective TEE in these patients.

PITFALLS OF ECHOCARDIOGRAPHY

A negative echocardiographic examination occurs in approximately 7% to 15% of IE cases.[20,31] This result most commonly occurs with very small lesions, with preexisting severe valvular lesions (eg, prolapse or degenerative mitral valve lesions) and with prosthetic valve endocarditis (PVE). Therefore, in the context of a high degree of suspicion of IE, repeat echocardiographic examination after 7 to 10 days to reassess

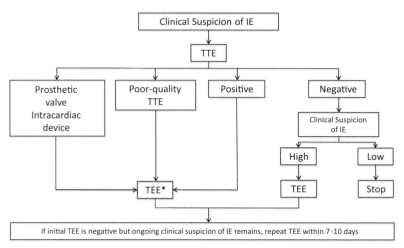

Fig. 1. An algorithm for the use of echocardiography in the diagnosis and assessment of extensiveness of IE disease; *denotes the need to consider additional TEE on the individual basis of the clinical context of the patient. (*Adapted from* Habib G, Badano L, Tribouilloy C, et al. Recommendations for the practice of echocardiography in infective endocarditis. Eur J Echocardiogr 2010;11(2):203; with permission.)

potential progression of vegetation may be warranted depending on the clinical status of the patient. Second, an echocardiographic false-positive diagnosis of IE may occur in certain patients. Examples of potential confounders include variants of normal cardiac structures (ie, Lambl excrescences), noninfective lesions (ie, marantic endo-carditis), or cardiac tumors. It is not possible to echographically distinguish infective from noninfective lesions, and repeat echocardiographic examination needs to be considered on an individual basis.

SUPPORTIVE AND ANTIMICROBIAL MANAGEMENT

The reader is also referred to articles by Keynan and colleagues elsewhere in this issue dealing with specific organisms. IE, which was formerly an invariably fatal disease, is associated with a 20% mortality. In IE caused by virulent organisms like SA, the mortality is still ∼30%, with many of the patients dying during their first hospitalization.[8]

CRITICAL CARE MANAGEMENT

Patients with IE can progress to critical illness requiring an admission to an ICU. Diligent clinical assessment, augmented with continuous invasive, and noninvasive ICU monitoring, are the cornerstones to effective management. Standard continuous monitoring includes electrocardiography, arterial pressure, and pulse oximetry. Although the use of pulmonary artery catheters remains of uncertain benefit,[37–40] central venous monitoring may be of value in central venous gas assessment and guiding fluid administration.[41]

Mourvillier and colleagues[42] reported a larger retrospective review of 228 consecutive patients meeting the Duke criteria for IE admitted to 2 regional, tertiary ICUs from 1993 to 2000. Approximately 64% of these patients (n = 146) suffered from NVE, with the remaining patients (n = 82) admitted with PVE. Approximately 50% of patients with NVE and 40% of patients with PVE were managed medically. SA was the most common cultured microbe (50%). Significant complications occurred frequently, with neurologic injury being the most frequent (40% of cases). The overall mortality was high in this cohort, at 45% (108/228). Clinical factors in patients with NVE who were independently associated with in-hospital mortality included (in descending strength of association) septic shock (odds ratio [OR] 4.81), cerebral emboli (OR 3.00), and immunocompromised state (OR 2.88). The investigators emphasized that cardiac surgery was protective (OR 0.475). In patients with prosthetic valve IE, the factors associated with mortality were septic shock (OR 4.07), neurologic complications (OR 3.1), and immunocompromised state (3.46), with higher survival rates with surgery compared with medical management alone.

TREATING SEVERE SEPSIS OR SEPTIC SHOCK IN THE PATIENT WITH IE

The patient with IE who is admitted to ICU requires prompt and protocolized care to maximize survival. In 2008, the update to the international guidelines for management of severe sepsis and septic shock provided the contemporary framework for management of patients with IE requiring admission to the ICU.[43] The key principles are: (1) Goal-directed resuscitation; (2) Diagnosis, including echo; (3) initiation of appropriate antimicrobial therapy; and (4) source control.

Goal-directed resuscitation: the current recommendation is that hypotension is treated aggressively once hypoperfusion is recognized. During the initial first 6 hours of resuscitation, the clinician should seek to achieve all of the following hemodynamic and clinical goals[44]:

- Central venous pressure 8 to 12 mm Hg
- Mean arterial pressure 65 mm Hg
- Urine output 0.5 mL/kg/h
- Central venous (superior vena cava) or mixed venous oxygen saturation 70% or 65%, respectively.[45]

The early initiation of antimicrobial therapy[42] and surgical consideration of repair/replacement of infected cardiac valves are necessary to improve outcomes in patients with IE.[46]

NATURAL VALVE IE

Results of blood cultures for accurate diagnosis are usually available within 1 to 3 days. Blood cultures are positive in most patients, and empirical antibiotic therapy should be administered only after at least 2 (preferably 3) sets of blood cultures have been obtained from separate venipunctures, and ideally spaced over 30 to 60 minutes. Empirical therapy pending blood culture results should cover methicillin-susceptible SA (MSSA) and MRSA as well as streptococci and enterococci. Appropriate agents are either vancomycin 30 mg/kg/24 h in 2 divided doses or a single daily dose of daptomycin 10 to 12 mg/kg. Most patients become afebrile within 3 to 5 days of appropriate therapy. Patients with SA IE may remain febrile for 5 to 7 days. Right-sided endocarditis with septic pulmonary emboli can lead to a longer febrile period. The initial microbiologic response to therapy should be assessed by repeat blood cultures 48 to 72 hours after antibiotics are begun. Thereafter, regular examinations should be performed to search for heart failure, emboli, and other complications. The length of therapy for patients with native valve IE depends on the organism and valve involved as well as on the presence of complications. Two-week therapy is suitable for patients with right-sided endocarditis and for patients with highly susceptible VGS (minimum inhibitory concentration [MIC] <0.1 μg/mL of penicillin) treated with antibiotic combination therapy. Most other patients are treated with 4 to 6 weeks of intravenous (IV) therapy. Patients with complications or when therapy has started late benefit from prolonged courses of IV therapy (6 weeks).

Combination therapy using a β-lactam agent, such as penicillin, with an aminoglycoside has been shown to be highly effective in streptococcal and enterococcal endocarditis, and of equivocal efficacy in patients with staphylococcal endocarditis.

Combination therapy with a penicillin and an aminoglycoside or ceftriaxone and an aminoglycoside for 2 weeks is highly effective in carefully selected patients with *Streptococcus viridans* endocarditis.[47]

Combination therapy with nafcillin or oxacillin or cloxacillin and an aminoglycoside for 2 weeks has been shown to be effective in patients with right-sided endocarditis caused by SA.[6] In contrast, combined therapy with vancomycin and an aminoglycoside administered for 2 weeks does not seem to be effective in these patients. In addition, combined therapy with nafcillin and an aminoglycoside is not effective in left-sided endocarditis if treatment is given for only 2 weeks.[48]

VIRIDANS STREPTOCOCCI AND *STREPTOCOCCUS GALLOLYTICUS* (FORMERLY *STREPTOCOCCUS BOVIS*)

Members of the viridans group (VGS) are responsible for half of all community-acquired mitral valve endocarditis; other members of the VGS include *Streptococcus mitis, Streptococcus mutans, Streptococcus oralis, Streptococcus sanguinis, Streptococcus sobrinus*, and the *Streptococcus milleri* group (*Streptococcus anginosus, Streptococcus constellatus*, and *Streptococcus intermedius*). Most VGS are highly penicillin susceptible, defined as an MIC of 0.12 μg/mL or less. Occasional strains have intermediate susceptibility to penicillin (MIC >0.12 μg/mL and ≤0.5 μg/mL), and rare strains are considered to be fully resistant, with a penicillin MIC greater than 0.5 μg/mL. For the VGS and *Streptococcus gallolyticus* IE treatment consists of crystalline penicillin G 12 to 18 million units/24 h divided into 4 or 6 equal doses for 4 weeks if the causative pathogen has an MIC less than 0.12 μg/mL. Ceftriaxone 2 g IV/24 h can substitute penicillin for the same treatment duration.

Penicillin-allergic patients can usually be treated with ceftriaxone, if their penicillin allergy consists of rash without other signs of immediate-type hypersensitivity. Patients with histories of immediate-type hypersensitivity may either be treated with vancomycin or desensitized to penicillin and treated with a standard regimen. Once penicillin therapy is stopped for more than 24 hours in desensitized patients, repeat desensitization is required. In patients with streptococcal endocarditis and a history of significant penicillin allergy, a combination of gentamicin with vancomycin (or teicoplanin) can be used.

For treatment of streptococci with intermediate penicillin susceptibility (MIC≥0.12 and ≤0.5 μg/mL), and for nutritionally deficient streptococci, 24 million units daily either continuously or in 4 to 6 equally divided doses) or ceftriaxone (2 g IV or intramuscularly once daily) for a total of 4 weeks should be used, gentamicin should be added to this regimen for the first 2 weeks.[49] IE caused by strains of VGS and streptococcallike organisms (eg, *Abiotrophia defectiva, Granulicatella* spp, and *Gemella* spp) that have penicillin MICs greater than 1 μg/mL are considered fully resistant to penicillin and should be treated with regimens used to treat enterococcal endocarditis. Other streptococcal species (eg, groups A, B, C, and G, and *Streptococcus pneumoniae*) should be treated according to their susceptibility; most of these strains are highly susceptible to penicillin, and an infectious diseases consultation is needed in such cases. Some strains of group B, C, and G streptococci are more resistant to penicillin than

Streptococcus pyogenes. Therefore, adding gentamicin to a penicillin or cephalo-sporin for the first 2 weeks of a 4-week to 6-week course of therapy is recommended.[50]

Pneumococcal IE is usually fulminant and causes severe valve damage, and embolic complications, valve perforation, and ring abscess are frequently detected.[51] In penicillin-susceptible strains, high-dose penicillin (24 million/24 h) is recommended. In other strains, therapy is similar to intermediate and resistant streptococci.

ENTEROCOCCAL IE

Members of the genus *Enterococcus* are all resistant to low concentrations of peni-cillin. They are also relatively resistant to expanded spectrum penicillins (eg, ampi-cillin, piperacillin), as well as to the cephalosporins. In addition, they are typically resistant to aminoglycosides at concentrations achieved using standard dosing reg-imens. However, many strains of enterococci are killed if penicillin, ampicillin, or vancomycin, which exert only bacteriostatic activity, are combined with an amino-glycoside such as gentamicin, the combination being bactericidal. However, there are exceptions to this suggested therapy: some enterococci produce β-lactamase, rendering them β-lactam resistant; others may have high-level resistance to amino-glycosides (>1000 μg/mL), rendering them resistant to the cidal activity of the com-bination. Some strains are vancomycin resistant; for more details the reader is referred to the article on vancomycin-resistant enterococci (VRE) elsewhere in this issue.

Most cases of enterococcal IE are caused by *Enterococcus faecalis*. Therapy for *E faecalis* with low-level penicillin resistance consists of a combination of IV aqueous penicillin G, or ampicillin, plus gentamicin. In penicillin-allergic patients, penicillin should be substituted with vancomycin administered together with gentamicin. Gentamicin should be given in patients with normal renal function in a dose of 1 mg/kg every 8 hours to achieve peak levels of 3 to 4 μg/mL. Although ampicillin is slightly more active than penicillin against *E faecalis*, clinical trials do not favor the use of ampicillin for enterococcal IE, because its use is associated with a higher rate of adverse events (mainly rash) than is penicillin. Antibiotic combination therapy should be administered for 4 weeks. Patients with a history of penicillin allergy should be treated with a combination of vancomycin (30 mg/kg/d) and gentamicin (3 mg/kg/d) for 6 weeks or considered for desensitization. The reason for longer therapy with the vancomycin combination is the decreased activity of vancomycin against enterococci, compared with penicillin.[36] Enterococcal IE caused by strains that are susceptible to penicillin, vancomycin, and streptomycin but resistant to gentamicin can be treated with ampicillin or penicillin plus streptomycin (15 mg/kg/d in 2 equally divided doses). Patients who have enterococcal IE caused by ampicillin-susceptible (MIC ≤4 mg/L) and high-level gentamicin and streptomycin resistance (MIC >128 mg/L) may be treated with high-dose ampicillin monotherapy. Enterococcal IE caused by strains with intrinsic high-level penicillin resistance (MIC >16 μg/mL) can be treated with a combination of gentamicin plus either ampicillin-sulbactam (12 g per day in 4 equally divided doses) (if the resistance is β-lactamase mediated) or vancomycin (30 mg/kg daily given IV in 2 divided doses) for 6 weeks. IE caused by VRE is limited to isolated case reports; in such cases, an infectious diseases consult is needed. The reader is also referred to the article on VRE elsewhere in this issue.

STAPHYLOCOCCAL IE

For a more detailed discussion of staphylococcal infections, the reader is referred to the relevant article elsewhere in this issue.

MSSA

NVE caused by MSSA is best treated with a semisynthetic penicillin, such as nafcillin, oxacillin, or flucloxacillin (12 g per day IV in 4 to 6 equally divided doses). Aminoglycosides should not be combined routinely with antistaphylococcal penicillins, vancomycin, or daptomycin for treatment of SA bacteremia. Although in vitro and experimental models of endocarditis have shown that combination therapy facilitates more rapid killing of MSSA than monotherapy, the evidence for clinically significant benefit is minimal and the potential for renal toxicity is substantial.[52,53] In adults, 6 weeks of therapy is recommended for complicated right-sided IE and for all left-sided IE; complicated IE is defined as metastatic infections or when the course is otherwise complicated by secondary cardiac problems (eg, heart failure). In patients with uncomplicated right-sided IE, the duration of therapy is 2 weeks if synergistic therapy can be given. In children, 6 weeks of therapy is recommended regardless of the site of infection or presence of complications. Patients allergic to penicillin can be treated with a first-generation cephalosporin, such as cefazolin (2 g IV every 8 hours), if there is no previous history of penicillin reaction that is typical of an immediate-type allergy. Vancomycin and daptomycin are acceptable alternatives in patients with immediate-type penicillin allergy; however, in MSSA, vancomycin is a less effective antistaphylococcal antibiotic.[49,54] Clindamycin and macrolides are not acceptable alternatives, because the clinical relapse rate is high.[49]

Selected patients with native valve right-sided endocarditis caused by SA with no evidence of renal failure, extrapulmonary metastatic infections, or simultaneous left-sided valvular infection, may be successfully treated with 2-week regimens using the combination of nafcillin/methicillin/oxacillin and gentamicin. Regimens that substitute vancomycin or teicoplanin for nafcillin (eg, for penicillin-allergic patients) are not considered to be reliably effective if only 2 weeks of therapy are given.[55]

MRSA IE

The reader is referred to the article dealing with MRSA infections elsewhere in this issue. NVE caused by either MRSA or CONS should be treated with vancomycin for 6 weeks. Gentamicin should not be combined with vancomycin for MRSA native valve IE. The addition of rifampin to vancomycin has not been proved to be clinically beneficial. Daptomycin is an acceptable alternative to vancomycin.[56] In a randomized trial of 246 patients, daptomycin (6 mg/kg IV per day) was not inferior to standard therapy for SA bacteremia or right-sided endocarditis. Daptomycin resistance (MIC ≥ 2 μg/mL) developed in 6 patients. Randomized controlled trials of the effectiveness of linezolid, telavancin, and quinupristin-dalfopristin in humans with IE have not yet been published but isolated case reports have reported clinical success.[57–59]

CONS

Treatment regimens for CONS are identical to those for coagulase-positive staphylococci. Most strains of CONS are methicillin resistant.

HACEK ORGANISMS

Organisms in this category include *Haemophilus aphrophilus*, *Actinobacillus actinomycetemcomitans* (subsequently called *Aggregatibacter actinomycetemcomitans*), *Cardiobacterium hominis*, *Eikenella corrodens*, and *Kingella kingae*. They usually grow late in blood culture media and are responsible for 5% to 10% of IE cases. Treatment of IE caused by these organisms should be 4 weeks of ceftriaxone.

CULTURE-NEGATIVE ENDOCARDITIS

The main reasons for culture-negative endocarditis are previous administration of anti-microbial agents, inadequate microbiological techniques, and infection with highly fastidious bacteria (eg, *Coxiella burnetti, Brucellae, Tropheryma whippelii*), nonbacterial pathogens (eg, fungi), or noninfectious causes. Empirical treatment of patients with culture-negative endocarditis should provide coverage for both gram-positive and gram-negative organisms.

PVE

For optimal management of PVE a regimen with proven efficacy combined with understanding of the underlying cardiac disease are necessary. Surgical interventions are frequently required in the context of complications, especially when infection extends beyond the valve. Patients with hemodynamic instability or acute disease should receive empirical antibiotics promptly after 3 sets of blood cultures have been obtained. Empirical antibiotic therapy should include vancomycin, gentamicin, and either cefepime or a carbapenem. Subsequent therapy should be adjusted based on culture results; if cultures remain negative, therapy as outlined for culture-negative PVE should be used. The length of therapy for PVE has not been studied, but experts agree that 6 weeks of therapy are needed.

STAPHYLOCOCCAL PVE

Antimicrobial treatment requires combination therapy. Major organizations (American Heart Association [AHA] and the European Society of Cardiology [ESC]) recommend a triple-drug regimen.

Nafcillin (or oxacillin) is the mainstay of therapy for isolates susceptible to methicillin (MSSA). If the organism is susceptible to gentamicin, this should be the second agent, with rifampin as the third agent. The aminoglycoside should be administered for the initial 2 weeks of treatment, and the remaining 2 agents continued for at least 4 additional weeks. If a fluoroquinolone is used in lieu of an aminoglycoside, the 3-drug regimen should continue for the course of treatment. When the isolate is resistant to all aminoglycosides and fluoroquinolones, linezolid, ceftaroline, or trimethoprim-sulfamethoxazole could be considered as a third drug for the initial 2 weeks of therapy.[60,61]

If breakthrough bacteremia or microbiologic failure occurs in patients receiving vancomycin, the isolate recovered should be tested for the development of both vancomycin and daptomycin resistance.

Optimal therapy for PVE caused by MRSA with reduced vancomycin susceptibility, or when failing vancomycin therapy, has not been established. High-dose daptomycin (if the isolate remains daptomycin susceptible), telavancin, ceftaroline, and linezolid is often used, although clinical experience in the treatment of PVE is limited.

Rifampin has the unique ability to kill staphylococci that are adherent to foreign material, and therefore is an essential component of the treatment of staphylococcal PVE. However, resistance to rifampin may develop during therapy, and toxicity may be significant. Susceptibility to rifampin should be reassessed when regimens containing rifampin fail.[62]

STREPTOCOCCAL PVE

Combination therapy with a β-lactam antibiotic and an aminoglycoside (if the isolate does not show high-level resistance to the aminoglycoside) is the preferred regimen for streptococcal PVE. Treatment is as delineated for native valve IE.

ENTEROCOCCI

Treatment of enterococcal PVE requires the synergistic interaction of a cell wall active agent (penicillin, ampicillin, or vancomycin) and an aminoglycoside in order to achieve a synergistic effect. The organisms should be tested for high-level aminoglycoside resistance. Cephalosporins are not active against enterococci and do not provide bactericidal synergy when combined with an aminoglycoside. If the enterococcus isolate has high-level resistance to streptomycin and gentamicin, synergy is not feasible, and an aminoglycoside should not be administered. In these cases, a prolonged course of 8 to 12 weeks of β-lactam or vancomycin should be administered instead, but few cases are clinically successful. In such cases, the combination of ampicillin (2 g every 4 hours) and ceftriaxone (2 g every 12 hours) for 6 weeks yielded acceptable clinical results in nonprosthetic valve infections with these organisms.[63] In the setting of progressive nephrotoxicity, the duration of aminoglycoside administration may be reduced to less than 6 weeks with no decrease in cure rates.[64]

In PVE caused by vancomycin-resistant *E faecium* (VRE), organisms that are often also resistant to penicillin and ampicillin, and highly resistant to gentamicin and streptomycin, treatment options are few. The reader is referred to the article on VRE elsewhere in this supplement. Surgical intervention during suppressive bacteriostatic therapy should be strongly considered when PVE is caused by highly resistant enterococci.

HACEK

See earlier discussion in the natural valve endocarditis section.

CORYNEBACTERIA (DIPHTHEROIDS)

If the strain is susceptible to gentamicin (MIC <4.0 μg/mL), penicillin plus gentamicin result in synergistic bactericidal activity and are the recommended therapy. Gentamicin resistance precludes bactericidal synergy.[65] Vancomycin is bactericidal against diphtheroids and is recommended for therapy when strains are resistant to gentamicin or in the context of allergic to penicillin.

GRAM-NEGATIVE BACILLI

Where possible, a synergistic bactericidal regimen should be used. Surgery to excise the infected valve is often required in gram-negative bacillary endocarditis, especially that caused by *Pseudomonas aeruginosa* or when infection involves the left-sided heart valves.

FUNGI

A combined approach that uses both antifungal agents and valve replacement is commonly used. Amphotericin B (daily doses ranging from 0.7 to 1.0 mg/kg per day or higher doses for mycelial fungi) is the antimicrobial of choice for treatment of fungal PVE; the greatest clinical experience in treating fungal PVE is with this agent.[66,67] Liposomal amphotericin B has not been assessed in fungal PVE. This treatment should be followed by suppressive second-phase oral therapy with fluconazole (200–400 mg daily or another triazole) for prolonged periods or indefinitely. Successful treatment of *Candida* PVE without surgery has been reported in a few case reports using a combination regimen of fluconazole and caspofungin or fluconazole and amphotericin B.[68,69]

CULTURE-NEGATIVE

With onset within the first year after valve surgery, therapy should include vancomycin, gentamicin, cefepime, and rifampin.[49] For initial therapy for PVE with onset greater than 1 year after surgery, the recommended treatment is with ampicillin-sulbactam plus gentamicin or vancomycin, gentamicin, and ciprofloxacin.[1,49,50] For patients with onset of PVE more than 12 months after valve implantation in whom *Bartonella* is suspected, treatment with ceftriaxone, gentamicin, and doxycycline should be administered.[49] If unexplained fever persists in the face of empirical therapy, surgery to obtain a vegetation for microbiological evaluation should be considered (for *Coxiella*, *Bartonella*, *Trephomyra*, and so forth).

INDICATIONS AND APPROACH TO THE SURGICAL MANAGEMENT OF IE

Surgical management of IE is challenging for the entire multidisciplinary team. One of the most important considerations in management of IE relates to the indications for and timing of surgical intervention. The primary indications for surgical intervention during antibiotic treatment of endocarditis (considered the active phase) relate to prevention of deterioration as a result of worsening CHF, systemic embolism, or uncontrolled infection. The principles of surgical therapy involve the widespread debridement of infected tissues with subsequent reconstruction and valve replacement. Choice of prosthesis and the possibility of repair need to be planned, and in the cases of significant destruction, complex reconstruction may be required.

Indications for Surgical Intervention

The latest comprehensive guidelines addressing surgical intervention come from the American College of Cardiology (ACC)/AHA and the ESC.[70,71] The indications in these documents are classified as I, II (a or b), and III according to the well-accepted system of assessing relative usefulness (of the intervention) from supportive literature.

The guidelines are reasonably matched in their assessment of class I indications for surgical intervention in IE (**Table 2**). The ESC guidelines are more explicit in their breakdown of the recommendations into 3 categories of consideration, which include heart failure, uncontrolled infection, and prevention of embolism. Furthermore, the ESC guidelines assign a relative urgency to the indications, which include emergent (surgery within 24 hours), urgent (surgery within a few days), and elective (surgery after 1 to 2 weeks of antibiotic therapy). The ACC/AHA guidelines do not address timing.

Multiple publications have shown that CHF is the most important predictor of mortality both in-hospital and at 6 months.[7,24,49,72-74] Higher levels of brain natriuretic peptide and troponin have been correlated with mortality as well.[75] The presence of heart failure is a class I indication in both sets of guidelines. The ESC suggests that refractory pulmonary edema or shock constitute emergencies in terms of timing. Furthermore, the ESC guidelines consider severe valve dysfunction without heart failure to be a IIa indication for surgery. This subject is not mentioned in the ACC/AHA guidelines. There is reasonable evidence to suggest that surgical intervention carries a better prognosis for patients with CHF in IE compared with nonsurgical management, and it is the most common indication for surgical intervention, occurring 60% to 70% of the time.[74,76-80]

Periannular extension of IE can lead to many complications involving the destruction of surrounding tissues, including abscess formation, pseudoaneurysms, fistulae, and heart block.[81-83] Periannular extension and fistulas are more common in PVE than in native valve IE, and in the aortic valve compared with the mitral.[49,83-85] Mortality for patients with periannular extension is high at 40%, even with surgery.[84,86] Both sets

---

Table 2
Indications for surgical intervention in IE according to the latest ESC and ACC/AHA guidelines

Indication for Surgical Intervention	Guidelines ACC/AHA	ESC	Timing (ESC Only)
Heart failure indications			
Refractory pulmonary edema or cardiogenic shock as a result of aortic or mitral IE causing severe acute valve regurgitation, valve obstruction, or fistula into a cardiac chamber	X	X	Emergency
Persisting heart failure or echocardiographic signs of poor hemodynamic tolerance as a result of aortic or mitral IE, causing severe acute regurgitation or valve obstruction	X	X	Urgent
Uncontrolled infection			
IE complicated by heart block, annular, or aortic abscess or destructive penetrating lesions (eg, fistula, false aneurysm)[a]	X	X	Urgent
IE with persisting fever and positive blood cultures >7–10 d		X	Urgent
IE caused by fungi or multiresistant organisms	X	X	Urgent/elective
Prevention of embolism			
Aortic or mitral IE with large vegetations (>10 mm) after ≥1 embolic episodes despite appropriate antibiotic therapy[b]		X	Urgent

[a] Heart block not specified by ESC guidelines.
[b] Class IIa recommendation in ACC/AHA guidelines.
 Data from Bonow RO, Carabello BA, Chatterjee K, et al. 2008 focused update incorporated into the ACC/AHA 2006 guidelines for the management of patients with valvular heart disease: a report of the American College of Cardiology/American Heart Association Task Force on Practice Guidelines (Writing Committee to Revise the 1998 Guidelines for the Management of Patients With Valvular Heart Disease): endorsed by the Society of Cardiovascular Anesthesiologists, Society for Cardiovascular Angiography and Interventions, and Society of Thoracic Surgeons. Circulation 2008;118(15):e596; and Vahanian A, Alfieri O, Andreotti F, et al. Guidelines on the management of valvular heart disease (version 2012): the Joint Task Force on the Management of Valvular Heart Disease of the European Society of Cardiology (ESC) and the European Association for Cardio-Thoracic Surgery (EACTS). Eur J Cardiothorac Surg 2012;42(4):S1–44.

of guidelines list uncontrolled infection by way of annular abscess, destructive, or penetrating lesions as class I indications for surgical intervention; however, the ESC guidelines address persistent fever and positive blood cultures (>7–10 days) in this category as well. Recently, an association between persistently positive blood cultures at 48 to 72 hours and poorer survival has been observed.[87] In such patients, it is reasonable to diagnose and treat extracardiac infection (eg. septic joint, indwelling lines) in case the persistent sepsis is on this basis; however, if vegetations are increasing in size, heart block develops, or new abscesses or other periannular abnormalities develop, the source of the ongoing sepsis is likely uncontrolled intracardiac infection.[1,88] TEE has been shown to be the best imaging modality for detection of these locally destructive complications of IE, especially when compared with TTE; however, TEE is still not 100% sensitive for detection of abscesses, particularly of the mitral valve.[85,89–92]

Fungal or multiresistant organisms are considered to be class I indications for intervention. An analysis of 270 cases of fungal endocarditis over 30 years showed a mortality of 72%.[93] Improved survival rates are associated with combined surgical-antifungal treatment. Thus surgical intervention is a standard in management of fungal IE.[94,95] Multidrug-resistant organisms such as MRSA and VRE require surgical intervention because of the inadequacy of antimicrobial treatment.[1,88] SA infections are virulent, destructive, and associated with mortality of 30% to 40% and therefore should be considered for early surgical intervention.[77,96–98]

Risk, outcome, and prevention of embolism is a subject of great importance, likely as a result of the greater level of equipoise of how and when to intervene for this indication when compared with CHF and periannular destruction. Embolic events occur in 22% to 50% of cases of IE, most commonly affect the CNS, and are associated with increased mortality.[22,25,72,99–103] The most consistent and powerful predictor of risk of embolism is the size of vegetation, which, when greater than 10 mm in diameter, are associated with higher rates of embolism.[72,91,104–107] One study further stratifies a higher incidence of embolism in 83% of patients with highly mobile vegetations of greater than 15 mm compared with 60% in patients with vegetations greater than 10 mm.[99] Other predictors of embolism include mitral location, enlarging vegetations despite antibiotics and SA or *Streptococcus gallolyticus* organism.[22,72,91,102,105,108,109] In particular, the risk decreases markedly from the first week to after the second week.[22,72] This situation was best identified by the ICE-PCS multicenter study analyzing 1437 consecutive patients with left-sided endocarditis, which showed that the incidence of embolism on appropriate antibiotics dropped from 4.82 per 1000 patient days in the first week to 1.71 per 1000 days in the second week and continued to decrease after that.[29] The ESC guidelines clearly categorize the presence of vegetations larger than 10 mm in the setting of 1 or more embolic episodes despite antibiotic therapy as a class I indication for surgery, whereas this is classified as class IIa in the ACC/AHA guidelines. Both sets consider large vegetations without clinical embolism to constitute a class IIb indication (the ESC use 15 mm, whereas the ACC/AHA use 10 mm). This situation has remained as a class IIb recommendation because of studies such as ICE and others, which have shown that antimicrobial therapy is an important mainstay in prevention of embolism. One can best conclude that surgery for prevention of embolism is likely to be most effective early in high-risk cases, as further discussed in the following section on timing.

Timing of Surgical Intervention

As surgery became an important tool in the treatment of endocarditis, multiple observational series were published that reported that patients who were operated on in an earlier time frame had better outcomes; these reports are subject to the biases inherent in analyses of retrospective cohorts.[77,110–112] Statistical methods including propensity matching and correction for all biases have been used to help answer the question.[43,76,78,113–118] These methods have been reviewed in 2 recent publications (**Table 3**); the impact of (early) surgery was positive in 5 studies and not beneficial in the other 4.[119,120] Both reviews conclude, based on analysis performed in the last 3 propensity studies, that the conflicting results of the earlier studies are most likely a result of differences in statistical methods and failure to account for all the biases. The largest and most recent of these studies is a multicenter analysis of 1238 patients in the propensity-matched model, with maximum accounting for selection, treatment, survivorship, and hidden biases, which found that early surgery conferred an in-hospital mortality benefit (absolute risk reduction 10.9%).[113] Benefits were most pronounced in the patients with the highest propensity for systemic embolization, SA infection, and stroke and seem to be derived mostly from patients in whom there is less controversy about the need for urgent surgery. Therefore, although the notion

Table 3
Review of studies examining the impact of early surgery on the prognosis of IE

Reference	Inclusion Period	Population	Number of Patients	Proportion Operated (%)	Outcome Measured	Bias Adjusted for	Effect of Surgery on Mortality (Propensity + Multivariable Analysis)
Vikram et al,[81] 2003	1990–1999	Complicated, left-sided NVE	513; 218 propensity-matched	45	6-mo all-cause mortality	Treatment selection bias	HR 0.40; 95% CI 0.18–0.91; P = .03
Mourvillier et al,[42] 2004	1993–1999	NVE or PVE hospitalized in an ICU	228 NVE; 54 propensity-matched	46	In-hospital mortality	Treatment selection bias	OR 0.47; 95% CI 0.22–1.00; P = .05
Cabell et al,[119] 2005	1985–1999	NVE	1516; 1497 in the propensity groups	40	In-hospital mortality	Treatment selection bias	Group 1 (lowest likelihood for surgery): medical therapy, 9.5%; surgical therapy, 20.0%; P = .16 Group 5 (strongest likelihood for surgery): medical therapy, 38.0%; surgical therapy, 11.2%; P<.001
Wang et al,[120] 2005	1985–1999	PVE	355; 136 propensity-matched	42	In-hospital mortality	Treatment selection bias	OR 0.56; 95% CI 0.23–1.36; P = .20
Aksoy et al,[83] 2007	1996–2002	Left-sided NVE or PVE without intracardiac device	333; 102 propensity-matched	23	5-y all-cause mortality	Treatment selection bias	HR 0.27; 95% CI 0.13–0.55; P = ?

Tleyjeh et al,[118] 2007	1980–1998	Left-sided NVE or PVE	546; 186 propensity-matched	24	6-mo all-cause mortality	Treatment selection bias; survivor bias	Matched cohort: HR 1.3; 95% CI 0.5–3.1; P = .56 Whole cohort, surgery as a time-dependent covariate: HR 1.9; 95% CI 1.1–3.2; P = .02 After adjustment for early (operative) mortality: HR 0.9; 95% CI 0.5–1.8; P = ?
Bannay et al,[117] 2011	1999	Left-sided NVE or PVE	449	53	5-y all-cause mortality	Treatment selection bias; survivor bias	Within 14 d after intervention, mortality was higher in the surgery group: adjusted HR 3.69; 95% CI 2.17–6.25; P<.0001 Thereafter, it was lower in the surgery group: adjusted HR 0.55; 95% CI 0.35–0.87; P = .01
Sy et al,[116] 2009	1996–2006	Left-sided NVE or PVE	223	28	5.2-y all-cause mortality	Treatment selection bias; survivor bias	After adjustment for baseline differences in propensity for surgery and risk of mortality: HR 0.50; 95% CI 0.28–0.88; P = .02 After time-dependent analysis: HR 0.77; 95% CI 0.42–1.40; P = .39
Lalani et al,[115] 2010	2000–2005	NVE	1552; 1238 in the propensity groups	46	In-hospital mortality	Treatment selection bias; survivor bias; hidden bias	ARR −11.2%; OR 0.44; 95% CI 0.33–0.59; P<.001

Abbreviations: ?, not available; ARR, absolute risk reduction; CI, confidence interval; HR, hazard ratio.
Data from Refs.[42,76,78,113–118], and *Adapted from* Delahaye F. Is early surgery beneficial in infective endocarditis? A systematic review. Arch Cardiovasc Dis 2011;104(1):37, with permission.

of early surgery for endocarditis is supported by these analyses, their statistical accounting does not generate data as robust as would be seen from a randomized controlled trial.

In 2012, Kang and colleagues[49] published 'Early surgery versus conventional treatment for infective endocarditis', a randomized controlled trial in which patients with left-sided endocarditis, severe valve disease, and large vegetations (>10 mm) either underwent urgent early surgery (within 48 hours, 37 patients) or conventional treatment (39 patients). The primary end point was a composite of in-hospital death and embolic events occurring within 6 weeks of randomization. The major finding of the study was an arrival at the end point in 23% of the conventional patients versus in only 3% of the early surgery group. There was no difference in death, and the major finding was driven by clinical embolic events. The investigators are careful not to use their findings as justification for a recommendation for early surgery in the broader population. This caveat is fair considering that the study was small, not blinded, did not use systematic imaging in both groups (relying only clinical determination), did not provide long-term disability or quality-of-life data, and 77% of patients in the control group required surgical intervention for complications of endocarditis or ongoing symptoms. This last point suggests that, although the population fits a IIa or IIb recommendation by the guidelines, they were a sick population, in whom some centers would already be inclined to intervene.[1,70] Decisions regarding the approach to large vegetation size are confounded by the other important inclusion criterion; severe valvular dysfunction. The timing of surgery with respect to patients having recent cerebrovascular accidents (CVAs) is particularly challenging. Embolism on its own confers an indication for surgery (if secondary to embolic phenomena) and yet raises a concern for exacerbation or worsening of the neurologic status with surgery. In particular, the massive dose of heparin required during surgery creates a concern about hemorrhagic transformation of these lesions, but cardiac operations in general create opportunities for additional injury to the vulnerable brain.[49,121] Most groups would attempt to wait 4 weeks in the case of intracranial hemorrhage but ischemic events are less clear.[122] This situation is reflected in the literature: some groups have advocated for early surgery based on their case series, whereas other groups have suggested a waiting period of 2 to 4 weeks.[72,123–126] These studies are all limited by their small numbers and retrospective nature and do not always use a time-dependent analysis. For example, Thuny and colleagues reported a neurologic deterioration in only 6% of patients (total 63 patients) with symptomatic CVAs in whom the median time to surgery was 9 days, but the range is from 0 to 2146 days. No stratification per amount of delay is offered.[72] Angstwurm and colleagues[127] combined their own patients with other groups to create a population of 240 patients with embolic stroke preceding cardiac surgery. They concluded that the risk of deterioration is 20% to 50% with surgery in the first 2 weeks, but less than 10% after 14 days and less than 1% after 4 weeks; and is likely the basis for many groups' desire to wait 2 to 4 weeks before operating on these patients. Recently, the ICE investigators published the data from their prospective registry including 198 patients who underwent surgery after ischemic CVA related to IE.[128] They analyzed the patients according to early surgery (1–7 days after CVA, 58 patients) and late surgery (>7 days, 140 patients) and after adjusting for risk factors found no difference in mortality either in-hospital or at 1 year. Although this study benefits from organized prospective data collection, the investigators acknowledge that referral bias relating to their tertiary-care centers and lack of preoperative data with respect to anatomy and severity of neurologic injury weaken their conclusion that there is no survival benefit to delaying surgery in these patients. Furthermore, no postoperative neurologic or quality of life data are presented. It becomes difficult, therefore, to make definitive recommendations, and the chance of seeing a randomized trial in this particular subset of patients is low.

There is increasing evidence that early surgery is beneficial for patients with endocarditis. It is apparent that this complex population is difficult to characterize in 1 study and that performance of randomized controlled trials is difficult. The randomized study by Kang and colleagues[49] is enlightening and yet generates more questions about who benefits and how with early intervention. Nevertheless, the studies have continued to push the notion, and it is becoming clear that patients with true indications for surgical treatment of IE need to be dealt with expeditiously. This time frame is still not clear, but until more data are available, the recommendations by the ESC with respect to timing (see **Table 1**) seem to be reasonable. There are a multitude of factors surrounding these critically ill patients that require individualization of treatment, but the plan must account for the urgency required to deal with the disease, and arbitrary waiting no longer seems to be justified, except perhaps with respect to patients with preexisting embolic CVA in whom the risk of delay of 2 to 4 weeks has to be balanced against the risk of early surgery. In these patients, features suggestive of higher risk of recurrent embolism and other accepted class I indications for surgery should likely be dealt with as soon as possible and even before 2 weeks, especially in the context of silent or small neurologic events.

OPERATIVE PROCEDURES

Thorough valve exploration, aggressive debridement, reconstruction or replacement choice, and adequate antimicrobial coverage remain the fundamental principles that guide operations for IE.

Although beneficial, preoperative optimization of patients with IE cannot always be achieved.[127] Ongoing heart failure, sepsis, and metabolic derangements can make the intraoperative period challenging. Anesthetic and cardiopulmonary bypass (CPB) may lead to significant hypotension. Patients may require complex surgical reconstruction further prolonging their CPB time, which can make separation from the heart-lung machine difficult. As a result, these patients are often markedly, critically ill on return to the ICU. With respect to coronary angiography, published guidelines suggest it should be performed in men older than 40 years, postmenopausal women or patients with at least 1 risk factor for or a history of coronary disease except if large aortic vegetations are present. In cases of the latter, CT angiography is acceptable to screen for severe proximal disease.

When the infectious process is isolated to the aortic valve leaflets, complete excision of the leaflets with implantation of a prosthesis is the standard approach.[129] There is no good evidence to suggest that any particular artificial valve is superior with respect to reinfection in the setting of isolated valvular endocarditis.[130] The choice between mechanical versus bioprosthetic depends on patient preference, age, and suitability for lifelong anticoagulation. Depending on the extent of involvement, vegetectomy ± leaflet repair may also be feasible.[131] When repair is required, autologous pericardial patches are favored.

For mitral valve endocarditis, because of the anticoagulation issues associated with mechanical valves, and the poor durability of bioprosthetic valves, vegetectomy ± repair has been advocated as the initial approach if feasible.[132,133] Tricuspid valve endocarditis has been associated with IV drug use.[134] Depending on pulmonary pressures, extent of involvement and patient profile, surgery can be performed in a staged manner.[135,136] The first stage involves valve excision to allow passive blood flow from the heart to the lungs. After the infection has resolved and the patient rehabilitated, a second stage involving valve replacement can be performed months later. In scenarios in which the infectious process is limited, a less invasive approach with vegetectomy ± repair as seen with the mitral valve can also be performed.

If the infectious process involves the periannular regions such as a root abscess or fistula, radical resection of the involved tissues is crucial.[137,138] Depending on the degree of debridement required, either autologous pericardium for small defects or glutaraldehyde-fixed bovine pericardium for larger defects can be used for reconstruction.[139] If there is significant aortic root involvement, complete resection with implantation of a homograft to aid with the reconstruction of the left ventricular outflow tract is often used.[140,141] Each operation must be tailored to the patient and the extent of endocarditis.

POSTCARDIAC SURGERY
General Considerations

The first 12 to 24 hours after a cardiac surgical procedure is the usual time frame in which the postoperative patients with IE experience dynamic changes in cardiac rhythm and hemodynamics.[142,143] Identifying and correcting the cause of postoperative hypoperfusion are tantamount to preserving organ function. Typical causes of hypotension and hypoperfusion in the postoperative patient with IE include (but are not limited to) hypovolemia, bleeding, cardiac tamponade, arrhythmias, poor myocardial contractility, new myocardial ischemia, and tension pneumothorax. Similarly, excessive blood pressure may lead to bleeding and disruption of surgical anastamotic sites. The establishment of appropriate hemodynamic and transfusion goals through a team-based, formal handover from the operating room to the ICU teams may be of benefit in these complex surgical patients.[144–146]

Heart Rhythm

Injury to the conductive tissue may occur with extensive valve annulus debridement during surgical management of IE cases. Subsequent alterations in heart rate or conduction may contribute to hypotension or hypoperfusion.[143] Attainment of sinus rhythm, or sinuslike rhythm with the dual-chamber pacing using epicardial-pacing wires, placed in the operating room, is preferred to maintain the atrial contraction contribution to cardiac output.

Bleeding

Postoperative bleeding via mediastinal and pleural drains needs to be monitored and hemodynamically assessed because clinically important anemia may require further medical (ie, blood product transfusion) or surgical (ie, mediastinal reexploration) therapy. Postoperative coagulopathy may arise from a variety of potential mechanisms, such as hypothermia, sepsis, hemodilution, and the use of CPB. Recommendations on the appropriate blood product use for the postoperative cardiac surgery patient were provided in 2007 by a joint practice guideline from the Society of Thoracic Surgery and Society of Cardiovascular Anesthesiologists.[147–152]

SUMMARY

IE is a disease with many facets and various expressions, depending on the site of infection, microorganism, underlying heart lesion, immune status of the host, and remote effects such as emboli, organ dysfunction, and the general condition of the host. Diagnosis is the first crucial step, which depends on meticulous clinical examination, blood cultures results, and echocardiographic findings. The management of the patient with endocarditis in the ICU is complex and needs a multidisciplinary team, including the intensivist, a cardiologist, an experienced echocardiologist, an infectious diseases specialist, and a cardiac surgeon. The medical and surgical management of such patients is complex, and timely decisions are important.

REFERENCES

1. Habib G, Hoen B, Tornos P, et al. Guidelines on the prevention, diagnosis, and treatment of infective endocarditis (new version 2009): the Task Force on the Prevention, Diagnosis, and Treatment of Infective Endocarditis of the European Society of Cardiology (ESC). Endorsed by the European Society of Clinical Microbiology and Infectious Diseases (ESCMID) and the International Society of Chemotherapy (ISC) for Infection and Cancer. Eur Heart J 2009;30(19): 2369–413.
2. Bayer AS. Infective endocarditis. Clin Infect Dis 1993;17(3):313–20 [quiz: 321–2].
3. Berlin JA, Abrutyn E, Strom BL, et al. Incidence of infective endocarditis in the Delaware Valley, 1988–1990. Am J Cardiol 1995;76(12):933–6.
4. Delahaye F, Goulet V, Lacassin F, et al. Characteristics of infective endocarditis in France in 1991. A 1-year survey. Eur Heart J 1995;16(3):394–401.
5. Hill EE, Herijgers P, Claus P, et al. Infective endocarditis: changing epidemiology and predictors of 6-month mortality: a prospective cohort study. Eur Heart J 2007;28(2):196–203.
6. Kourany WM, Miro JM, Moreno A, et al. Influence of diabetes mellitus on the clinical manifestations and prognosis of infective endocarditis: a report from the International Collaboration on Endocarditis-Merged Database. Scand J Infect Dis 2006;38(8):613–9.
7. Miro JM, Anguera I, Cabell CH, et al. Staphylococcus aureus native valve infective endocarditis: report of 566 episodes from the International Collaboration on Endocarditis Merged Database. Clin Infect Dis 2005;41(4):507–14.
8. Fowler VG Jr, Miro JM, Hoen B, et al. Staphylococcus aureus endocarditis: a consequence of medical progress. J Am Med Assoc 2005;293(24):3012–21.
9. Duval X, Delahaye F, Alla F, et al. Temporal trends in infective endocarditis in the context of prophylaxis guideline modifications: three successive population-based surveys. J Am Coll Cardiol 2012;59(22):1968–76.
10. Selton-Suty C, Celard M, Le Moing V, et al. Preeminence of Staphylococcus aureus in infective endocarditis: a 1-year population-based survey. Clin Infect Dis 2012;54(9):1230–9.
11. Tleyjeh IM, Steckelberg JM, Murad HS, et al. Temporal trends in infective endocarditis: a population-based study in Olmsted County, Minnesota. J Am Med Assoc 2005;293(24):3022–8.
12. Correa de Sa DD, Tleyjeh IM, Anavekar NS, et al. Epidemiological trends of infective endocarditis: a population-based study in Olmsted County, Minnesota. Mayo Clin Proc 2010;85(5):422–6.
13. Gill SR, McIntyre LM, Nelson CL, et al. Potential associations between severity of infection and the presence of virulence-associated genes in clinical strains of Staphylococcus aureus. PLoS One 2011;6(4):e18673.
14. Murdoch DR, Corey GR, Hoen B, et al. Clinical presentation, etiology, and outcome of infective endocarditis in the 21st century: the International Collaboration on Endocarditis-Prospective Cohort Study. Arch Intern Med 2009;169(5): 463–73.

15. Kokoglu OF, Hosoglu S, Geyik MF, et al. Clinical and laboratory features of brucellosis in two university hospitals in Southeast Turkey. Trop Doct 2006; 36(1):49–51.

16. Erbay AR, Erbay A, Canga A, et al. Risk factors for in-hospital mortality in infective endocarditis: five years' experience at a tertiary care hospital in Turkey. J Heart Valve Dis 2010;19(2):216–24.

17. Chu VH, Woods CW, Miro JM, et al. Emergence of coagulase-negative staphylococci as a cause of native valve endocarditis. Clin Infect Dis 2008;46(2):232–42.

18. Liang M, Mansell C, Wade C, et al. Unusually virulent coagulase-negative *Staphylococcus lugdunensis* is frequently associated with infective endocarditis: a Waikato series of patients. N Z Med J 2012;125(1354):51–9.

19. Patel R, Piper KE, Rouse MS, et al. Frequency of isolation of *Staphylococcus lugdunensis* among staphylococcal isolates causing endocarditis: a 20-year experience. J Clin Microbiol 2000;38(11):4262–3.

20. Karth G, Koreny M, Binder T, et al. Complicated infective endocarditis necessitating ICU admission: clinical course and prognosis. Crit Care 2002;6(2):149–54.

21. Sonneville R, Mirabel M, Hajage D, et al. Neurologic complications and outcomes of infective endocarditis in critically ill patients: the ENDOcardite en RE-Animation prospective multicenter study. Crit Care Med 2011;39(6):1474–81.

22. Pankey GA. Subacute bacterial endocarditis at the University of Minnesota Hospital, 1939 through 1959. Ann Intern Med 1961;55:550–61.

23. Heiro M, Nikoskelainen J, Engblom E, et al. Neurologic manifestations of infective endocarditis: a 17-year experience in a teaching hospital in Finland. Arch Intern Med 2000;160(18):2781–7.

24. Hoen B, Alla F, Selton-Suty C, et al. Changing profile of infective endocarditis: results of a 1-year survey in France. J Am Med Assoc 2002;288(1):75–81.

25. Hasbun R, Vikram HR, Barakat LA, et al. Complicated left-sided native valve endocarditis in adults: risk classification for mortality. J Am Med Assoc 2003; 289(15):1933–40.

26. Thuny F, Avierinos JF, Tribouilloy C, et al. Impact of cerebrovascular complications on mortality and neurologic outcome during infective endocarditis: a prospective multicentre study. Eur Heart J 2007;28(9):1155–61.

27. Cooper HA, Thompson EC, Laureno R, et al. Subclinical brain embolization in left-sided infective endocarditis: results from the evaluation by MRI of the brains of patients with left-sided intracardiac solid masses (EMBOLISM) pilot study. Circulation 2009;120(7):585–91.

28. Lefort A, Lortholary O, Casassus P, et al. Comparison between adult endocarditis due to beta-hemolytic streptococci (serogroups A, B, C, and G) and *Streptococcus milleri*: a multicenter study in France. Arch Intern Med 2002;162(21): 2450–6.

29. Pierrotti LC, Baddour LM. Fungal endocarditis, 1995–2000. Chest 2002;122(1): 302–10.

30. Dickerman SA, Abrutyn E, Barsic B, et al. The relationship between the initiation of antimicrobial therapy and the incidence of stroke in infective endocarditis: an analysis from the ICE Prospective Cohort Study (ICE-PCS). Am Heart J 2007; 154(6):1086–94.

31. Anguera I, Miro JM, Evangelista A, et al. Periannular complications in infective endocarditis involving native aortic valves. Am J Cardiol 2006;98(9):1254–60.

32. Anguera I, Miro JM, Vilacosta I, et al. Aorto-cavitary fistulous tract formation in infective endocarditis: clinical and echocardiographic features of 76 cases and risk factors for mortality. Eur Heart J 2005;26(3):288–97.

33. Graupner C, Vilacosta I, SanRoman J, et al. Periannular extension of infective endocarditis. J Am Coll Cardiol 2002;39(7):1204–11.
34. American College of Cardiology Foundation Appropriate Use Criteria Task Force, American Society of Echocardiography, American Heart Association, et al. ACCF/ASE/AHA/ASNC/HFSA/HRS/SCAI/SCCM/SCCT/SCMR 2011 Appropriate Use Criteria for Echocardiography. A Report of the American College of Cardiology Foundation Appropriate Use Criteria Task Force, American Society of Echocardiography, American Heart Association, American Society of Nuclear Cardiology, Heart Failure Society of America, Heart Rhythm Society, Society for Cardiovascular Angiography and Interventions, Society of Critical Care Medicine, Society of Cardiovascular Computed Tomography, Society for Cardiovascular Magnetic Resonance American College of Chest Physicians. J Am Coll Cardiol 2011;24:229–67.
35. Habib G, Badano L, Tribouilloy C, et al. Recommendations for the practice of echocardiography in infective endocarditis. Eur J Echocardiogr 2010;11:202–19.
36. Greaves K, Mou D, Patel A, et al. Clinical criteria and the appropriate use of transthoracic echocardiography for the exclusion of infective endocarditis. Heart 2003;89(3):273–5.
37. Palraj BR, Sohail MR. Appropriate use of echocardiography in managing *Staphylococcus aureus* bacteremia. Expert Rev Anti Infect Ther 2012;10(4):501–8.
38. Reynolds HR, Jagen MA, Tunick PA, et al. Sensitivity of transthoracic versus transesophageal echocardiography for the detection of native valve vegetations in the modern era. J Am Soc Echocardiogr 2003;16(1):67–70.
39. Field LC, Guldan GJ, Finley AC. Echocardiography in the intensive care unit. Semin Cardiothorac Vasc Anesth 2011;15(1–2):25–39.
40. Shively BK, Gurule FT, Roldan CA, et al. Diagnostic value of transesophageal compared with transesophageal echocardiography in infective endocarditis. J Am Call Cardiol 1991;18:391–7.
41. Evangelista A, Gonzalez-Alujas MT. Echocardiography in infective endocarditis. Heart 2004;90(6):614–7.
42. Mourvillier B, Trouillet JL, Timsit JF, et al. Infective endocarditis in the intensive care unit: clinical spectrum and prognostic factors in 228 consecutive patients. Intensive Care Med 2004;30(11):2046–52.
43. Bellomo R, Uchino S. Cardiovascular monitoring tools: use and misuse. Curr Opin Crit Care 2003;9(3):225–9.
44. Karkouti K, Wijeysundera DN, Beattie SW. Pulmonary-artery catheters in high-risk surgical patients. N Engl J Med 2003;348(20):2035–7 [author reply: 2035–7].
45. Sandham JD, Hull RD, Brant RF, et al. A randomized, controlled trial of the use of pulmonary-artery catheters in high-risk surgical patients. N Engl J Med 2003; 348(1):5–14.
46. Dellinger RP, Levy MM, Carlet JM, et al. Surviving Sepsis Campaign: international guidelines for management of severe sepsis and septic shock: 2008. Crit Care Med 2008;36(1):296–327.
47. Rivers E, Nguyen B, Havstad S, et al. Early goal-directed therapy in the treatment of severe sepsis and septic shock. N Engl J Med 2001;345(19):1368–77.
48. Kumar A, Roberts D, Wood KE, et al. Duration of hypotension before initiation of effective antimicrobial therapy is the critical determinant of survival in human septic shock. Crit Care Med 2006;34(6):1589–96.
49. Kang DH, Kim YJ, Kim SH, et al. Early surgery versus conventional treatment for infective endocarditis. N Engl J Med 2012;366(26):2466–73.

50. Francioli P, Ruch W, Stamboulian D. Treatment of streptococcal endocarditis with a single daily dose of ceftriaxone and netilmicin for 14 days: a prospective multicenter study. Clin Infect Dis 1995;21(6):1406–10.

51. Chambers HF, Miller RT, Newman MD. Right-sided *Staphylococcus aureus* endocarditis in intravenous drug abusers: two-week combination therapy. Ann Intern Med 1988;109(8):619–24.

52. Baddour LM, Wilson WR, Bayer AS, et al. Infective endocarditis: diagnosis, antimicrobial therapy, and management of complications: a statement for healthcare professionals from the Committee on Rheumatic Fever, Endocarditis, and Kawasaki Disease, Council on Cardiovascular Disease in the Young, and the Councils on Clinical Cardiology, Stroke, and Cardiovascular Surgery and Anesthesia, American Heart Association: endorsed by the Infectious Diseases Society of America. Circulation 2005;111(23):e394–434.

53. Baddour LM. Infective endocarditis caused by beta-hemolytic streptococci. The Infectious Diseases Society of America's Emerging Infections Network. Clin Infect Dis 1998;26(1):66–71.

54. Lefort A, Mainardi JL, Selton-Suty C, et al. *Streptococcus pneumoniae* endocarditis in adults. A multicenter study in France in the era of penicillin resistance (1991-1998). The Pneumococcal Endocarditis Study Group. Medicine 2000; 79(5):327–37.

55. Korzeniowski O, Sande MA. Combination antimicrobial therapy for *Staphylococcus aureus* endocarditis in patients addicted to parenteral drugs and in nonaddicts: a prospective study. Ann Intern Med 1982;97(4):496–503.

56. Cosgrove SE, Vigliani GA, Fowler VG Jr, et al. Initial low-dose gentamicin for *Staphylococcus aureus* bacteremia and endocarditis is nephrotoxic. Clin Infect Dis 2009;48(6):713–21.

57. Levine DP, Fromm BS, Reddy BR. Slow response to vancomycin or vancomycin plus rifampin in methicillin-resistant *Staphylococcus aureus* endocarditis. Ann Intern Med 1991;115(9):674–80.

58. DiNubile MJ. Short-course antibiotic therapy for right-sided endocarditis caused by *Staphylococcus aureus* in injection drug users. Ann Intern Med 1994; 121(11):873–6.

59. Fowler VG Jr, Boucher HW, Corey GR, et al. Daptomycin versus standard therapy for bacteremia and endocarditis caused by *Staphylococcus aureus*. N Engl J Med 2006;355(7):653–65.

60. Batard E, Jacqueline C, Boutoille D, et al. Combination of quinupristin-dalfopristin and gentamicin against methicillin-resistant *Staphylococcus aureus*: experimental rabbit endocarditis study. Antimicrobial Agents Chemother 2002; 46(7):2174–8.

61. Dailey CF, Dileto-Fang CL, Buchanan LV, et al. Efficacy of linezolid in treatment of experimental endocarditis caused by methicillin-resistant *Staphylococcus aureus*. Antimicrobial Agents Chemother 2001;45(8):2304–8.

62. Nace H, Lorber B. Successful treatment of methicillin-resistant *Staphylococcus aureus* endocarditis with telavancin. J Antimicrob Chemother 2010;65(6):1315–6.

63. Rouse MS, Wilcox RM, Henry NK, et al. Ciprofloxacin therapy of experimental endocarditis caused by methicillin-resistant *Staphylococcus epidermidis*. Antimicrobial Agents Chemother 1990;34(2):273–6.

64. Souli M, Pontikis K, Chryssouli Z, et al. Successful treatment of right-sided prosthetic valve endocarditis due to methicillin-resistant teicoplanin-heteroresistant *Staphylococcus aureus* with linezolid. Eur J Clin Microbiol Infect Dis 2005; 24(11):760–2.

65. Karchmer AW, Longworth DL. Infections of intracardiac devices. Infect Dis Clin North Am 2002;16(2):477–505, xii.

66. Karchmer AW. Nosocomial bloodstream infections: organisms, risk factors, and implications. Clin Infect Dis 2000;31(Suppl 4):S139–43.

67. Karchmer AW, Longworth DL. Infections of intracardiac devices. Cardiology 2003;21(2):253–71, vii.

68. Gavalda J, Len O, Miro JM, et al. Brief communication: treatment of *Enterococcus faecalis* endocarditis with ampicillin plus ceftriaxone. Ann Intern Med 2007;146(8):574–9.

69. Olaison L, Schadewitz K. Enterococcal endocarditis in Sweden, 1995–1999: can shorter therapy with aminoglycosides be used? Clin Infect Dis 2002;34(2):159–66.

70. Murray BE, Karchmer AW, Moellering RC Jr. Diphtheroid prosthetic valve endocarditis. A study of clinical features and infecting organisms. Am J Med 1980; 69(6):838–48.

71. Rubinstein E, Noriega ER, Simberkoff MS, et al. Fungal endocarditis: analysis of 24 cases and review of the literature. Medicine 1975;54(4):331–4.

72. Pappas PG, Kauffman CA, Andes D, et al. Clinical practice guidelines for the management of candidiasis: 2009 update by the Infectious Diseases Society of America. Clin Infect Dis 2009;48(5):503–35.

73. Lye DC, Hughes A, O'Brien D, et al. *Candida glabrata* prosthetic valve endocarditis treated successfully with fluconazole plus caspofungin without surgery: a case report and literature review. Eur J Clin Microbiol Infect Dis 2005;24(11):753–5.

74. Aaron L, Therby A, Viard JP, et al. Successful medical treatment of *Candida albicans* in mechanical prosthetic valve endocarditis. Scand J Infect Dis 2003; 35(5):351–2.

75. Bonow RO, Carabello BA, Chatterjee K, et al. 2008 focused update incorporated into the ACC/AHA 2006 guidelines for the management of patients with valvular heart disease: a report of the American College of Cardiology/American Heart Association Task Force on Practice Guidelines (Writing Committee to Revise the 1998 Guidelines for the Management of Patients With Valvular Heart Disease): endorsed by the Society of Cardiovascular Anesthesiologists, Society for Cardiovascular Angiography and Interventions, and Society of Thoracic Surgeons. Circulation 2008;118(15):e523–661.

76. Vahanian A, Alfieri O, Andreotti F, et al. Guidelines on the management of valvular heart disease (version 2012): the Joint Task Force on the Management of Valvular Heart Disease of the European Society of Cardiology (ESC) and the European Association for Cardio-Thoracic Surgery (EACTS). G Ital Cardiol (Rome) 2013;14(3):167–214.

77. Thuny F, Di Salvo G, Belliard O, et al. Risk of embolism and death in infective endocarditis: prognostic value of echocardiography: a prospective multicenter study. Circulation 2005;112(1):69–75.

78. Bouza E, Menasalvas A, Munoz P, et al. Infective endocarditis–a prospective study at the end of the twentieth century: new predisposing conditions, new etiologic agents, and still a high mortality. Medicine (Baltimore) 2001;80(5): 298–307.

79. Kiefer T, Park L, Tribouilloy C, et al. Association between valvular surgery and mortality among patients with infective endocarditis complicated by heart failure. J Am Med Assoc 2011;306(20):2239–47.

80. Shiue AB, Stancoven AB, Purcell JB, et al. Relation of level of B-type natriuretic peptide with outcomes in patients with infective endocarditis. Am J Cardiol 2010;106(7):1011–5.

81. Vikram HR, Buenconsejo J, Hasbun R, et al. Impact of valve surgery on 6-month mortality in adults with complicated, left-sided native valve endocarditis: a propensity analysis. J Am Med Assoc 2003;290(24):3207–14.

82. Remadi JP, Habib G, Nadji G, et al. Predictors of death and impact of surgery in *Staphylococcus aureus* infective endocarditis. Ann Thorac Surg 2007;83(4): 1295–302.

83. Aksoy O, Sexton DJ, Wang A, et al. Early surgery in patients with infective endocarditis: a propensity score analysis. Clin Infect Dis 2007;44(3):364–72.

84. Tornos P, Iung B, Permanyer-Miralda G, et al. Infective endocarditis in Europe: lessons from the Euro heart survey. Heart 2005;91(5):571–5.

85. Revilla A, Lopez J, Vilacosta I, et al. Clinical and prognostic profile of patients with infective endocarditis who need urgent surgery. Eur Heart J 2007;28(1):65–71.

86. Seo MS, Fukamizu A, Nomura T, et al. The human renin gene in transgenic mice. J Cardiovasc Pharmacol 1990;16(Suppl 4):S8–10.

87. Leung DY, Cranney GB, Hopkins AP, et al. Role of transoesophageal echocardiography in the diagnosis and management of aortic root abscess. Br Heart J 1994;72(2):175–81.

88. David TE, Regesta T, Gavra G, et al. Surgical treatment of paravalvular abscess: long-term results. Eur J Cardiothorac Surg 2007;31(1):43–8.

89. Lopez J, Sevilla T, Vilacosta I, et al. Prognostic role of persistent positive blood cultures after initiation of antibiotic therapy in left-sided infective endocarditis. Eur Heart J 2013;34(23):1749–54.

90. Prendergast BD, Tornos P. Surgery for infective endocarditis: who and when? Circulation 2010;121(9):1141–52.

91. Lengyel M. The impact of transesophageal echocardiography on the management of prosthetic valve endocarditis: experience of 31 cases and review of the literature. J Heart Valve Dis 1997;6(2):204–11.

92. Karalis DG, Bansal RC, Hauck AJ, et al. Transesophageal echocardiographic recognition of subaortic complications in aortic valve endocarditis. Clinical and surgical implications. Circulation 1992;86(2):353–62.

93. Mugge A, Daniel WG, Frank G, et al. Echocardiography in infective endocarditis: reassessment of prognostic implications of vegetation size determined by the transthoracic and the transesophageal approach. J Am Coll Cardiol 1989; 14(3):631–8.

94. Hill EE, Herijgers P, Claus P, et al. Abscess in infective endocarditis: the value of transesophageal echocardiography and outcome: a 5-year study. Am Heart J 2007;154(5):923–8.

95. Ellis ME, Al-Abdely H, Sandridge A, et al. Fungal endocarditis: evidence in the world literature, 1965–1995. Clin Infect Dis 2001;32(1):50–62.

96. Nguyen MH, Nguyen ML, Yu VL, et al. *Candida* prosthetic valve endocarditis: prospective study of six cases and review of the literature. Clin Infect Dis 1996;22(2):262–7.

97. Garzoni C, Nobre VA, Garbino J. *Candida parapsilosis* endocarditis: a comparative review of the literature. Eur J Clin Microbiol Infect Dis 2007; 26(12):915–26.

98. San Roman JA, Lopez J, Vilacosta I, et al. Prognostic stratification of patients with left-sided endocarditis determined at admission. Am J Med 2007;120(4): 369.e1–7.

99. Yoshinaga M, Niwa K, Niwa A, et al. Risk factors for in-hospital mortality during infective endocarditis in patients with congenital heart disease. Am J Cardiol 2008;101(1):114–8.

100. Bishara J, Leibovici L, Gartman-Israel D, et al. Long-term outcome of infective endocarditis: the impact of early surgical intervention. Clin Infect Dis 2001; 33(10):1636–43.
101. Di Salvo G, Habib G, Pergola V, et al. Echocardiography predicts embolic events in infective endocarditis. J Am Coll Cardiol 2001;37(4):1069–76.
102. De Castro S, Magni G, Beni S, et al. Role of transthoracic and transesophageal echocardiography in predicting embolic events in patients with active infective endocarditis involving native cardiac valves. Am J Cardiol 1997; 80(8):1030–4.
103. Heinle S, Wilderman N, Harrison JK, et al. Value of transthoracic echocardiography in predicting embolic events in active infective endocarditis. Duke Endocarditis Service. Am J Cardiol 1994;74(8):799–801.
104. Vilacosta I, Graupner C, San Roman JA, et al. Risk of embolization after institution of antibiotic therapy for infective endocarditis. J Am Coll Cardiol 2002;39(9): 1489–95.
105. Rohmann S, Erbel R, Gorge G, et al. Clinical relevance of vegetation localization by transoesophageal echocardiography in infective endocarditis. Eur Heart J 1992;13(4):446–52.
106. Durante Mangoni E, Adinolfi LE, Tripodi MF, et al. Risk factors for "major" embolic events in hospitalized patients with infective endocarditis. Am Heart J 2003;146(2):311–6.
107. Cabell CH, Pond KK, Peterson GE, et al. The risk of stroke and death in patients with aortic and mitral valve endocarditis. Am Heart J 2001;142(1):75–80.
108. Tischler MD, Vaitkus PT. The ability of vegetation size on echocardiography to predict clinical complications: a meta-analysis. J Am Soc Echocardiogr 1997; 10(5):562–8.
109. Sanfilippo AJ, Picard MH, Newell JB, et al. Echocardiographic assessment of patients with infectious endocarditis: prediction of risk for complications. J Am Coll Cardiol 1991;18(5):1191–9.
110. Pergola V, Di Salvo G, Habib G, et al. Comparison of clinical and echocardiographic characteristics of Streptococcus bovis endocarditis with that caused by other pathogens. Am J Cardiol 2001;88(8):871–5.
111. Rohmann S, Erbel R, Darius H, et al. Prediction of rapid versus prolonged healing of infective endocarditis by monitoring vegetation size. J Am Soc Echocardiogr 1991;4(5):465–74.
112. Thuny F, Beurtheret S, Mancini J, et al. The timing of surgery influences mortality and morbidity in adults with severe complicated infective endocarditis: a propensity analysis. Eur Heart J 2011;32(16):2027–33.
113. Castillo JC, Anguita MP, Ramirez A, et al. Long term outcome of infective endocarditis in patients who were not drug addicts: a 10 year study. Heart 2000; 83(5):525–30.
114. Bogers AJ, van Vreeswijk H, Verbaan CJ, et al. Early surgery for active infective endocarditis improves early and late results. Thorac Cardiovasc Surg 1991; 39(5):284–8.
115. Lalani T, Cabell CH, Benjamin DK, et al. Analysis of the impact of early surgery on in-hospital mortality of native valve endocarditis: use of propensity score and instrumental variable methods to adjust for treatment-selection bias. Circulation 2010;121(8):1005–13.
116. Sy RW, Bannon PG, Bayfield MS, et al. Survivor treatment selection bias and outcomes research: a case study of surgery in infective endocarditis. Circ Cardiovasc Qual Outcomes 2009;2(5):469–74.

117. Bannay A, Hoen B, Duval X, et al. The impact of valve surgery on short- and long-term mortality in left-sided infective endocarditis: do differences in methodological approaches explain previous conflicting results? Eur Heart J 2011; 32(16):2003–15.

118. Tleyjeh IM, Ghomrawi HM, Steckelberg JM, et al. The impact of valve surgery on 6-month mortality in left-sided infective endocarditis. Circulation 2007;115(13): 1721–8.

119. Cabell CH, Abrutyn E, Fowler VG Jr, et al. Use of surgery in patients with native valve infective endocarditis: results from the International Collaboration on Endocarditis Merged Database. Am Heart J 2005;150(5):1092–8.

120. Wang A, Pappas P, Anstrom KJ, et al. The use and effect of surgical therapy for prosthetic valve infective endocarditis: a propensity analysis of a multicenter, international cohort. Am Heart J 2005;150(5):1086–91.

121. Delahaye F. Is early surgery beneficial in infective endocarditis? A systematic review. Arch Cardiovasc Dis 2011;104(1):35–44.

122. Hedberg M, Engstrom KG. Stroke after cardiac surgery–hemispheric distribution and survival. Scand Cardiovasc J 2013;47(3):136–44.

123. Wolman RL, Nussmeier NA, Aggarwal A, et al. Cerebral injury after cardiac surgery: identification of a group at extraordinary risk. Multicenter Study of Perioperative Ischemia Research Group (McSPI) and the Ischemia Research Education Foundation (IREF) Investigators. Stroke 1999;30(3):514–22.

124. Derex L, Bonnefoy E, Delahaye F. Impact of stroke on therapeutic decision making in infective endocarditis. J Neurol 2010;257(3):315–21.

125. Ruttmann E, Willeit J, Ulmer H, et al. Neurological outcome of septic cardioembolic stroke after infective endocarditis. Stroke 2006;37(8):2094–9.

126. Piper C, Wiemer M, Schulte HD, et al. Stroke is not a contraindication for urgent valve replacement in acute infective endocarditis. J Heart Valve Dis 2001;10(6): 703–11.

127. Angstwurm K, Borges AC, Halle E, et al. Timing the valve replacement in infective endocarditis involving the brain. J Neurol 2004;251(10):1220–6.

128. Eishi K, Kawazoe K, Kuriyama Y, et al. Surgical management of infective endocarditis associated with cerebral complications. Multi-center retrospective study in Japan. J Thorac Cardiovasc Surg 1995;110(6):1745–55.

129. Barsic B, Dickerman S, Krajinovic V, et al. Influence of the timing of cardiac surgery on the outcome of patients with infective endocarditis and stroke. Clin Infect Dis 2013;56(2):209–17.

130. Landoni G, Rodseth RN, Santini F, et al. Randomized evidence for reduction of perioperative mortality. J Cardiothorac Vasc Anesth 2012;26(5):764–72.

131. Nishimura RA, Carabello BA, Faxon DP, et al. ACC/AHA 2008 guideline update on valvular heart disease: focused update on infective endocarditis: a report of the American College of Cardiology/American Heart Association Task Force on Practice Guidelines: endorsed by the Society of Cardiovascular Anesthesiologists, Society for Cardiovascular Angiography and Interventions, and Society of Thoracic Surgeons. Circulation 2008;118(8):887–96.

132. Shapiro SM, Young E, De Guzman S, et al. Transesophageal echocardiography in diagnosis of infective endocarditis. Chest 1994;105(2):377–82.

133. Moon MR, Miller DC, Moore KA, et al. Treatment of endocarditis with valve replacement: the question of tissue versus mechanical prosthesis. Ann Thorac Surg 2001;71(4):1164–71.

134. Newton S, Hunter S. What type of valve replacement should be used in patients with endocarditis? Interact Cardiovasc Thorac Surg 2010;11(6):784–8.

135. Mayer K, Aicher D, Feldner S, et al. Repair versus replacement of the aortic valve in active infective endocarditis. Eur J Cardiothorac Surg 2012;42(1):122–7.
136. Feringa HH, Shaw LJ, Poldermans D, et al. Mitral valve repair and replacement in endocarditis: a systematic review of literature. Ann Thorac Surg 2007;83(2):564–70.
137. Ruttmann E, Legit C, Poelzl G, et al. Mitral valve repair provides improved outcome over replacement in active infective endocarditis. J Thorac Cardiovasc Surg 2005;130(3):765–71.
138. Demin AA, Drobysheva VP, Vel'ter O. Infectious endocarditis in intravenous drug abusers. Klin Med (Mosk) 2000;78(8):47–51 [in Russian].
139. Arneborn P, Bjork VO, Rodriguez L, et al. Two-stage replacement of tricuspid valve in active endocarditis. Br Heart J 1977;39(11):1276–8.
140. Wright JS, Glennie JS. Excision of tricuspid valve with later replacement in endocarditis of drug addiction. Thorax 1978;33(4):518–9.
141. Hwang HY, Kim KH, Kim KB, et al. Mechanical tricuspid valve replacement is not superior in patients younger than 65 years who need long-term anticoagulation. Ann Thorac Surg 2012;93(4):1154–60.
142. Spiliopoulos K, Haschemi A, Fink G, et al. Infective endocarditis complicated by paravalvular abscess: a surgical challenge. An 11-year single center experience. Heart Surg Forum 2010;13(2):E67–73.
143. d'Udekem Y, David TE, Feindel CM, et al. Long-term results of surgery for active infective endocarditis. Eur J Cardiothorac Surg 1997;11(1):46–52.
144. d'Udekem Y, David TE, Feindel CM, et al. Long-term results of operation for paravalvular abscess. Ann Thorac Surg 1996;62(1):48–53.
145. Glazier JJ, Verwilghen J, Donaldson RM, et al. Treatment of complicated prosthetic aortic valve endocarditis with annular abscess formation by homograft aortic root replacement. J Am Coll Cardiol 1991;17(5):1177–82.
146. Musci M, Weng Y, Hubler M, et al. Homograft aortic root replacement in native or prosthetic active infective endocarditis: twenty-year single-center experience. J Thorac Cardiovasc Surg 2010;139(3):665–73.
147. Masud F, Zainab A, Ratnani I, et al. Updates on critical care management of cardiovascular patients. Methodist Debakey Cardiovasc J 2011;7(4):28–32.
148. St André AC, DelRossi A. Hemodynamic management of patients in the first 24 hours after cardiac surgery. Crit Care Med 2005;33(9):2082–93.
149. Stamou S, Camp S, Stiegel R, et al. Quality improvement program decreases mortality after cardiac surgery. J Thorac Cardiovasc Surg 2008;136(2):494–499.e498.
150. Cohen MD, Hilligoss B, Kajdacsy-Balla Amaral AC. A handoff is not a telegram: an understanding of the patient is co-constructed. Crit Care 2012;16(1):303.
151. Joy BF, Elliott E, Hardy C, et al. Standardized multidisciplinary protocol improves handover of cardiac surgery patients to the intensive care unit. Pediatric Crit Care Med 2011;12(3):304–8.
152. Society of Thoracic Surgeons Blood Conservation Guideline Task Force, Ferraris VA, Ferraris SP, et al. Perioperative blood transfusion and blood conservation in cardiac surgery: the Society of Thoracic Surgeons and The Society of Cardiovascular Anesthesiologists clinical practice guideline. Ann Thorac Surg 2007;83(Suppl 5):S27–86.

Life-Threatening Infection in Transplant Recipients

Daire T. O'Shea, MB BCh, MSc, MRCPI, Atul Humar, MD, MSc, FRCPC*

KEYWORDS

- Transplant infection • Critical care • Immunosuppression • Opportunistic infection
- Microbiological diagnosis

KEY POINTS

- Transplant patients represent a heterogeneous and rapidly growing patient group requiring a high index of suspicion for infection.
- Infection is a major posttransplant cause of morbidity and mortality, and new threats continually emerge.
- Individualized assessments of net state of immunosuppression and infection risk are important.
- Aggressive pursuit of an early microbiological diagnosis is crucial; invasive procedures should be used if necessary.
- In the setting of life-threatening infection, reduction or cessation of immunosuppressive therapy whenever possible is an important adjunct to therapy.

INTRODUCTION

Transplant recipients constitute an increasingly diverse and complex patient cohort. They comprise a heterogeneous patient group undergoing solid organ transplantation (SOT), hematopoietic stem cell transplantation (HSCT), or pancreatic islet cell transplantation, and now also include the emerging group of individuals undergoing vascularized composite allotransplantation, such as limb transplants. Infection remains a major cause of morbidity and mortality in transplant recipients; for example, approximately 17% to 20% of the mortality following allogeneic HSCT can be attributed to infection.[1–3]

In SOT where immunosuppressants are prescribed indefinitely, transplant physicians and their patients perpetually negotiate the delicate balance between the risk of graft rejection and infection. Advances in techniques and in modern immunosuppression have improved graft survival but continually unveil new infection challenges

Disclosures: A. Humar has received grant support from Roche and consulting fees from Astellas.
Transplant Infectious Diseases, Alberta Transplant Institute, University of Alberta, 6–030 Katz Center for Health Research, 11361–87 Ave, Edmonton, Alberta T6G 2E1, Canada
* Corresponding author.
E-mail address: ahumar@ualberta.ca

for the patient.[4–6] The pharmacology of immunosuppression has evolved dramatically in recent years with a plethora of agents now available for physicians to use (**Box 1**).[7] Specific agents vary greatly in their mode, intensity, and duration of immunosuppression, adding yet another layer of complexity to the management and prevention of infectious morbidity and mortality in transplant recipients.[8]

The risk of infection in transplant recipients is a dynamic process and numerous influencing factors must be considered during the evaluation of patients (**Box 2**). The net state of immunosuppression is a central concept in transplantation medicine and represents a key determinant of infectious risk.[1,9] The net state is a measure of an individual's unique susceptibility to infection and incorporates assessment of several important contributing factors

- Pretransplant diagnosis or treatment (eg, myeloablative conditioning before HSCT)
- Induction therapy used at time of transplantation
- Nature of organ or stem cell transplant received (eg, lung vs liver organ transplant or umbilical cord blood, T-cell-depleted stem cell transplants)
- Dose, duration, and choice of maintenance immunosuppression
- Comorbidities (eg, viral coinfection [hepatitis C virus (HCV), cytomegalovirus (CMV)], malnutrition, end-organ failure [cirrhosis, chronic kidney disease])
- Breaches of the mucocutaneous barrier: indwelling devices, mucositis

The time after transplant is also of key importance (**Fig. 1, Table 1**). It directly influences the potential pathogens from which an individual patient is at risk.[1] Following periods of intensification of immunosuppression (eg, due to graft rejection or flare of Graft-versus-host disease [GVHD]) the patient's infection risk is adjusted to reflect earlier time points again after transplantation. In the absence of chronic GVHD requiring ongoing immunosuppression in HSCT recipients, immune restitution can in general be considered complete at 2 years after stem cell transplant.[3]

The authors' learning objective is to review significant posttransplant infections that can necessitate critical care support. For ease of description this discussion is divided into infections presenting early after transplantation and those occurring later after transplantation. A more detailed discussion of specific pathogens will then follow.

Early infections are classified here as

- SOT: those encountered between the transplant procedure and 4 weeks after transplantation
- HSCT: infection occurring in the preengraftment phase

Box 1
Immunosuppressant therapies and mechanism of action

Corticosteroids—multiple anti-inflammatory effects

Anti-proliferative agents: mycophenolate mofetil—inhibit nucleotide synthesis and prevent T-cell and B-cell proliferation

Calcineurin inhibitors: cyclosporine, tacrolimus—inhibits T-cell activation

mTor inhibitors: sirolimus—inhibits T-cell activation and proliferation

Monoclonal antibodies: basiliximab (IL-2 receptor antagonist), alemtuzumab (anti-CD52: prolonged T-cell, B-cell depletion), belatacept (binds CD80/86 to prevent T-cell costimulatory signal)

Antilymphocyte antibodies: anti-thymocyte globulin—prolonged T-cell depletion

---

Box 2
Infection risk assessment after transplantation

Net state of immunosuppression

Time after transplantation

Type of transplant (highest risk in SOT is lung transplant; in HSCT is T-cell depleted grafts or cord blood stem cell transplants)

HLA mismatch, episodes of graft rejection

Prior antimicrobial exposure: prophylactic/therapeutic

Prior colonization with drug resistant organisms

Prolonged hospitalization

Ongoing neutropenia, lymphopenia, or hypogammaglobulinemia

Infectious entities unique to transplant recipients, and emerging pathogens of importance, are emphasized with the understanding that many more frequently observed infections (dealt with in other articles) are equally applicable to this cohort of patients.

GENERAL PRINCIPLES OF ASSESSMENT

Transplant recipients are frequent users of critical care services, and the intensivist forms an integral part of posttransplant care pathways. Following SOT, many patients routinely receive their initial period of postoperative care in the critical care setting. In later posttransplant periods these patients can require critical care support for the management of infections manifesting as severe septic shock or in the setting of severe compromise of a vital organ function (eg, pneumonia) or disease affecting the central nervous system (CNS).

Recognition of infection in transplant recipients is notoriously difficult and maintaining a high index of suspicion is of paramount importance. The presentation of infection is frequently altered due to impaired innate and adaptive immune responses. The absence of fever does not preclude the possibility of serious infection and localizing signs may be absent or only identifiable late in the disease process. A multidisciplinary approach is essential to achieve optimal outcomes for patients. This approach involves transplant physicians, transplant surgeons, critical care clinicians, clinical pharmacists, and allied health specialists all working together.

At the core of successful diagnosis and management is a thorough assessment of infectious risk, and a detailed history and physical examination inclusive of cutaneous and ophthalmologic examinations, which can frequently provide subtle but vital diagnostic clues.

Microbiological diagnosis is crucial in this patient group. In the context of extensive differential diagnoses, the value of early and specific diagnostics with the use of invasive procedures if necessary (bronchoscopy, tissue biopsy, or aspiration of collections) to obtain specimens cannot be overemphasized (**Box 3**). After transplantation, serologic techniques are of limited use because transplant recipients may not mount timely serologic responses. Antigen detection or molecular nucleic acid detection assays are preferred. Adoption of newer microbiological techniques for pathogen identification carries the potential to improve the ability to achieve a definitive diagnosis, greatly enabling the prompt commencement of specific antimicrobials.[10,11]

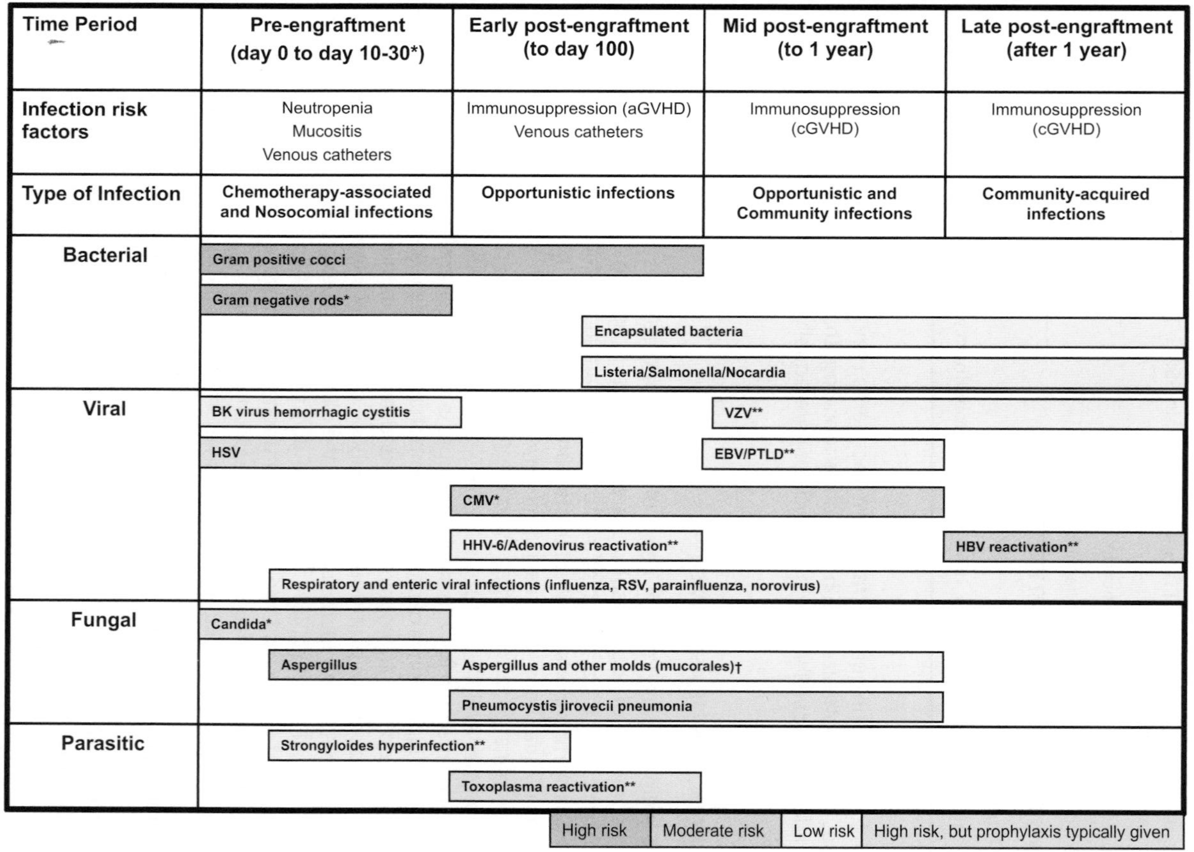

Fig. 1. Timeline of infections after hematopoietic stem cell transplant. *Some centers mitigate this risk with prophylaxis. **In previously exposed recipients. †High risk in those with severe GVHD. §Timeline described is primarily for those undergoing myeloablative conditioning. (*From* Marty FM, Baden LR. Infection in the hematopoetic stem cell transplant recipient. In: Soiffer RJ, editor. Hematopoetic stem cell transplantation. Totowa (NJ): Humana Press, 2008. p. 423; with kind permission from Springer Science and Business Media.)

Table 1
Timeline of infections after organ transplant

Time Period	0–1 mo Posttransplant	1–6 mo Posttransplant	>6 mo Posttransplant
Type of infection	Nosocomial infections: pneumonia, catheter-related, UTI Postsurgical infections: wound, anastomotic leaks, abscesses Donor-derived infection	Opportunistic infection Reactivation of recipient or donor-latent infections (prophylaxis may shift further)	Community-acquired infections In the absence of prophylaxis: reactivation of latent infections during intense immunosuppression for acute graft rejection
Bacterial	C difficile colitis Antimicrobial-resistant bacteria (MRSA, VRE, ESBL, multi-drug resistant (MDR) gram-negative rods) Postsurgical infections (infected biliomas in liver transplant, pneumonia in lung transplant, UTI in renal transplant)	Listeria, Nocardia (if no TMP/sulfamethoxazole) M. tuberculosis, Legionella	Ongoing risk for Listeria, Nocardia, M tuberculosis, Legionella if ongoing intense immunosuppression Graft-related infections (cholangitis in liver, pneumonia in lung, UTI in kidney) Community-acquired pneumonia pathogens
Viral	In the absence of anti-herpes virus prophylaxis: HSV Donor-derived: lymphocytic choriomeningitis virus, rhabdovirus, West Nile virus, HIV	BK nephropathy (kidney), HCV reactivation (liver), adenovirus, respiratory viruses CMV, EBV, HSV, VZV (after discontinuation of prophylaxis)	Late-onset CMV (postprophylaxis), EBV-related PTLD, recurrent HSV, VZV, HCV progression, JC polyomavirus Respiratory viruses, enteric viruses, West Nile virus
Fungal	Candida spp Early Aspergillus only in some settings	Cryptococcus, Aspergillus, atypical molds, Zygomycetes species Pneumocystis only if no prophylaxis	During intense immunosuppression in the absence of antifungal prophylaxis: Aspergillus, atypical molds, Zygomycetes species Geographically restricted endemic fungi
Parasitic	Uncommon	Toxoplasma, Strongyloides, Trypanosoma, Leishmania	Ongoing risk if intense immunosuppression

From Deepali K, Humar A, editors. The AST handbook of transplant infections. Hoboken (NJ): Wiley Blackwell; p. 3; with permission.

Box 3
Initial infectious diagnostic evaluation in transplant recipients

Multiple blood cultures (from periphery and central vascular catheters if present)

Urine culture

Respiratory specimen for culture

Radiological imaging: chest radiograph, CT

Specific diagnostics (see later) according to site of infection/potential pathogens/ epidemiologic risk (eg, CMV PCR, CSF sampling, bronchoalveolar lavage)

Detailed radiological examinations using computed tomography (CT) scan or magnetic resonance imaging (MRI) allow the early identification of occult sites of infection.

However, in most instances, following the collection of initial specimens for culture, immediate institution of empiric broad antimicrobial coverage targeting the likely pathogens is imperative.

Noninfectious entities can also precipitate illness requiring critical care support in transplant recipients and may mimic infection; these should always be borne in mind. Transplant recipients are susceptible to episodes of graft rejection, GVHD flares, or even recurrence of their primary disease. In addition, adverse effects arising from drug toxicity or drug-drug interactions, which can resemble infectious entities, may be observed (eg, Sirolimus-induced pneumonitis).[12,13]

Effective management of infection after transplantation often necessitates a reduction in immunosuppression if possible. This management alters the net state of immunosuppression in favor of enabling a more robust host immune response. Adjuvant immunotherapy using immunoglobulin is used for certain infections.[14] Additional therapeutic concerns relate to drug interactions between antimicrobials and immunosuppressant drugs, and appropriate dosing and delivery in the critically ill patient with vital organ dysfunction.[13] Surgical intervention may be required to aid diagnosis or to effect definitive management.

Early Posttransplantation Period

In the early period posttransplantation, bacterial infections predominate. Frequent issues arising relate to common nosocomial infectious complications, such as[2,15,16]

- Bloodstream infection (BSI), catheter-associated BSI[17]
- Health care/ventilator-associated pneumonia
- Urinary tract infections (UTI)
- Surgical site infections
- Clostridium difficile-associated diarrhea

The risk of these infections relates to the technical difficulty of the transplant procedure, as well as the pretransplant status of the recipient. The usual nosocomial pathogens prevail, such as Staphylococcus aureus, coagulase-negative staphylococci, enterococci, enterobacteriaceae, and Pseudomonas aeruginosa. As a consequence of significant health care exposure antimicrobial-resistant pathogens (methicillin-resistant S aureus [MRSA], vancomycin-resistant Enterococcus [VRE], extended spectrum β-lactamase [ESBL] -producing gram-negative organisms) are encountered with increased frequency in transplant recipients.[18–25] In addition, antimicrobial prophylaxis and prior treatment episodes can markedly alter an individual's commensal flora. Thus a heightened awareness of organisms less frequently encountered is required and in certain circumstances empiric therapy should take these organisms into consideration (eg. *Stenotrophomonas maltophila, Acinetobacter baumannii* complex) given the mortality associated with delayed therapy.[17,26,27]

Candida infections and candidemia are frequently encountered in the critical care setting. The prevalence of non-*albicans Candida* species continues to increase and in transplant recipients this shift can be further promoted by the use of antifungal prophylaxis following HSCT or solid-organ transplantation.[28]

C difficile

Transplant recipients have an increased incidence of infection because of *C difficile* and experience more severe disease. The highest incidence is in the first 3 months after transplant. Relapsing disease is common and prolonged courses of therapy are often required.[29,30]

Specific to SOT are the risks of donor-derived infection and infections originating within the operative field.

Donor-derived infection A broad range of potential infecting pathogens can be transmitted by organ transplantation.[31] These infecting pathogens include the following:

- Known latent infections (eg, CMV, Epstein-Barr virus [EBV])
- Unknown latent infections (eg, tuberculosis, endemic mycoses)
- Infections that are not manifest or detected in the donor at the time of transplantation (eg, bloodstream infections, viral infections such as West Nile virus,[32] lymphocytic choriomeningitis virus, human immunodeficiency virus [HIV], HCV).[33,34]

Unexplained fever early after transplant with altered mental status or signs of unexplained multiorgan failure despite thorough investigations raises the possibility of donor-derived infection.[35] Open communication with the relevant organ procurement organizations is vital when such situations arise.

Operative field infections Early posttransplant residual fluid collections or hematomas in conjunction with devitalized tissues or leaking anastomoses can provide the ideal conditions for the establishment of deep-seated infection. Vascular complications such as thrombosis of vessels may also occur, leading to graft ischemia, dysfunction, and necrosis. Early radiological diagnosis and intervention are critical and the approach to diagnosis and management often necessitates surgical intervention for microbiological diagnosis and to perform effective debridement.

ISSUES SPECIFIC TO CERTAIN TRANSPLANT TYPES
Cardiothoracic Recipients

Lung transplant recipients experience the highest frequency of infections among SOT recipients and infection incidence is double that of heart transplant recipients.[36,37] Contributory factors include

- Donor lung colonization[38]
- Extended periods of intubation
- Disruption of lymphatic drainage
- Reduced cough reflex and ciliary function
- More intensive immunosuppression

Particular attention is paid to the bronchial anastomoses, which can be susceptible to ischemia, breakdown, and infection. Mediastinitis and pleural-based disease are prevalent in cardiothoracic transplant recipients and early imaging with CT is indicated when clinical concern exists.[39] Occasionally culture-negative surgical site infections may be attributable to unusual pathogens such as *Mycoplasma hominis.*[40]

Cystic fibrosis patients undergoing lung transplantation deserve particular mention.[41] They often come to transplant colonized with resistant and fastidious organisms; 52% to 75% are colonized with multi-drug-resistant *Pseudomonas*, and 6% to 9% are colonized with *Burkholderia* spp.[42–44] These patients require individualized antimicrobial prophylactic regimens but breakthrough infection can still occur. This breakthrough infection can manifest as sepsis, empyema, lung abscess, or central venous catheter—associated BSI early or late after transplant. Close surveillance and early aggressive therapy are essential. Antimicrobial therapy should be optimized based on susceptibility testing. Source control, entailing catheter removal or drainage of sites of infection, should be pursued.

Abdominal Organ Transplantation: Liver, Pancreas, Kidney, Intestinal

In critical care settings, early posttransplantation nosocomial infections again prevail.[16] Gram-negative bacilli, enterococci, and anaerobic organisms represent the predominant pathogens. Infections related to technical complications are common. These infections may be due to vascular or nonvascular anastomotic problems and a thorough understanding of the transplanted organ anatomy is important. For example, in liver transplant recipients the biliary anastomosis may leak or stricture. Biliary leaks or bilomas represent common sites for the initiation of infection. Thrombosis of the hepatic artery is uncommon but may lead to devastating complications, including hepatic abscesses, necrosis, and sepsis. Early imaging and diagnosis are essential in this setting.

Liver, pancreas, and intestinal recipients are at particular risk for fungal infection most often caused by *Candida* species.[28] Close surveillance is required and antifungal prophylaxis is recommended for patients at high risk (intestinal recipient, reoperation, retransplantation, renal failure, massive transfusion, *Candida* colonization).[45,46]

HSCT Recipients

During the pre-engraftment phase HSCT recipients most commonly require critical care support due to sepsis or pneumonia.[15]

BSI

Severe mucositis predisposes to the establishment of BSI by skin, oral, or gastrointestinal (GI) tract flora. Catheter-associated BSI is also common. The spectrum of BSI pathogens has altered over time. Following the introduction of fluroquinolone prophylaxis, the incidence of GNB infection declined but was replaced with increasing incidence of gram-positive organisms.[47,48] The spectrum reflects the prevailing organisms present within an institution but common to all is a rising incidence of drug-resistant organisms that carry an increased risk of mortality (eg, VRE, ESBL-producing enterobacteriaceae).[22] Akin to SOT recipients, due consideration should be given to the possibility of unusual bacterial pathogens.

Candida BSI is also increasingly due to non-albicans species reflecting the use of antifungal prophylaxis. Candidemia in transplant recipients should prompt a search for end-organ sites of infection, such as endocarditis, endophthalmitis, renal abscesses, or hepatosplenic candidiasis, depending on the clinical setting.[28]

Pneumonia

Severe pneumonia occurring pre-engraftment can precipitate the requirement for critical care support. Nosocomial organisms or respiratory viruses cause most pneumonias in this setting; however, these patients are also particularly susceptible to invasive fungal infections (IFI).[49] Prolonged periods of neutropenia pre-HSCT contribute to a substantially increased risk of IFI early post-HSCT. *Aspergillus* is the most common pathogen encountered with an overall incidence of 5% to 30% in allogeneic HSCT recipients.[50] Other molds, namely *Fusarium*, Zygomycetes, and *Scedosporium* spp, are emerging as important causes of IFI in HSCT recipients.[28] All can manifest with pulmonary and/or disseminated extrapulmonary disease (see more detailed discussion later).

The diverse approaches required to manage pneumonia appropriately due to bacterial, viral, or fungal pathogens in this setting emphasize the importance of early microbiological diagnosis using invasive procedures if necessary.

Typhlitis/neutropenic enterocolitis

Typhlitis occurs in approximately 5% of patients with hematologic malignancies.[51–53] Mucosal injury and profound neutropenia allow secondary bowel wall infection and transmural inflammation. The cecum is most often involved and patients present with right lower quadrant pain or peritoneal signs. Progression to septicemia and/or bowel perforation can occur. Typhlitis is a clinical diagnosis supplemented by CT to confirm and establish the extent of disease or the presence of perforation. Conservative management is the mainstay of therapy with bowel rest, total parenteral nutrition, and broad spectrum antimicrobials to cover gut flora (ie, gram-positive, gram-negative, anaerobic organisms, and fungi while awaiting neutrophil recovery).[53] Surgery is recommended only in the case of complications or where conservative management has failed.

LATE INFECTIOUS COMPLICATIONS POSTTRANSPLANTATION

Late post transplantation, infections which are observed in the early posttransplant period continue to be encountered, but opportunistic pathogens and community-acquired infections tend to dominate.[1,9] Again, the intensity of ongoing immunosuppression dictates the breadth of pathogens an individual is susceptible to. To maintain relevance to critical care clinicians, common and emerging infection syndromes unique to transplant recipients are discussed and the approach to diagnosis and initial management is reviewed.

Common community infections, which can require critical care support, such as invasive pneumococcal or staphylococcal disease, urosepsis, meningococcal disease, and influenza, have been reviewed elsewhere. Transplant recipients can present at more advanced stages of illness but the management is broadly in keeping with that in immunocompetent individuals. Decisions to adjust immunosuppression or use adjunctive immunoglobulin therapy are based on the patient's individual clinical circumstances.

Pneumonia

Pulmonary infection is the most common form of documented invasive infection observed in transplant recipients. It will frequently cause sufficient compromise in respiratory function to require critical care support. The differential diagnosis in transplant recipients is very broad (**Box 4**) and definitive diagnosis is crucial to effective therapy and resolution.

Chest radiograph may often underestimate the true extent of disease and CT thorax can provide further information regarding the extent and pattern of pulmonary involvement, such as the presence of cavitation or nodular infiltrates. Routine diagnostic evaluation with blood cultures remains important but specific tests for opportunistic

---

Box 4
Differential diagnosis of pneumonia in transplant recipients

Bacterial:

Community-acquired pathogens: *S pneumoniae, H influenzae, M catarrhalis, S aureus, Mycoplasma pneumoniae, Chlamydia pneumoniae*

Nosocomial: gram-negative bacilli (*E coli, P aeruginosa, K pneumoniae*), MRSA

Legionella

Nocardia

Rhodoccus equi

Viral:

Respiratory viruses: influenza, parainfluenza, RSV, human metapneumovirus, adenovirus, coronavirus, entero/rhinovirus

CMV, Herpes simplex virus (HSV), Varicella-zoster virus (VZV)

Mycobacteria:

Tuberculosis

Nontuberculous mycobacteria: *Mycobacterium avium* complex (MAC), *M abscessus* (CF patients)

Fungal:

Invasive molds: *Aspergillus, Zygomycetes, Fusarium, Scedosporium*

P jirovecii pneumonia (PJP/PCP)

Cryptococcus (neoformans, gattii)

Endemic mycoses: histoplasmosis, coccidiomycosis, blastomycosis

Parasitic:

Strongyloides hyperinfection syndrome

Toxoplasmosis

---

pathogens are equally important (eg, plasma CMV viral load estimation by polymerase chain reaction [PCR], serum galactomannan).

Bronchoalveolar lavage (BAL) yields representative specimens of an adequate quality more reliably than sputum collection. Performing a bronchoscopy and BAL should be considered early with specimens processed for the potential bacterial, mycobacterial, fungal, and viral pathogens (see specific pathogens). Clinicians should also maintain a low threshold for performing a biopsy of involved lung tissue for histology and culture.

Central Nervous System Infection

Infection of the CNS in transplant recipients can vary from indolent presentations with chronic low-grade headache, to a more fulminant meningoencephalitic presentation requiring admission to critical care. The CNS may be the only site of infection (isolated intracerebral abscess) or it may be involved as part of a disseminated infectious process. In transplant recipients the differential diagnoses for such presentations are diverse and again cover the spectrum from common community acquired to opportunistic pathogens (**Box 5**).

Box 5
Differential diagnosis of CNS infection in transplant recipients
Intracerebral abscess/space occupying lesion:
Bacterial: embolic or contiguous disease from local site
Nocardia; Listeria monocytogenes
Fungal: *Aspergillus*; zygomycetes; *Cryptococcus*
EBV associated posttransplant lymphoproliferative disorder (PTLD)
Tuberculosis
Toxoplasmosis
Meningoencephalitis:
Bacterial: *S pneumoniae; Neisseria meningitides; Listeria*
Viral: CMV; EBV; HSV; VZV; HHV6; Enterovirus; JC virus
Fungal: Cryptococcus, Coccidioides, Histoplasma capsulatum
Tuberculosis
Treponema pallidum; Borrelia burgdorferi

MRI is the neuroimaging modality of choice providing better resolution of the brain parenchyma and improved diagnostic specificity.[54] Lumbar puncture should be performed if safe, and cerebrospinal fluid (CSF) should be processed for specific pathogen testing (eg, viral PCR, cryptococcal antigen; see specific pathogens).

Enteritis/Colitis

Occasionally severe enterocolitis may require admission to critical care due to cardiovascular compromise or as a consequence of perforation/bleeding. In transplant recipients the predominant infectious etiologies to consider are

- *C difficile*
- CMV, EBV (posttransplant lymphoproliferative disorder [PTLD])
- Norovirus, rotavirus: both can cause protracted diarrheal illnesses
- *Cryptosporidium, isospora, Giardia lamblia*
- *Strongyloides stercoralis* (hyperinfection syndrome)

Specific diagnostic tests include stool specimens for culture, ova/parasite examination, and *C difficile* toxin. Enteric virus PCR on stool samples can be performed if available often with improved sensitivity compared with electron microscopy.[55] Colonoscopy and tissue biopsy may be required to diagnose CMV definitively because in the setting of CMV colitis, CMV may not be detected in plasma by PCR.

SPECIFIC PATHOGENS

Following is a discussion of selected pathogens that are particularly common causes of life-threatening or severe illness in transplant recipients.

CMV

CMV is one of the most prevalent opportunistic pathogens posttransplant. Before the development of sensitive diagnostic tests and the advent of prophylactic/preemptive strategies, CMV reactivation rates of 70% to 80% were observed with significant attributable morbidity and mortality.[56,57] Currently, with the widespread use of prophylaxis and preemptive prevention strategies, mortality due to CMV has declined substantially. Despite these advances, CMV remains an important pathogen after transplantation. Seronegative SOT recipients of CMV-seropositive organs are the group at highest risk for severe CMV disease.[58] In HSCT, seropositive recipients receiving stem cells from a seronegative donor represent the highest risk group.[59]

CMV after transplantation can manifest clinically in several ways

- Fever alone
- CMV syndrome: fever with evidence of myelosuppression, arthralgias, myalgias
- Invasive disease: pneumonitis, enterocolitis, encephalitis, hepatitis (retinitis is rare)

CMV is most frequently detected 1 to 4 months after transplant but late-onset disease is being increasingly reported, the natural history being altered by the use of antiviral prophylaxis.[60,61]

Diagnosis

CMV DNA in plasma can be rapidly detected by quantitative PCR. Alternatively, an antigen-detection assay (pp65 antigenemia test) is available. Histology remains the gold standard to prove tissue invasive disease but is often only necessary to diagnose colitis when occasionally CMV DNA can be undetectable in the plasma by PCR.[58] CMV PCR can also be performed on clinical samples from other sites of infection, such as CSF.

Treatment

Severe disease is best treated initially with intravenous ganciclovir 5 mg/kg every 12 hours.[62,63] Initial oral valganciclovir is only an option in patients with mild or no symptoms.[64] The dose of both agents requires adjustment in the setting of renal impairment. Patients often require a reduction in immunosuppression if possible. CMV immunoglobulin (cytogam) may have additive benefit in severe disease and in particular for CMV pneumonitis.[14] Recommended dosing is 100 to 150 mg/kg 3 times per week.[62] Treatment is continued until resolution of viremia.

EBV-associated PTLD

EBV and associated PTLD cause a wide spectrum of clinical conditions ranging from uncomplicated infectious mononucleosis to true malignant disorders.[65] The estimated incidence of PTLD is 3% to 10% in SOT recipients and up to 18% in high-risk HSCT recipients (HLA mismatch, GVHD, T-cell-depleted transplants).[66–68] Attributable mortality approaches 40% to 60%. This entity most often manifests as a nonspecific febrile illness. Approximately 25% of patients have involvement of the GI tract. CNS disease can on occasion lead to a fulminant course and dramatic presentations requiring critical care support.

Diagnosis

Quantitative EBV viral load testing can be performed on whole blood, plasma, and CSF if indicated.[69,70] Radiological assessment/staging requires positron emission tomography -CT scanning and brain MRI. Adequate tissue sampling and histologic staining for morphology and in situ hybridization studies confirm the diagnosis.

Treatment

Many different modalities can be used for treatment.

- Reduction of immunosuppression
- Surgical excision of localized lesions (eg, GI tract masses)

- Ganciclovir/valganciclovir have variable efficacy
- Adoptive immunotherapy
- Anti-CD20 monoclonal antibody (Rituximab)
- Cytotoxic chemotherapy

Respiratory Viruses

Respiratory syncytial virus (RSV), parainfluenza, influenza, human metapneumovirus, adenovirus, entervirus, rhinovirus, coronavirus

These common respiratory viruses are frequently encountered in transplant recipients and attack rates follow the usual seasonal pattern.[71] In immunocompetent individuals most cause only mild symptoms but progression to involvement of the lower respiratory tract and more severe disease occurs with increased frequency in transplant recipients.[72,73] Pediatric patients are at higher risk for both infection and severe disease.[74]

Diagnosis

Specific viruses can be detected by direct fluorescence antibody, culture, or multiplex PCR from nasopharyngeal swabs or BAL specimens.[71]

Treatment

Aside from antiviral therapy for influenza, no consensus exists for the treatment of other respiratory viruses.[75] Early treatment in certain patients (lung transplant recipients, HSCT patients preengraftment) can be used to reduce the risk of lower tract disease and limit severity.[76,77] Treatments reported to demonstrate efficacy are detailed below.

- RSV: aerosolized Ribavirin ± intravenous immunoglobulin (IVIg).[77] Palivizumab (anti-RSV monoclonal antibody) has also provided additive benefit to Ribavirin[78]
- Parainfluenza: aerosolized Ribavirin ± IVIg[79]
- Human metapneumovirus: an emerging respiratory pathogen that has been associated with severe, often fatal disease in HSCT recipients.[80] Aerosolized Ribavirin and IVIg have also been used with some success in case reports[81,82]
- Adenoviridae can cause a wide range of clinical syndromes; self-limited fever, pneumonitis, hepatitis, hemorrhagic colitis.[83,84] Rarely, adenovirus can cause a severe disseminated disease with multi-organ failure. This manifestation occurs more frequently in pediatric recipients and carries a high mortality.[85] Treatment options include cidofovir and ribavirin or the experimental drug CMX001.[86,87]

Aspergillus spp

Aspergillus is the most common cause of IFI in allogeneic HSCT recipients with an incidence of 5% to 30%.[49,50,88] In SOT recipients the incidence is considerably lower, 1% to 15%.[89,90] Mortality attributable to invasive aspergillosis (IA) has varied from 65% to 92% in transplant recipients, although it may be lower in the current era.[90] Risk factors for IA include prolonged neutropenia, lung transplantation, CMV infection, Aspergillus colonization, graft rejection/failure, GVHD, and iron overload.

The lungs and sinuses are the most common sites of disease involvement. Patients can present with fever, chest pain, hemoptysis, or dyspnea. Pulmonary disease can involve lung parenchyma only or present as a more diffuse tracheobronchitis. Sinus disease can cause facial pain and seizures, or focal neurologic signs with extensive disease.

Pulmonary radiologic appearances are best appreciated using CT and include nodules with or without cavitation, or patchy segmental areas of consolidation or ground glass change. Disease outside of the respiratory tract can occur with cutaneous involvement or solitary intracerebral abscesses.

Diagnosis

Sputum culture lacks sensitivity and the isolation of *Aspergillus* alone does not reflect disease. The gold standard for diagnosis is the demonstration of the organism and angio-invasive disease in tissue biopsies (lung or sinus tissue).[90] Fungal stain and culture of such specimens to confirm genus and species remain very important in diagnosis particularly now in the era of prophylaxis using second-generation triazoles (voriconazole, posaconazole), which have altered the spectrum of species encountered.[91,92]

Galactomannan is a constituent of the *Aspergillus* cell wall and is released during hyphal growth. Estimation of galactomannan in serum is widely used but lacks sensitivity. This test appears to perform better in hematological patients than SOT recipients.[93] Estimating galactomannan in BAL demonstrates superior sensitivity,[94] and it can also be performed on CSF specimens but has not been widely standardized. The evolution of molecular assays using PCR should add to the ability to achieve a definitive diagnosis.[95]

Treatment

Voriconazole is now the accepted treatment of choice.[96] A loading dose of 6 mg/kg every 12 hours is administered on day 1 followed by maintenance of 4 mg/kg 12 hourly thereafter. The measurement of trough levels is advised after approximately 1 week of therapy (target range, 1–5.5 µg/mL).[97] Voriconazole interacts significantly with calcineurin inhibitors and thus levels of these agents must also be closely monitored. A minimum of 12 weeks of therapy is advised and duration can be guided by clinico-radiologic resolution and surveillance galactomannan assays.

Again species confirmation is vital to guide therapy because the susceptibility of different species (*Aspergillus terreus, Aspergillus calidoustus*) can vary considerably, and novel antifungal combinations may be required.[98] Surgical intervention is indicated in the context of significant hemoptysis or extensive sinonasal disease.

Other Molds Causing IFI

These pathogens cause disease that mimics IA and represent a considerable emerging threat in the era of posaconazole/voriconazole prophylaxis.[5,28,99] Pathogens of note include zygomycetes, *fusarium*, and *scedosporium*.[100–103]

Pneumocystis Jirovecci Pneumonia/PCP

Effective prophylaxis has dramatically reduced the incidence of *Pneumocystis jirovecci* pneumonia (PJP) in transplant recipients.[104] However, it remains a pathogen of note and is an important diagnostic consideration in a transplant patient presenting acutely with respiratory failure.[105] Classically patients present with subacute fever, cough, and dyspnea. The hallmark of PJP remains profound hypoxia with a relative paucity of clinical findings. Chest radiographs may reveal bihilar infiltrates or pneumothoraces but are often quite unremarkable, and CT thorax is more sensitive for diagnosis.

Diagnosis

Diagnosis is best achieved via the demonstration of the organism in BAL or lung biopsy specimens.[106] Several specific staining methods can be used including monofluorescent antibody stains, gomori-methanamine silver stain, or Giemsa and Wright stains. The infectious burden is generally less in SOT recipients; thus, the diagnostic sensitivity is lower than the 98% reported in patients with HIV.[106]

Treatment

Trimethoprim (TMP)/sulfamethoxazole remains the treatment of choice. Recommended dosing is 15 to 20 mg/kg/d of the TMP component in 3 to 4 divided doses.[105] Adverse effects are frequent (rash, nausea, renal impairment) and alternatives include clindamycin (600–900 mg 6–8 hourly) and primaquine (15–30 mg daily); or dapsone (100 mg daily) and TMP (15 mg/kg/d in 3 divided doses). As in HIV, adjunctive corticosteroids are an important consideration and are generally recommended in cases with severe hypoxemia (Pao_2 <70 mm Hg).[107] Doses in the region of 40 to 60 mg twice daily for 1 week followed by a taper over 2 weeks are used.

Strongyloides Hyperinfection Syndrome

Strongyloides hyperinfection syndrome is a rare but particularly severe manifestation of latent *Strongyloides* infection primarily reported in SOT recipients.[108–110] Massive dissemination of filariform larvae to the lungs, liver, heart, and CNS occurs. Concomitant gram-negative BSI or bacterial meningitis is recognized. Patients present with a severe systemic illness and mortality is high. Diagnosis is achieved via detection of the larvae in stool, respiratory secretions, or CSF. Treatment is with ivermectin 200 μg/kg/d or albendazole 400 mg twice daily. Extended courses are advised in the setting of hyperinfection in transplant recipients.

SUMMARY

Transplant recipients represent a complex, heterogenous patient population who often require periods of critical care support. Infectious complications precipitate the majority of admissions to critical care post-transplantation, and patients are susceptible to an increasingly diverse array of common and opportunistic infecting pathogens. Clinicians must maintain a high index of suspicion for infection, and conduct early, thorough diagnostic work-up coupled with prompt institution of antimicrobial therapy. Detailed individualized infection risk assessments are central to guiding therapeutic care pathways and optimizing clinical outcomes.

REFERENCES

1. Fishman JA. Infection in solid-organ transplant recipients. N Engl J Med 2007; 357(25):2601–14.
2. Patel R, Paya CV. Infections in solid-organ transplant recipients. Clin Microbiol Rev 1997;10(1):86–124.
3. Tomblyn M, Chiller T, Einsele H, et al. Guidelines for preventing infectious complications among hematopoietic cell transplantation recipients: a global perspective. Bone Marrow Transplant 2009;15(10):1143–238.
4. Vincenti F, Charpentier B, Vanrenterghem Y, et al. A phase III study of belatacept-based immunosuppression regimens versus cyclosporine in renal transplant recipients (BENEFIT study). Am J Transplant 2010;10(3):535–46.
5. Nishi SP, Valentine VG, Duncan S. Emerging bacterial, fungal, and viral respiratory infections in transplantation. Infect Dis Clin North Am 2010;24(3):541–55.
6. Peleg AY, Husain S, Kwak EJ, et al. Opportunistic infections in 547 organ transplant recipients receiving alemtuzumab, a humanized monoclonal CD-52 antibody. Clin Infect Dis 2007;44(2):204–12.

7. Halloran PF. Immunosuppressive drugs for kidney transplantation. N Engl J Med 2004;351(26):2715–29.
8. Issa NC, Fishman JA. Infectious complications of antilymphocyte therapies in solid organ transplantation. Clin Infect Dis 2009;48(6):772–86.
9. Fishman JA. Introduction: infection in solid organ transplant recipients. Am J Transplant 2009;9(Suppl 4):S3–6.
10. Mitsuma SF, Mansour MK, Dekker JP, et al. Promising new assays and technologies for the diagnosis and management of infectious diseases. Clin Infect Dis 2013;56:996–1002.
11. Clerc O, Prod'hom G, Vogne C, et al. Impact of Matrix-Assisted Laser Desorption Ionization Time-Of-Flight Mass Spectrometry (MALDI-TOF) on the clinical management of patients with Gram-negative bacteremia: a prospective observational study. Clin Infect Dis 2012;56:1101–7.
12. Champion L, Stern M, Israel-Biet D, et al. Brief communication: sirolimus-associated pneumonitis: 24 cases in renal transplant recipients. Ann Intern Med 2006;144(7):505–9.
13. Thomas LD, Miller GG. Interactions between antiinfective agents and immunosuppressants. Am J Transplant 2009;9(Suppl 4):S263–6.
14. Reed EC, Bowden RA, Dandliker PS, et al. Treatment of cytomegalovirus pneumonia with ganciclovir and intravenous cytomegalovirus immunoglobulin in patients with bone marrow transplants. Ann Intern Med 1988;109(10): 783–8.
15. Dettenkofer M, Wenzler-Rottele S, Babikir R, et al. Surveillance of nosocomial sepsis and pneumonia in patients with a bone marrow or peripheral blood stem cell transplant: a multicenter project. Clin Infect Dis 2005; 40(7):926–31.
16. Razonable RR, Findlay JY, O'Riordan A, et al. Critical care issues in patients after liver transplantation. Liver Transpl 2011;17(5):511–27.
17. Moreno A, Cervera C, Gavalda J, et al. Bloodstream infections among transplant recipients: results of a nationwide surveillance in Spain. Am J Transplant 2007; 7(11):2579–86.
18. Fishman JA. Vancomycin-resistant Enterococcus in liver transplantation: what have we left behind? Transpl Infect Dis 2003;5(3):109–11.
19. Linares L, Cervera C, Cofan F, et al. Risk factors for infection with extended-spectrum and AmpC beta-lactamase-producing gram-negative rods in renal transplantation. Am J Transplant 2008;8(5):1000–5.
20. Russell DL, Flood A, Zaroda TE, et al. Outcomes of colonization with MRSA and VRE among liver transplant candidates and recipients. Am J Transplant 2008; 8(8):1737–43.
21. Patel R, Allen SL, Manahan JM, et al. Natural history of vancomycin-resistant enterococcal colonization in liver and kidney transplant recipients. Liver Transpl 2001;7(1):27–31.
22. Weinstock DM, Conlon M, Iovino C, et al. Colonization, bloodstream infection, and mortality caused by vancomycin-resistant enterococcus early after allogeneic hematopoietic stem cell transplant. Biol Blood Marrow Transplant 2007; 13(5):615–21.
23. van Delden C, Blumberg EA. Multidrug resistant gram-negative bacteria in solid organ transplant recipients. Am J Transplant 2009;9(Suppl 4):S27–34.
24. Munoz P. Multiply resistant gram-positive bacteria: vancomycin-resistant enterococcus in solid organ transplant recipients. Am J Transplant 2009;9(Suppl 4): S50–6.

25. Garzoni C. Multiply resistant gram-positive bacteria methicillin-resistant, vanco-mycin-intermediate and vancomycin-resistant Staphylococcus aureus (MRSA, VISA, VRSA) in solid organ transplant recipients. Am J Transplant 2009; 9(Suppl 4):S41–9.

26. Sopirala MM, Pope-Harman A, Nunley DR, et al. Multidrug-resistant Acineto-bacter baumannii pneumonia in lung transplant recipients. J Heart Lung Trans-plant 2008;27(7):804–7.

27. Playford EG, Craig JC, Iredell JR. Carbapenem-resistant acinetobacter bau-mannii in intensive care unit patients: risk factors for acquisition, infection and their consequences. J Hosp Infect 2007;65(3):204–11.

28. Person AK, Kontoyiannis DP, Alexander BD. Fungal infections in transplant and oncology patients. Infect Dis Clin North Am 2010;24(2):439–59.

29. Riddle DJ, Dubberke ER. Clostridium difficile infection in solid organ transplant recipients. Curr Opin Organ Transplant 2008;13(6):592–600.

30. Albright JB, Bonatti H, Mendez J, et al. Early and late onset Clostridium difficile-associated colitis following liver transplantation. Transpl Int 2007;20(10):856–66.

31. Grossi PA, Fishman JA. Donor-derived infections in solid organ transplant recip-ients. Am J Transplant 2009;9(Suppl 4):S19–26.

32. Iwamoto M, Jernigan DB, Guasch A, et al. Transmission of West Nile virus from an organ donor to four transplant recipients. N Engl J Med 2003;348(22): 2196–203.

33. Fischer SA, Graham MB, Kuehnert MJ, et al. Transmission of lymphocytic choriomeningitis virus by organ transplantation. N Engl J Med 2006;354(21): 2235–49.

34. Humar A, Fishman JA. Donor-derived infection: old problem, new solutions? Am J Transplant 2008;8(6):1087–8.

35. Morris MI, Fischer SA, Ison MG. Infections transmitted by transplantation. Infect Dis Clin North Am 2010;24(2):497–514.

36. Speich R, van der Bij W. Epidemiology and management of infections after lung transplantation. Clin Infect Dis 2001;33(Suppl 1):S58–65.

37. Mattner F, Fischer S, Weissbrodt H, et al. Post-operative nosocomial infections after lung and heart transplantation. J Heart Lung Transplant 2007;26(3):241–9.

38. Avlonitis VS, Krause A, Luzzi L, et al. Bacterial colonization of the donor lower airways is a predictor of poor outcome in lung transplantation. Eur J Cardio-thorac Surg 2003;24(4):601–7.

39. Abid Q, Nkere UU, Hasan A, et al. Mediastinitis in heart and lung transplanta-tion: 15 years experience. Ann Thorac Surg 2003;75(5):1565–71.

40. Hopkins PM, Winlaw DS, Chhajed PN, et al. Mycoplasma hominis infection in heart and lung transplantation. J Heart Lung Transplant 2002;21(11):1225–9.

41. Flume PA, Egan TM, Paradowski LJ, et al. Infectious complications of lung trans-plantation. Impact of cystic fibrosis. Am J Respir Crit Care Med 1994;149(6): 1601–7.

42. Dobbin C, Maley M, Harkness J, et al. The impact of pan-resistant bacterial pathogens on survival after lung transplantation in cystic fibrosis: results from a single large referral centre. J Hosp Infect 2004;56(4):277–82.

43. Boussaud V, Guillemain R, Grenet D, et al. Clinical outcome following lung trans-plantation in patients with cystic fibrosis colonised with Burkholderia cepacia complex: results from two French centres. Thorax 2008;63(8):732–7.

44. Zaidi S, Elidemir O, Heinle JS, et al. Mycobacterium abscessus in cystic fibrosis lung transplant recipients: report of 2 cases and risk for recurrence. Transpl Infect Dis 2009;11(3):243–8.

45. Cruciani M, Mengoli C, Malena M, et al. Antifungal prophylaxis in liver transplant patients: a systematic review and meta-analysis. Liver Transpl 2006;12(5): 850–8.
46. Eschenauer GA, Lam SW, Carver PL. Antifungal prophylaxis in liver transplant recipients. Liver Transpl 2009;15(8):842–58.
47. Cullen M, Steven N, Billingham L, et al. Antibacterial prophylaxis after chemotherapy for solid tumors and lymphomas. N Engl J Med 2005;353(10):988–98.
48. Bucaneve G, Micozzi A, Menichetti F, et al. Levofloxacin to prevent bacterial infection in patients with cancer and neutropenia. N Engl J Med 2005;353(10): 977–87.
49. Neofytos D, Horn D, Anaissie E, et al. Epidemiology and outcome of invasive fungal infection in adult hematopoietic stem cell transplant recipients: analysis of Multicenter Prospective Antifungal Therapy (PATH) Alliance registry. Clin Infect Dis 2009;48(3):265–73.
50. Wald A, Leisenring W, van Burik JA, et al. Epidemiology of aspergillus infections in a large cohort of patients undergoing bone marrow transplantation. J Infect Dis 1997;175(6):1459–66.
51. Morgan C, Tillett T, Braybrooke J, et al. Management of uncommon chemotherapy-induced emergencies. Theoria 2011;12(8):806–14.
52. Davila ML. Neutropenic enterocolitis. Curr Treat Options Gastroenterol 2006; 22(1):44–7.
53. Nesher L, Rolston KV. Neutropenic enterocolitis, a growing concern in the era of widespread use of aggressive chemotherapy. Clin Infect Dis 2012;56: 711–7.
54. Erdogan C, Hakyemez B, Yildirim N, et al. Brain abscess and cystic brain tumor: discrimination with dynamic susceptibility contrast perfusion-weighted MRI. J Comput Assist Tomogr 2005;29(5):663–7.
55. Pang XL, Preiksaitis JK, Lee B. Multiplex real time RT-PCR for the detection and quantitation of norovirus genogroups I and II in patients with acute gastroenteritis. J Clin Virol 2005;33(2):168–71.
56. Hodson EM, Craig JC, Strippoli GF, et al. Antiviral medications for preventing cytomegalovirus disease in solid organ transplant recipients. Cochrane Database Syst Rev 2008;(2):CD003774.
57. Gluckman E, Traineau R, Devergie A, et al. Prevention and treatment of CMV infection after allogeneic bone marrow transplant. Ann Hematol 1992; 64(Suppl):A158–61.
58. Humar A, Snydman D. Cytomegalovirus in solid organ transplant recipients. Am J Transplant 2009;9(Suppl 4):S78–86.
59. George B, Pati N, Gilroy N, et al. Pre-transplant cytomegalovirus (CMV) serostatus remains the most important determinant of CMV reactivation after allogeneic hematopoietic stem cell transplantation in the era of surveillance and preemptive therapy. Transpl Infect Dis 2010;12(4):322–9.
60. Limaye AP, Bakthavatsalam R, Kim HW, et al. Late-onset cytomegalovirus disease in liver transplant recipients despite antiviral prophylaxis. Transplantation 2004;78(9):1390–6.
61. Boeckh M, Leisenring W, Riddell SR, et al. Late cytomegalovirus disease and mortality in recipients of allogeneic hematopoietic stem cell transplants: importance of viral load and T-cell immunity. Blood 2003;101(2):407–14.
62. Kotton CN, Kumar D, Caliendo AM, et al. International consensus guidelines on the management of cytomegalovirus in solid organ transplantation. Transplantation 2010;89(7):779–95.

63. Asberg A, Humar A, Rollag H, et al. Oral valganciclovir is noninferior to intravenous ganciclovir for the treatment of cytomegalovirus disease in solid organ transplant recipients. Am J Transplant 2007;7(9):2106–13.
64. Humar A, Siegal D, Moussa G, et al. A prospective assessment of valganciclovir for the treatment of cytomegalovirus infection and disease in transplant recipients. J Infect Dis 2005;192(7):1154–7.
65. Green M, Webber S. Posttransplantation lymphoproliferative disorders. Pediatr Clin North Am 2003;50(6):1471–91.
66. Preiksaitis JK. New developments in the diagnosis and management of posttransplantation lymphoproliferative disorders in solid organ transplant recipients. Clin Infect Dis 2004;39(7):1016–23.
67. Allen U, Preiksaitis J. Epstein-Barr virus and posttransplant lymphoproliferative disorder in solid organ transplant recipients. Am J Transplant 2009;9(Suppl 4): S87–96.
68. Gerritsen EJ, Stam ED, Hermans J, et al. Risk factors for developing EBV-related B cell lymphoproliferative disorders (BLPD) after non-HLA-identical BMT in children. Bone 1996;18(2):377–82.
69. Tsai DE, Nearey M, Hardy CL, et al. Use of EBV PCR for the diagnosis and monitoring of post-transplant lymphoproliferative disorder in adult solid organ transplant patients. Am J Transplant 2002;2(10):946–54.
70. Green M, Webber SA. EBV viral load monitoring: unanswered questions. Am J Transplant 2002;2(10):894–5.
71. Ison MG, Michaels MG. RNA respiratory viral infections in solid organ transplant recipients. Am J Transplant 2009;9(Suppl 4):S166–72.
72. Machado CM, Boas LS, Mendes AV, et al. Low mortality rates related to respiratory virus infections after bone marrow transplantation. Bone 2003;31(8): 695–700.
73. Palmer SM Jr, Henshaw NG, Howell DN, et al. Community respiratory viral infection in adult lung transplant recipients. Chest 1998;113(4):944–50.
74. Lee JH, Jang JH, Lee SH, et al. Respiratory viral infections during the first 28 days after transplantation in pediatric hematopoietic stem cell transplant recipients. Clinic 2012;26(5):736–40.
75. Kumar D, Michaels MG, Morris MI, et al. Outcomes from pandemic influenza A H1N1 infection in recipients of solid-organ transplants: a multicentre cohort study. Lancet Infect Dis 2010;10(8):521–6.
76. Sparrelid E, Ljungman P, Ekelof-Andstrom E, et al. Ribavirin therapy in bone marrow transplant recipients with viral respiratory tract infections. Bone 1997; 19(9):905–8.
77. Li L, Avery R, Budev M, et al. Oral versus inhaled ribavirin therapy for respiratory syncytial virus infection after lung transplantation. J Heart Lung Transplant 2012; 31(8):839–44.
78. Shah JN, Chemaly RF. Management of RSV infections in adult recipients of hematopoietic stem cell transplantation. Blood 2011;117(10):2755–63.
79. Wendt CH, Weisdorf DJ, Jordan MC, et al. Parainfluenza virus respiratory infection after bone marrow transplantation. N Engl J Med 1992;326(14):921–6.
80. Egli A, Bucher C, Dumoulin A, et al. Human metapneumovirus infection after allogeneic hematopoietic stem cell transplantation. Infection 2012;40(6): 677–84.
81. Bonney D, Razali H, Turner A, et al. Successful treatment of human metapneumovirus pneumonia using combination therapy with intravenous ribavirin and immune globulin. Br J Haematol 2009;145(5):667–9.

82. Oliveira R, Machado A, Tateno A, et al. Frequency of human metapneumovirus infection in hematopoietic SCT recipients during 3 consecutive years. Bone 2008;42(4):265–9.
83. Ison MG, Green M. Adenovirus in solid organ transplant recipients. Am J Transplant 2009;9(Suppl 4):S161–5.
84. Chakrabarti S. Adenovirus infections after hematopoietic stem cell transplantation: still unravelling the story. Clin Infect Dis 2007;45(8):966–8.
85. Hoffman JA. Adenoviral disease in pediatric solid organ transplant recipients. Pediatrician 2006;10(1):17–25.
86. Howard DS, Phillips IG, Reece DE, et al. Adenovirus infections in hematopoietic stem cell transplant recipients. Clin Infect Dis 1999;29(6):1494–501.
87. La Rosa AM, Champlin RE, Mirza N, et al. Adenovirus infections in adult recipients of blood and marrow transplants. Clin Infect Dis 2001;32(6):871–6.
88. Marr KA, Carter RA, Crippa F, et al. Epidemiology and outcome of mould infections in hematopoietic stem cell transplant recipients. Clin Infect Dis 2002;34(7): 909–17.
89. Cahill BC, Hibbs JR, Savik K, et al. Aspergillus airway colonization and invasive disease after lung transplantation. Chest 1997;112(5):1160–4.
90. Singh N, Husain S. Invasive aspergillosis in solid organ transplant recipients. Am J Transplant 2009;9(Suppl 4):S180–91.
91. Cornely OA, Maertens J, Winston DJ, et al. Posaconazole vs. fluconazole or itraconazole prophylaxis in patients with neutropenia. N Engl J Med 2007;356(4): 348–59.
92. Ullmann AJ, Lipton JH, Vesole DH, et al. Posaconazole or fluconazole for prophylaxis in severe graft-versus-host disease. N Engl J Med 2007;356(4): 335–47.
93. Pfeiffer CD, Fine JP, Safdar N. Diagnosis of invasive aspergillosis using a galactomannan assay: a meta-analysis. Clin Infect Dis 2006;42(10):1417–27.
94. Maertens J, Maertens V, Theunissen K, et al. Bronchoalveolar lavage fluid galactomannan for the diagnosis of invasive pulmonary aspergillosis in patients with hematologic diseases. Clin Infect Dis 2009;49(11):1688–93.
95. Mengoli C, Cruciani M, Barnes RA, et al. Use of PCR for diagnosis of invasive aspergillosis: systematic review and meta-analysis. Lancet Infect Dis 2009; 9(2):89–96.
96. Herbrecht R, Denning DW, Patterson TF, et al. Voriconazole versus amphotericin B for primary therapy of invasive aspergillosis. N Engl J Med 2002;347(6): 408–15.
97. Pascual A, Calandra T, Bolay S, et al. Voriconazole therapeutic drug monitoring in patients with invasive mycoses improves efficacy and safety outcomes. Clin Infect Dis 2008;46(2):201–11.
98. Egli A, Fuller J, Humar A, et al. Emergence of Aspergillus calidoustus infection in the era of posttransplantation azole prophylaxis. Transplantation 2012;94(4): 403–10.
99. Imhof A, Balajee SA, Fredricks DN, et al. Breakthrough fungal infections in stem cell transplant recipients receiving voriconazole. Clin Infect Dis 2004;39(5): 743–6.
100. Lanternier F, Sun HY, Ribaud P, et al. Mucormycosis in organ and stem cell transplant recipients. Clin Infect Dis 2012;54(11):1629–36.
101. Kubak BM, Huprikar SS. Emerging & rare fungal infections in solid organ transplant recipients. Am J Transplant 2009;9(Suppl 4):S208–26.

102. Nucci M, Anaissie E. Fusarium infections in immunocompromised patients. Clinic 2007;20(4):695–704.
103. Husain S, Munoz P, Forrest G, et al. Infections due to Scedosporium apiospermum and Scedosporium prolificans in transplant recipients: clinical characteristics and impact of antifungal agent therapy on outcome. Clin Infect Dis 2005; 40(1):89–99.
104. Rodriguez M, Fishman JA. Prevention of infection due to Pneumocystis spp. in human immunodeficiency virus-negative immunocompromised patients. Clinic 2004;17(4):770–82 table of contents.
105. Martin SI, Fishman JA. Pneumocystis pneumonia in solid organ transplant recipients. Am J Transplant 2009;9(Suppl 4):S227–33.
106. Huang L, Morris A, Limper AH, et al. An Official ATS workshop summary: recent advances and future directions in pneumocystis pneumonia (PCP). Proc Am Thorac Soc 2006;3(8):655–64.
107. Briel M, Bucher HC, Boscacci R, et al. Adjunctive corticosteroids for Pneumocystis jiroveci pneumonia in patients with HIV-infection. Cochrane Database Syst Rev 2006;(3):CD006150.
108. Patel G, Arvelakis A, Sauter BV, et al. Strongyloides hyperinfection syndrome after intestinal transplantation. Transpl Infect Dis 2008;10(2):137–41.
109. Safdar A, Malathum K, Rodriguez SJ, et al. Strongyloidiasis in patients at a comprehensive cancer center in the United States. Cancer 2004;100(7):1531–6.
110. Marty FM. Strongyloides hyperinfection syndrome and transplantation: a preventable, frequently fatal infection. Transpl Infect Dis 2009;11(2):97–9.

Bacterial Meningitis and Other Nonviral Infections of the Nervous System

Thomas P. Bleck, MD

KEYWORDS

- Central nervous system • Meningitis • Spinal cord • Bacteria • Fungi

KEY POINTS

- Bacteria and fungi, owing to their intrinsic properties and the host responses they produce, result in relatively specific clinical syndromes when they infect the central nervous system.
- The infecting organism may produce symptoms and signs by interfering with the function of the nervous system tissue being invaded or compressed.
- The major impediments to the movement of both microorganisms and inflammatory substances from the systemic circulation into the central nervous system are the blood-brain and blood–cerebrospinal fluid barriers.
- The natural history of spinal cord compression caused by an epidural abscess highlights the need for alacrity in diagnosis and treatment.
- The definitive treatment of central nervous system infection depends on correct identification and antimicrobial treatment of the infecting organism, relief of excessive pressure or mass effect that it exerts, and modulation of the host's immune response to allow clearance of the organism while minimizing excessive inflammation.

HISTORY AND NOMENCLATURE

Infections of the central nervous system (CNS) were well known to the ancients; descriptions of meningitis date back to the 16th century. The major syndromes of neurologic infection were described by the great 19th century pathologists. Quincke's lumbar puncture needle, introduced in 1891, and more recently, computed tomography (CT) and magnetic resonance imaging (MRI), round out the current understanding of these disorders.

To understand CNS infections, one requires knowledge of anatomy, because the consequences of infection vary with both the anatomic spaces involved and the functions of the tissues located within them.[1] Although a few organisms can cross tissue planes, most infections initially manifest in a single space.

Disclosures: The author has nothing to disclose.
Rush Medical College, Rush University Medical Center, 600 South Paulina Street, 544 AF, Chicago, IL 60612, USA
E-mail address: tbleck@gmail.com

Epidural infections are usually excluded from direct extension into, or immunologic effects compromising, CNS structures.[2] Their manifestations are primarily due to compression of adjacent tissues. Cranial epidural abscesses cause signs and symptoms corresponding to the increase in intracranial pressure (ICP) produced by the additional volume of alien tissue (eg, headache and altered consciousness), and to the compression of the brain beneath the abscess. Spinal epidural abscesses, in contrast, cause local pain, then nerve root compression, and finally spinal cord compression. Subdural empyema typically incites an inflammatory response in the underlying brain or spinal cord, causing findings out of proportion to the volume of inflammatory exudates produced.[3] Although either the dura mater or the pia mater may become infected, the term meningitis usually refers to infection in the subarachnoid space (SAS).[4] Rarely, infection is confined to the lining tissues themselves, producing pachymeningitis or arachnoiditis. When the infection is predominantly within the ventricular system, ventriculitis or ependymitis isdiagnosed.

The brain or spinal cord may develop focal bacterial or fungal infections, initially in the form of cerebritis or myelitis, which then typically evolve into a parenchymal abscess.[5] The blood vessels may also become infected, producing an arteritis (also termed vasculitis). When veins or venous sinuses are involved, the pathophysiologic consequences are typically due to thrombosis, called septic venous thrombosis or sinus thrombosis.[6] Although not truly parts of the nervous system, infections of the cranium or spinal column (osteomyelitis) or the bony sinuses (sinusitis) are important predecessors of CNS infection.[7]

ETIOLOGY

Bacteria and fungi, owing to their intrinsic properties and the host responses they produce, result in relatively specific clinical syndromes when they infect the CNS. Because the host's defenses play such an important part in shaping the signs and symptoms, abnormalities of host response may cause different syndromes in different patients infected with the same organism. The major infecting organisms are grouped by their syndromes and host characteristics in **Table 1**.

PATHOGENESIS

The infecting organism must first gain entry into the target tissue. The usual paths of infection include (1) hematogenous spread via the arterial blood, or (2) direct extension from another site of infection, such as infected bones or sinuses.[8] Direct extension occurs when trauma results in a direct communication between the external environment and the CNS. Once the organism has invaded, it must elude or subvert the local host defenses to survive and reproduce. These local host defense mechanisms may then invoke a more systemic response. These defensive responses are intended to clear the infection, but their effects are often deleterious to the nervous system tissue itself; many of the signs and symptoms of infection are consequences of the inflammatory response and its aftermath. The use of corticosteroids in the treatment of bacterial meningitis arose from the recognition that the host response was often the cause of further tissue damage.

PATHOPHYSIOLOGY

The infecting organism may produce symptoms and signs by interfering with the function of the nervous system tissue being invaded or compressed, but many findings

Table 1
Common organisms and syndromes of central nervous system infection

Organism	Syndrome	Typical Patient Age	Initial Treatment Pending Sensitivities	Common Host Characteristics
Bacteria				
Streptococcus pneumoniae	Acute bacterial meningitis	Adult	Ceftriaxone and vancomycin	Normal; may be impaired
Neisseria meningitidis	Acute bacterial meningitis	Adolescent	Ceftriaxone	Normal
Hemophilus influenzae type B	Acute bacterial meningitis	Child	Ceftriaxone or ampicillin/ gentamicin	Normal
Listeria monocytogenes[25]	Acute bacterial meningitis	Infant	Ampicillin/gentamicin or trimethoprim/ sulfamethoxazone	Normal, associated with maternal infection
	Brain abscess (typically involving the pons, termed rhombencephalitis)	Any	Ampicillin/gentamicin or trimethoprim/ sulfamethoxazone	Normal
	Acute or subacute bacterial meningitis	Older adult	Ampicillin/gentamicin or trimethoprim/ sulfamethoxazone	Often immunocompromised
Staphylococcus aureus (coagulase-positive staphylococcus)	Acute bacterial meningitis	Any	Vancomycin	Anatomic or surgical defect in skull or meninges
	Brain abscess	Any	Vancomycin	Hematogenous dissemination (eg, endocarditis)
	Epidural abscess	Any	Vancomycin	Direct extension from osteomyelitis
Staphylococcus epidermidis (coagulase-negative staphylococcus)	Subacute bacterial meningitis	After neurosurgical procedures	Vancomycin	
Streptococcus agalactiae (group B streptococcus)	Acute or subacute bacterial meningitis	Newborns and older adults	Ampicillin	Colonization during delivery; gastrointestinal source of bacteremia

(continued on next page)

Table 1
(continued)

Organism	Syndrome	Typical Patient Age	Initial Treatment Pending Sensitivities	Common Host Characteristics
Escherichia coli	Acute bacterial meningitis	Newborns or patients with anatomic or surgical defects	Ceftriaxone or cefotaxime	
Other gram-negative rods	Meningitis	Any	Cefepime	After neurosurgical procedures
	Brain abscess	Any	Ceftriaxone (or cefepime), vancomycin, and metronidazole	After neurosurgical procedures
Streptococcus milleri group	Brain abscess	Any	Ceftriaxone (or cefepime), vancomycin, and metronidazole	
Bacteroides species and other anaerobes	Brain abscess	Any	Ceftriaxone (or cefepime), vancomycin, and metronidazole	
Bacillus anthracis[26]	Meningitis	Any	Penicillin or ciprofloxacin	
Treponema pallidum[27]	Meningitis (secondary syphilis; later, meningovascular syphilis)	Any	Penicillin	Accelerated course in HIV patients
	Encephalitis (general paresis)	Older adults	Penicillin	
	Parenchymal neurosyphilis	Older adults	Penicillin	
	Tabes dorsalis	Older adults	Penicillin	
	Congenital neurosyphilis	Neonates	Penicillin	
Borrelia burgdorferi	Meningitis	Any	Ceftriaxone or doxycycline	
	Peripheral neuropathy	Any	Ceftriaxone or doxycycline	
Rickettsii (eg, *Rickettsia rickettsii*, Rocky Mountain spotted fever)	Encephalitis	Any	Doxycycline	

Organism	Manifestation	Age	Host factors
Higher bacteria			
Nocardia	Brain abscess	Any	Cell-mediated immunity defects
Actinomyces	Brain abscess	Any	
Mycobacteria			
Mycobacterium tuberculosis[28]	Meningitis	More severe in children	
	Brain abscess (tuberculoma)	Any	
	Epidural abscess (Potts disease)	Any	
Mycobacterium avium complex	Meningitis	Any	HIV patients most commonly affected
	Encephalitis	Any	HIV patients most commonly affected
Mycobacterium leprae	Peripheral neuropathy	Any	
Fungi[29]			
Aspergillus spp[30]	Brain abscess	Any	Granulocytopenic patients
	Meningitis	Any	
Cryptococcus neoformans[31]	Meningitis	Any	Patients with HIV infection and others with cell-mediated immune defects (especially steroids)
	Brain abscess	Any	Patients with HIV infection and others with cell-mediated immune defects (especially steroids)
Coccidioides immitis	Meningitis	Any	Geographically limited
	Brain abscess		
Candida albicans (and other species)	Meningitis	Any	
	Brain abscess	Any	
Rhizopus, Mucor, and related fungi	Meningitis with vasculitis	Any (usually adults)	Acidotic patients

reflect the inflammatory response produced by the host in response to the infection. In bacterial meningitis, the structural barriers imposed by the dura and the arachnoid provide substantial protection from bacterial invasion. However, infection by direct extension, usually from the skull (including the sinuses), does occur, presumably because the inoculum of the infecting organism is too large for containment by the extradural defenses. Whether the organisms reach the SAS by traversing these membranes, or via hematogenous spread, the SAS itself provides a relatively favorable location for bacterial or fungal replication. The SAS and the brain are often considered immunologically "privileged" sites, because they are extensively protected by anatomic barriers, but at the same time they partially exclude many of the cells and substances (eg, complement); when infection does occur, they are in part immunologically deprived.[9]

The major impediments to the movement of both microorganisms and inflammatory substances from the systemic circulation into the CNS are the blood-brain and blood-cerebrospinal fluid (CSF) barriers. Anatomically, these barriers reside in the investment of cerebral capillaries (which themselves have tight junctions) by astrocytic foot processes, which completely envelop the cerebral microvasculature. These barriers normally regulate the transit of molecules from the bloodstream into the brain. However, inflammation and trauma can damage the barrier, making it much less selective; matrix metalloproteinase-9 is probably a major mediator of this effect, which is not completely deleterious, because it allows many antimicrobial agents to enter the CNS in higher concentrations when an infection is present. Endogenous substances, such as complement, also cross in higher concentrations, but generally less than those of the blood. Antibodies needed to combat infection also cross, but as the inflammatory response continues, local plasma cells will produce considerably more immunoglobulin locally.[10]

The cellular components of the immune response are less dependent on changes in blood-brain and blood-CSF barrier function than the humoral components. About half of the resident macrophages of the CNS, microglia, are derived from bone marrow precursors and easily pass in and out of these otherwise protected spaces. When inflamed, the CNS releases activated complement components, cytokines (eg, tumor necrosis factor, interleukin (IL)-1β, IL-6, IL-8, and IL-10), and chemokines, which attract neutrophils and other inflammatory cells. The initial response to infection causes neutrophils in small vessels to begin rolling along the endothelial surface due to the effect of selectins; these cells are then attached to the vessel wall by integrins and soon migrate through the vessel wall under the influence of IL-8. The initial neutrophilic response to most infections is followed by other components of the macrophage/monocyte system, and the eventual arrival of lymphocytes, some of which will become plasma cells and produce antibody locally.

The CNS lacks lymphatics, so the debris of inflammation exits the parenchyma via the perivascular (Virchow-Robin) space. This space is actually a continuation of the SAS along penetrating blood vessels. Inflammatory infiltrate in this space is one of the pathologic criteria of many types of infection.[11] The accumulation of this debris in the SAS contributes to the development of cerebral arterial vasculitis and cerebral venous thrombosis, common complications of diseases such as bacterial meningitis. This observation has led to a resurgence of interest in continuous lumbar CSF drainage to decrease inflammation.[12]

Neuronal damage is partially mediated by the effects of nitric oxide (NO) and excitatory amino acids. NO is released by inflammatory cells and by neurons in the course of normal function, but when inflammatory cells undergo an oxidative burst to kill micro-organisms, the excessive NO triggers apoptosis in neurons, particularly in the hippocampi.[13] The involvement of microglia via toll-like receptors in this process indicates that the innate immune system of the brain also participates in this potentially deleterious process.[14] Understanding of the role of excitatory amino acids continues to evolve; blocking their effects may stop seizures but not apoptosis.[15]

Foreign bodies in the CNS provide locales for bacteria to multiply, with some protection from immune surveillance and attack. The bacteria involved are often less pathogenic than the usual causes of meningitis (eg, infection of ventriculo-peritoneal shunt tubing often involves *Staphylococcus epidermidis*, which produces a disease that is initially much less severe than *Staphylococcus aureus*). However, the presence of the foreign body also makes both the host immune attack and the antibiotic treatment incompletely effective; foreign bodies must often be removed to cure such an infection.

Increased ICP causes 2 major problems: interference with cerebral blood flow, and shift of structures within the cranium.

Seizures are a common manifestation of supratentorial intracranial infections, except for epidural abscesses.

NATURAL HISTORY

In the pre-antibiotic era, the natural history of most CNS infections was dismal. A few patients would recover spontaneously from bacterial meningitis, but the mortality often exceeded 90%. Epidural abscesses of the cranium or spine could be drained surgically and thus had some possibility of improvement, and brain abscesses could sometimes be treated by resection.

The prognosis of these conditions changed drastically with the availability of antimicrobial agents. The mortality of bacterial meningitis has fallen to about 30%. This percentage has remained relatively constant over the past 6 decades, which probably reflects the coincidence of more effective drugs with the development of antibiotic resistance among bacteria and the increasing number of immunocompromised patients. Data for the other, less numerous, infections are less clear but generally show a substantial benefit of antibiotic treatment.

The survivors of CNS infections are frequently left with serious neurologic compromise. Seizures and neurologic deficits are common following the otherwise successful treatment of brain abscesses and subdural empyemas. Patients who have recovered from bacterial meningitis, including tuberculous meningitis, frequently have chronic problems related to vascular complications; cranial nerve deficits are also common. Meninigitis in children may result in developmental delay; in these patients, one should exclude hearing loss as a contributor to a decline in school performance after meningitis, because auditory nerve problems are very frequent.

Tubercular and fungal meningitides generally develop signs and symptoms more chronically. Hydrocephalus, due to impairment of CSF flow at the base of the brain, and strokes, as a consequence of arterial inflammation in the circle of Willis, may be the initial manifestations. In patients with T-cell defects, cryptococcal meningitis is relatively common.

Brain abscesses may arise either by contiguous extension from a paranasal mastoid sinus or by hematogenous dissemination. The presentation depends on the organism, the location of the abscess, and the host response. About half of brain abscess patients are afebrile and have normal peripheral white blood cell counts. Seizures are a common presentation, with headache also common but often mild. Abscesses that appear to be mature, with a well-defined capsule and a core of nectrotic material on CT or MRI scans, may still be in a phase of cerebritis pathologically.

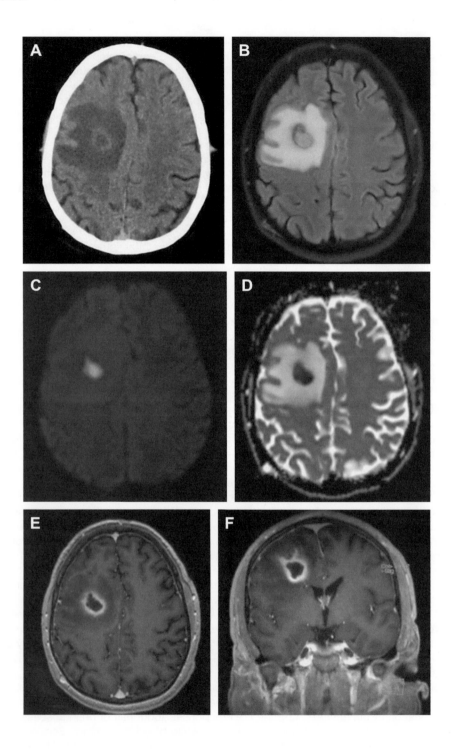

The natural history of spinal cord compression caused by an epidural abscess highlights the need for alacrity in diagnosis and treatment. When the condition is diagnosed and treated at the stage of local pain, complete recovery is typical, but if intervention is delayed until radicular symptoms are present, the spinal cord is spared but the nerve roots may not recover. When long tract findings appear, permanent disability may develop within hours; this constitutes a medical and surgical emergency, which must be managed immediately.

DIAGNOSIS

The diagnosis of acute bacterial meningitis with virulent organisms such as *Streptococcus pneumoniae* in a normal host is rarely unsuspected. The previously healthy patient who presents with headache, fever, and nuchal rigidity but without coma or focal neurologic signs should undergo a lumbar puncture as quickly as possible. If this test is delayed for other diagnostic studies, empiric antibiotic treatment for the most rapidly fatal organisms should be given, after blood cultures are obtained but before the patient undergoes radiologic studies.

CSF analysis is the cornerstone of diagnosis in the meningitides. The CSF of the typical patient with bacterial meningitis will have a neutrophilic pleocytosis, a low-glucose concentration (less than 30% of the contemporaneous plasma glucose), and an elevated protein concentration. However, antibiotic therapy, even oral antibiotics given for another reason, may shift the pleocytosis to lymphocytes within hours; this same shift may be seen early in the course of viral encephalitides and rarely with brain abscesses.

The Gram stain of the CSF often yields clues that are important both diagnostically and therapeutically, but in some bacterial meningitides the Gram stain may not demonstrate an organism; *Listeria monocytogenes* is the most important example of this phenomenon. If listeriosis is suspected, the therapeutic regimen should be expanded (see below in the Treatment section).

CSF analysis rarely yields useful microbiologic information in patients with epidural abscesses or subdural empyemas and should not be performed routinely in these patients.

◀──

Fig. 1. Different imaging studies of a brain abscess. (*A*) Unenhanced CT scan of a brain abscess. The hypodense central portion of the abscess revealed cerebritis on histologic examination, rather than necrotic material. The larger hypodense area is edema surrounding the isodense wall of the abscess itself. (*B*) Fluid attenuation inversion recovery image of the brain abscess. The edema surrounding the abscess has a high T2 signal. The fluid attenuation inversion recovery sequence suppresses the CSF signal, improving the recognition of vasogenic (extracellular) edema around the abscess. Note the midline shift. The patient presented with a single seizure without other complaints and had only subtle signs of right hemisphere dysfunction. (*C*) Diffusion-weighted image of a brain abscess. The white area indicates restricted diffusion, reflecting cytotoxic (intracellular) edema. (*D*) Apparent diffusion coefficient (ADC) map of a brain abscess. Although the ADC map has poorer spatial resolution than the diffusion-weighted image (*C*), the dark center of the lesion confirms that the bright area seen on the diffusion-weighted image reflects restricted diffusion rather than vasogenic edema. (*E*) Axial T1-weighted postinfusion image showing enhancement in the wall of the abscess corresponding to the area of new blood vessel growth; these vessels lack a mature blood-brain barrier and allow the diffusion of gadolinium into the tissue. (*F*) Coronal T1-weighted image of a brain abscess. Note the contralateral shift of the falx; this can compress the anterior cerebral arteries, resulting in ipsilateral or bilateral infarction in these territories. Also note the effacement of the right lateral ventricle.

If cryptococcal meningitis is suspected, an India ink preparation of the CSF may reveal budding yeast. More commonly, though, the diagnosis is confirmed by the presence of cryptococcal antigen in serum and CSF.

Fungal and tubercular meningitides will usually present with a lymphocytic pleocytosis. Because obstruction to CSF flow is a major problem with some of these infections, the CSF protein concentration may be very high. The CSF glucose concentration may be exceptionally low in patients with advanced tubercular meningitis. The initial differential diagnosis of patients with these more chronic meningitides is quite broad, and noninfectious causes need to be considered.[16]

Localized infections may present with focal neurologic findings, in which case the signs and symptoms will dictate the appropriate imaging study. **Fig. 1** shows the appearance of a *Fusobacterium* brain abscess on CT and with varying MR sequences. Although it is tempting to infer that the MR appearance of a lesion can definitively exclude a neoplasm, this is not yet the case, and pathologic confirmation remains a necessity.

TREATMENT

The definitive treatment of CNS infection depends on the correct identification and antimicrobial treatment of the infecting organism, relief of excessive pressure or mass effect that it exerts, and modulation of the host's immune response to allow clearance of the organism while minimizing the deleterious consequences of excessive inflammation. Empiric therapy is based on knowing the local epidemiology and antibiotic sensitivities of the organisms likely causing meningitis, and understanding the particular risk factors of the patient.[17] For example, patients with T-cell defects are at increased risk for *Listeria* meningitis, so their initial therapy should include ampicillin (perhaps with an aminoglycoside) or trimethoprim/sulfamethoxazole. If the differential diagnosis includes viral encephalitis, empiric treatment with acyclovir should be added until either another diagnosis is proven or a polymerase chain reaction study for herpes simplex virus is negative.

The emergence of penicillin and, to a lesser extent, cephalosporin resistance in pneumococci led to several changes in the empiric treatment of meningitis. Thus, empiric therapy for acute bacterial meningitis now includes a third-generation cephalosporin (eg, ceftriaxone) as well as vancomycin. Unfortunately, corticosteroid administration decreases the penetration of vancomycin into the CSF; this has limited enthusiasm for the use of steroids before antibiotic administration.[18] Nosocomial meningitides are more likely to involve resistant gram-negative rods, and the empiric regimen should include a fourth-generation cephalosporin (eg, cefepime) or a carbapenem, perhaps in concert with intrathecal or intraventricular aminoglycoside.[19]

Patients with meningitis often have nonconvulsive seizures, and their altered consciousness may be the consequence of nonconvulsive status epilepticus. Such patients should undergo continuous electroencephalogram monitoring for at least 3 days to exclude this phenomenon and guide its therapy.[20]

The use of antibiotics alone is usually inadequate in the treatment of abscesses. Thus, cranial and spinal epidural abscesses and subdural empyemas almost always require surgical or CT-guided drainage in addition to antibiotics for resolution. The situation with brain abscesses is more problematic. At the point in time when the abscess appears to have developed a capsule when viewed by CT or MR imaging, the tissue is usually still in the histologic state of cerebritis, rather than having a necrotic center that could be drained. Obtaining a sample of the infected tissue for microbiologic studies as soon as possible is important regardless of the age of the abscess, but it may be necessary to drain or resect the abscess later when it has become more mature. Second, one must choose antimicrobial agents that will achieve a useful concentration in the infected tissue. Epidural abscesses, for example, are outside of the CNS and can be treated with antibiotics that do not penetrate with brain. Clindamycin does not achieve useful concentrations in the CSF and should not be used to treat meningitis. Third, potent drugs, such as the third-generation cephalosporins, are very effective in sterilizing the CSF of many organisms causing meningitis, but the rapid release of bacterial cell wall components into the CSF prompts a profound inflammatory response, and this response is a cause of some of the complications of meningitis, such as seizures and sensorineural hearing loss. Treatment with corticosteroids before or just after the first dose of the antibiotic decreases this inflammatory response and seems to lower the incidence of some of these complications, and may provide a survival benefit.[21]

Because many brain abscesses are caused by anaerobic or mixed aerobic-anaerobic infection, empiric treatment should include metronidazole or meropenem. If metronidazole is used, the patient should also receive ceftriaxone (or cefepime if indicated based on exposure to resistant gram-negative rods), and vancomycin until Gram stain and culture results are available.

Osmotic therapy with either mannitol or hypertonic saline remains the mainstay of treatment of increased ICP.[22] Steroids may be useful in the treatment of brain abscesses, once appropriate antibiotic therapy is initiated. Hyperventilation works by reducing cerebral blood flow and should be reserved for extreme situations, such as the reversal of herniation, while waiting for osmotic agents to work, or to keep the patient alive until surgical treatment can be performed emergently.

Cranial and spinal epidural abscesses compress the CNS tissue below them and may produce permanent neurologic damage or death if the pressure is not relieved surgically in a timely manner. Subdural empyemas generally produce less mass effect, but the inflammatory response they incite damages the underlying cortex; they too should be removed expeditiously.

Fungal meningitides and abscesses should generally be treated with amphotericin pending identification of the organism and determination of its sensitivities. Tubercular infections may need empiric treatment with up to 5 agents until sensitivities are known.[23] When these infections occur in the setting of the acquired immunodeficiency syndrome, antiretroviral therapy should usually be delayed until the patient shows improvement in the signs and symptoms of infection to decrease the likelihood and severity of the immune reconstitution syndrome.[24]

REFERENCES

1. Tunkel AR. Approach to the patient with central nervous system infection. In: Mandell GM, Bennett JE, Dolin R, editors. Principles and practice of infectious diseases. 7th edition. Philadelphia: Elsevier; 2010. p. 1183–8.
2. Bleck TP, Greenlee JE. Epidural abscess. In: Mandell GM, Bennett JE, Dolin R, editors. Principles and practice of infectious diseases. 5th edition. New York: Churchill, Livingstone; 2000. p. 1031–4.
3. Bleck TP, Greenlee JE. Subdural empyema. In: Mandell GM, Bennett JE, Dolin R, editors. Principles and practice of infectious diseases. 5th edition. New York: Churchill, Livingstone; 2000. p. 1028–31.
4. Roos KL, Tunkel AR, Scheld WM. Acute bacterial meningitis. In: Scheld WM, Whitley RJ, Marra CM, editors. Infections of the central nervous system. 3rd edition. New York: LWW; 2004. p. 347–422.

5. Kastenbauer S, Pfister HW, Wispelwey B, et al. Brain abscess. In: Scheld WM, Whitley RJ, Marra CM, editors. Infections of the central nervous system. 3rd edition. New York: LWW; 2004. p. 479–508.

6. Bleck TP, Greenlee JE. Suppurative intracranial phlebitis. In: Mandell GM, Bennett JE, Dolin R, editors. Principles and practice of infectious diseases. 5th edition. New York: Churchill, Livingstone; 2000. p. 1034–6.

7. Gullipalli D, Bleck TP. Bacterial infections of the central nervous system. In: Asbury AK, McKhann GM, McDonald WI, et al, editors. Diseases of the nervous system: clinical neurobiology. 3rd edition. Philadelphia: WB Saunders; 2002. p. 1728–44.

8. Leib SL, Täuber MG. Pathogenesis and pathophysiology of bacterial infections. In: Scheld WM, Whitley RJ, Marra CM, editors. Infections of the central nervous system. 3rd edition. New York: LWW; 2004. p. 331–46.

9. Lucas SM, Rothwell NJ, Gibson RM. The role of inflammation in CNS injury and disease. Br J Pharmacol 2006;147(Suppl 1):S232–40.

10. Pfister H-W, Bleck TP. Bacterial infections. In: Brandt T, Caplan LR, Dichgans J, et al, editors. Neurological disorders: course and treatment. 2nd edition. San Diego (CA): Academic Press; 2003. p. 529–44.

11. Roberts M, Carmichael A, Martin P. Cerebral vasculitis caused by Aspergillus species in an immunocompetent adult. Infection 2004;32:360–3.

12. Abulhasan YB, Al-Jehani H, Valiquette MA, et al. Lumbar drainage for the treatment of severe bacterial meningitis. Neurocrit Care 2013;19:199–205.

13. Yamaguchi A, Tamatani M, Matsuzaki H, et al. Akt activation protects hippocampal neurons from apoptosis by inhibiting transcriptional activity of p53. J Biol Chem 2001;276:5256–64.

14. Iliev AI, Stringaris AK, Nau R, et al. Neuronal injury mediated via stimulation of microglial toll-like receptor-9 (TLR9). FASEB J 2004;18:412–4.

15. Kolarova A, Ringer R, Täuber MG, et al. Blockade of NMDA receptor subtype NR2B prevents seizures but not apoptosis of dentate gyrus neurons in bacterial meningitis in infant rats. BMC Neurosci 2003;4:21.

16. Zunt JR, Baldwin KJ. Chronic and subacute meningitis. Continuum 2012;18:1290–318.

17. Bartt R. Acute bacterial and viral meningitis. Continuum 2012;18:1255–70.

18. Bleck TP. Therapy for bacterial infections. In: Johnson RT, Griffin JW, McArthur JC, editors. Current therapy in neurologic disease. 6th edition. Chicago: Mosby-Year Book; 2002. p. 151–3.

19. Laxmi S, Tunkel AR. Healthcare-associated bacterial meningitis. Curr Infect Dis Rep 2011;13:367–73.

20. Bleck TP. Status epilepticus and the use of continuous EEG monitoring in the intensive care unit. Continuum 2012;18:560–78.

21. Fritz D, Brouwer MC, van de Beek D. Dexamethasone and long-term survival in bacterial meningitis. Neurology 2012;79:2177–9.

22. Koenig MA, Bryan M, Lewin JL 3rd, et al. Reversal of transtentorial herniation with hypertonic saline. Neurology 2008;70:1023–9.

23. Thwaites GE. Advances in the diagnosis and treatment of tuberculous meningitis. Curr Opin Neurol 2013;26:295–300.

24. Longley N, Harrison TS, Jarvis JN. Cryptococcal immune reconstitution inflammatory syndrome. Curr Opin Infect Dis 2013;26:26–34.

25. Gerner-Smidt P, Ethelberg S, Schiellerup P, et al. Invasive listeriosis in Denmark 1994-2003: a review of 299 cases with special emphasis on risk factors for mortality. Clin Microbiol Infect 2005;11:618–24.

26. Sejvar JJ, Tenover FC, Stevens DS. Management of anthrax meningitis. Lancet Infect Dis 2005;5:287–95.
27. Marra C. Neurosyphilis. In: Scheld WM, Whitley RJ, Marra CM, editors. Infections of the central nervous system. 3rd editon. New York: LWW; 2004. p. 649–58.
28. Almeida A. Tuberculosis of the spine and spinal cord. Eur J Radiol 2005;55: 193–201.
29. Perfect JR. Fungal meningitis. In: Scheld WM, Whitley RJ, Marra CM, editors. Infections of the central nervous system. 3rd edition. New York: LWW; 2004. p. 691–712.
30. Singh N. Invasive aspergillosis in organ transplant recipients: new issues in epidemiologic characteristics, diagnosis, and management. Med Mycol 2005; 43(Suppl 1):S267–70.
31. Lee SC, Dickson DW, Casadevall A. Pathology of cryptococcal meningoencephalitis: analysis of 27 patients with pathogenetic implications. Hum Pathol 1996;27: 839–47.

Catheter-Related and Infusion-Related Sepsis

Anand Kumar, MD, FRCPC[a],*, Shravan Kethireddy, MD[b],
Gloria Oblouk Darovic, RN[a]

KEYWORDS

- Intravascular cannulation • Fluid infusion • Colonization • Infection • Bacteremia
- Central venous catheter

KEY POINTS

- Although continuous vascular access is one of the most pervasive modalities in modern medicine, there is a substantial potential for producing iatrogenic complications, the most important of which is blood-borne infection.
- Clinicians often fail to consider the diagnosis of infusion-related sepsis because clinical signs and symptoms are indistinguishable from bloodstream infections arising from other sites.
- Understanding and consideration of the risk factors predisposing patients to infusion-related infections may guide the development and implementation of control measures for prevention.
- The importance of meticulously following sepsis prophylaxis in all aspects of patient care cannot be overstated.

The proliferation of increasingly complex medical and surgical therapies for the management of critically ill patients over the last 30 years is associated with tremendous technological advances during this time. Among the most important advances have been improvements in vascular access for continuous hemodynamic monitoring as well as infusion therapy for the administration of fluids, drugs, total parenteral nutrition (TPN), and blood products. Although continuous vascular access is one of the most pervasive and essential modalities in modern-day medicine, there is a substantial and generally underappreciated potential for producing iatrogenic complications, the most important of which is blood-borne infection.

Disclosures: The authors have nothing to disclose.
[a] Section of Critical Care Medicine, University of Manitoba, Winnipeg, Manitoba, Canada;
[b] Department of Critical Care and Infectious Diseases, Geisinger Health System, 100 N.Academy Road, Danville, PA 17820, USA
* Corresponding author. Section of Critical Care Medicine, Departments of Medicine, Medical Microbiology and Pharmacology/Therapeutics, Health Sciences Centre, 700 William Avenue, Winnipeg, Manitoba, R3E-0Z3 Canada.
E-mail address: akumar61@yahoo.com

Crit Care Clin 29 (2013) 989–1015
http://dx.doi.org/10.1016/j.ccc.2013.07.002
0749-0704/13/$ – see front matter © 2013 Elsevier Inc. All rights reserved.

This review focuses on the pathogenesis, diagnosis, prevention, and management of infectious complications of intravascular cannulation and fluid infusion. In this article, the term colonization refers to the presence and growth of viable microorganisms on the mucosa, skin, or in situ catheter in the absence of infection. Colonization may or may not be a precursor of infection. Infection represents a microbial phenomenon characterized by an inflammatory response to the presence of microorganisms or the invasion of normally sterile host tissue by microorganisms. Bacteremia is the presence of viable bacteria in the blood (usually demonstrated by positive blood culture). The term catheter colonization refers to the growth of significant numbers of organisms from the catheter surface in the absence of accompanying clinical symptoms. Catheter infection implies catheter colonization with accompanying clinical manifestations suggestive of infection. Health care–associated infection is any infection acquired in the hospital or health care environment. Sepsis represents the systemic response to infection (usually including various combinations of fever, tachycardia, tachypnea, and leukocytosis), typically associated with the presence of bacterial toxins and/or endogenous inflammatory mediators in the circulation. Central line–associated infection is the specific term for infection of central venous catheters whether or not it is associated with bacteremia. The general term catheter-related sepsis (CRS) relates to sepsis and septic complications, specifically attributable to the presence of intravascular catheters. Catheter-related bloodstream infection (CR-BSI) is a related term that indicates the isolation of identical infectious organisms from a catheter segment and from blood in a patient with CRS. Another related formal term, infusate-related bloodstream infection (IR-BSI), is more specific, indicating isolation of the same organism from infusate and percutaneous blood cultures. By contrast, infusion device–related sepsis (IRS) is a highly inclusive general term that relates to all sepsis and septic complications secondary to invasive monitoring and therapeutic devices including vascular catheters, fluid delivery systems, and infused solutions. Several of these terms are more precisely defined in the section on standardized microbiologic definitions of intravascular device-related infections.

EPIDEMIOLOGY

More than one-half of the 40 million patients hospitalized in the United States each year receive some form of infusion therapy.[1] Earlier estimates have suggested that nearly a million vascular device–related infections occur annually.[2] Although the prevalence of device–related infections has not been determined in the United States, in 1992 the European Prevalence of Infection in Intensive Care Study reported that 12% of patients in the intensive care unit (ICU) during a point prevalence study had a bloodstream infection.[3] The 2007 follow-up of this same study found in the 13,000 ICU patients observed, 15% had a bloodstream infection.[4] Mermel[5] estimated 80,000 to 200,000 cases of central line–associated bloodstream infections (CLA-BSIs) occur in United States ICUs annually. CLA-BSIs are an important and deadly cause of hospital-acquired infection, with a reported mortality of 12% to 25%.[6] Encouragingly, recent national initiatives have resulted in a decrease in the incidence of CLA-BSIs.

Analyzing data from several national registries, the Centers for Disease Control and Prevention (CDC) recently reported a 58% reduction (from 3.64 infections per 1000 central-line days to 1.65 infections per 1000 central-line days) in the incidence of ICU-related CLA-BSIs from 2001 to 2009, representing nearly 6000 lives saved.[6] The total cost of CLA-BSIs in the United States has been estimated at between $500 million and over $2 billion annually.[7–9] Although there has been improvement in recent years, a substantial number of CLA-BSIs continue to occur among hemo-dialysis patients both in the inpatient and outpatient setting.

The CDC has published guidelines for the prevention of intravascular device–related infections.[10] These guidelines also provide standardized microbiological definitions for catheter-related infections. Definitions are not necessarily mutually exclusive. Infusion device–related infections are classified according to the following criteria and correlate with 4 main clinical syndromes.

Contamination

Contamination is the presence of microorganisms on the catheter taken for culture, inadvertently introduced while collecting the sample. Although a colony-forming unit (CFU) count of fewer than 15 colonies on semiquantitative culture suggests contamination, there is no definitive means of differentiating a contaminated specimen from a colonized or infected specimen.

Catheter Colonization

A positive semiquantitative (>15 CFU) or quantitative (>1000 CFU) culture of either the proximal or distal catheter segment in the absence of accompanying signs of inflammation at the catheter site is considered to be synonymous with colonization of the catheter.[10–18] Some investigators have suggested that a quantitative culture of more than 100 CFU is sufficient to define colonization rather than contamination.[9,10] Colonization may occur in the complete absence of notable clinical signs or symptoms. Positive semiquantitative cultures have a 15% to 40% concordance with concomitant bacteremia and are usually, but not invariably, associated with inflammation at the insertion site.

In hospitalized patients, between 5% and 25% of intravascular catheters cultured after removal demonstrate evidence of colonization. This clinical condition is also occasionally referred to as asymptomatic catheter infection. Although this condition itself is intrinsically benign, it provides the biological substrate necessary for bacteremia.

Catheter Infection

The term catheter infection indicates a positive semiquantitative or quantitative culture of the catheter in association with accompanying signs of local inflammation (eg, erythema, warmth, swelling, or tenderness) at the device site.[10] In the absence of positive quantitative or semiquantitative cultures of a catheter segment, catheter infection can still be diagnosed when there is purulent drainage from the skin-catheter junction.

Exit-Site Infection

Erythema, tenderness, induration, and/or purulence within 2 cm of the catheter exit site that may be associated with other signs of infection, including fever, indicates an exit-site infection (infection at the catheter-insertion site).[10] This infection is usually associated with catheter colonization and may be associated with CR-BSI.

Tunnel Infection

Erythema, tenderness, and induration in the tissues overlying the catheter tract and greater than 2 cm from the catheter exit site indicate a tunnel infection. Associated signs of infection, including fever, may be present.[10]

The clinical syndrome of symptomatic local infection occurs when the colonized microorganisms have invaded and infected the tissue. An inflammatory response may be evident as local redness, pain, swelling, heat, and/or purulence at the vascular access site. However, in severely debilitated or immune-compromised patients, these classic clinical findings may be minimal or absent. The infection may primarily involve the skin and surface soft tissue (exit-site infection) or may involve the catheter tract (tunnel infection) with expressible purulence. Catheter cultures are positive, although infusate cultures may be negative. Local infection may resolve, or may become blood-borne and progress to systemic infection.

Catheter-Related Bloodstream Infection

CR-BSI is formally defined as isolation of the same organism (ie, identical species, antibiogram) from a semiquantitative or quantitative catheter-segment culture and from blood culture (preferably drawn from a peripheral vein) of a patient with clinical manifestations of bloodstream infection. Direct culture of the infusate should be nega-tive. Clinical or autopsy microbiological data should disclose no other apparent source of bacteremia. In the absence of laboratory confirmation, defervescence after catheter removal may serve as indirect evidence of CR-BSI.[10,11,13–15,19]

Infusate-Related Bloodstream Infection

IR-BSI is formally defined as isolation of the same organism from infusate and from separate percutaneous blood cultures, with no other identifiable source of infec-tion.[10–12,19] Typically the patient has clinical and laboratory evidence of sepsis. Culture of the catheter is negative or isolates an unrelated organism. This term is much more specific than the term IRS as used in this article.

Sepsis from an infected catheter or contaminated infusate is a clinical condition whereby the signs of local inflammation may or may not be present. Symptoms and/or signs of systemic infection are invariably present. Low-grade fever is a common presenting symptom of patients with systemic infusion-related infection involving *Staphylococcus epidermidis*. Other organisms may produce marked hyper-thermia (pyrexia/fever) or hypothermia, depending on the organism and the patient's overall health, and nutritional and immune status. Blood cultures may be positive and, if so, should match the catheter or infusate culture. Septic shock is rare; contaminated infusate is more likely to be associated with shock than is catheter infection or CR-BSI.

Septic thrombophlebitis or endarteritis is a severe complication of an infected cath-eter. Each produces high-grade and unremitting bacteremia or fungemia with fulmi-nant signs of overwhelming infection, which persist even after the catheter has been removed.[20–22] These forms of catheter-related infection are the most serious, and usually originate from central venous catheters that have been used for prolonged periods in patients at high risk of health care–associated infection.[20,21] The cannulated segment of the vessel becomes filled by an infected thrombus. The clinical course is predictable: unremitting bloodstream infection that often proves fatal. Of interest, patients with suppuration of the infected thrombus (suppurative phlebitis) may develop signs and symptoms of systemic infection only after the catheter has been removed.[20] Culture of the catheter is positive. Organisms isolated from the blood, thrombus, or adjacent resected parts of the vessel should match those isolated from the catheter.

PATHOGENESIS OF INFUSION-RELATED SEPSIS

When a catheter is placed in a blood vessel, a fibrin sheath quickly develops around the catheter. The clot generally produces no circulatory problem, but serves as a nidus for bacterial or fungal colonization.[20] Bacterial or fungal colonization of the intravas-cular device may occur via several mechanisms.

Migration of Cutaneous Flora Down the Skin Tract to the Intravascular Catheter

Aerobic microorganisms of cutaneous origin, such as coagulase-negative *Staphylococcus* (usually *S epidermidis*), *Staphylococcus aureus*, enterococci, or *Candida*, gain intravascular access through the insertion wound. The insertion site is commonly colonized heavily by the patient's endogenous cutaneous flora or becomes colonized by microorganisms from the hands of the medical personnel inserting or manipulating the catheter.[11,12,20,21,23–25] Maki and colleagues,[12] in a prospective study of 234 central venous catheters, found that the majority of early infections of percutaneously inserted central venous catheters originated from the skin at the insertion site rather than contamination of the hub. Overall, in venous catheters there is a strong correlation between skin microorganisms present on the catheter-insertion site and microorganisms implicated in CRS based on molecular typing.[11,12,24,25] The most common organism found in catheter-related infection is *S epidermidis*, the predominant aerobic species on the human skin. The risk of other, more pathogenic organisms rises with the presence and duration of severe illness.

Bloodstream Dissemination and Catheter Colonization from a Distant Septic Focus

The vascular catheter may become colonized by hematogenous seeding from remote sites of infection. For example, if patients have *Escherichia coli* bacteremia from an intra-abdominal source, vascular catheters may become seeded and colonized with *E coli*. The infected catheter may then, in turn, reseed the blood, thus propagating systemic infection even if the original septic focus has been eliminated. It has been suggested that CRS from certain organisms (yeast, enterococci, and enteric gram negatives) may often result from hematogenous spread.[26,27]

Manipulation and Contamination of the Catheter Hub

The hub of the catheter also may be a potential source of CRS. Sitges-Serra and colleagues[28] have suggested that the hub of the central venous catheter, rather than the intracutaneous tract, is the most important source of microorganisms that infect the catheter and bloodstream. These investigators reported little correlation between organisms found on the patient's skin and organisms found on the hub and on the catheter, but frequent contamination of catheter hubs and correlation with bacteremia. It was suggested that hubs became colonized during manipulation by clinicians. Maki and colleagues[12] have confirmed the occurrence of hub contamination, but were unable to demonstrate a major role in early CRS. Through the use of electron microscopy, Raad and colleagues[29] were able to demonstrate that hub contamination was the more likely mechanism of infection for long-term catheters (>30 days). Skin contamination was more likely in catheters in place for fewer than 10 days.

Contamination of the Delivery System

The catheter and hub are not the only elements of a vascular infusion that can produce infection. The delivery system, consisting of the fluid (infusate), stopcock, pressure transducer, and tubing, also can be a source of contamination, particularly epidemic nosocomial bacteremia (especially gram-negative bacteremia).[1,22,30,31]

Ostensibly closed delivery systems are frequently disrupted for the addition of medications and electrolytes, as well as withdrawal of blood for specific hemodynamic studies by members of the ICU staff. Accidental disconnection or leaks in the closed system may also occur. Overall, any disruption of the closed system and manipulation of infusion fluids may introduce microorganisms into the system.

Arterial lines are particularly vulnerable to contamination because they are so heavily manipulated. In all monitoring systems, meticulous care of stopcocks, replacing the sterile caps (deadheads) after withdrawal of blood, and flushing the sampling port of remaining blood are essential in the prevention of delivery-system contamination.

Infusate Contamination

Infusate contamination may also be a source of bacteremia or fungemia, but infusate-related infection can be identified only if the solution is cultured. This action is rarely taken in clinical practice because despite occasional epidemics, endemic bacteremia caused by extrinsically contaminated fluid during administration seems to be rare.[11,12,21] Based on anecdotal data, risk of infusate contamination may be higher with TPN and intravenous lipid emulsion–based medications such as propofol.[32–34]

DIAGNOSIS OF INFUSION-RELATED SEPSIS

Clinicians too often fail to consider the diagnosis of infusion-related sepsis, because clinical signs and symptoms are generally indistinguishable from bloodstream infections arising from other sites, such as the urinary tract or lung. Inflammation at the insertion site is not predictive of CR-BSI with short-term uncuffed catheters.[35] Sepsis from infected catheters and contaminated infusate also produce similar clinical features.[20] In general, the diagnosis of catheter-related or infusate-related infection should be considered whenever the patient has systemic or catheter-insertion site signs or symptoms of infection, particularly if the patient has no other identifiable septic focus. Maki[21,36] has listed 6 clinical and 3 microbiological findings that should alert the clinician to the possibility of infusion-related sepsis and prompt appropriate cultures and, in most cases, discontinuation of the infusion and removal of the catheter (**Box 1**).

Box 1
Findings suggestive of infusion-related sepsis

Clinical

1. Intravascular device in place at time of onset of sepsis, bacteremia, or candidemia (especially central venous catheter)

2. Patient is an unlikely candidate for sepsis, being young or without underlying predisposing diseases

3. Inflammation or expressible purulence at the catheter insertion site

4. Primary bacteremia or candidemia without apparent source of local infection

5. Precipitous onset of overwhelming sepsis with shock (often indicating massively contaminated infusate or intravascular suppuration)

6. Sepsis refractory to appropriate antimicrobial therapy or substantial improvement following removal of catheter or discontinuation of infusion

Microbiological

1. Bacteremia caused by staphylococci (especially coagulase-negative staphylococci), *Bacillus* species, *Corynebacterium* species, *Candida* species, and certain fungi or mycobacteria

2. Clusters of institutional outbreaks of sepsis due to *Enterobacter* species, *Serratia marcescens,* or *Pseudomonas* species other than *P aeruginosa*

3. High-grade candidemia (greater than 25 CFU/mL peripheral blood)

When CRS or IRS is suspected, ideally several cultures should be obtained, which should include a blood culture drawn from the suspected catheter, one or more peripheral blood cultures (from separate venipuncture sites) and, if the clinical presentation warrants, culture of the infusate in broth. If the suspected catheter is removed, semiquantitative tip culture should be performed. Blood cultures should be drawn before antibiotic administration whenever possible.

A firm diagnosis of IRS can be made only by demonstrating a colonized intravascular catheter or contamination of infusion solution, associated with culture-determined bacteremia or fungemia caused by the same microbial strain.[21] Negative catheter tip and infusion solution culture findings in the presence of bacteremia or fungemia strongly suggest that the intravenous device and solution are not the septic source.

When IRS is suspected, the catheter should be removed if possible (exceptions include limited situations involving surgically tunneled catheters or catheters that are unquestionably necessary and would be extremely risky to replace; in such situations, treatment of the catheter in situ may be attempted). The intravascular segment of the catheter is severed aseptically and then cultured.[20,21] Catheter segments may be cultured semiquantitatively rather than using broth cultures (qualitative culture). The clinical interpretation of a positive catheter culture in liquid media is uncertain because a single contaminating organism acquired from the skin as the catheter is being removed can produce a positive culture.[13] Positive broth-culture findings have not correlated well with signs of catheter-site inflammation either. The percentage of catheters showing positive cultures in broth is often many times higher than the true rate of CRS.[13]

The semiquantitative culture technique described by Maki and colleagues is now widely used to diagnose catheter-related infection. The proper method in obtaining the relevant catheter segments is crucial in ensuring reliable results.[14,15,24,31] For short catheters (arterial, peripheral venous): following catheter removal, aseptically cut the portion of the catheter that was within the vessel and transport it to the laboratory in a sterile container. For long catheters (central venous or pulmonary artery), obtain 2 segments for culture: a proximal segment that began several millimeters inside the former skin-catheter interface and the tip of the catheter. In the laboratory, the catheter segment is rolled or smeared (if unable to be rolled) back and forth across the plate. The plate is then incubated. Detecting 15 or more colonies growing on a semiquantitative plate is regarded as a positive culture. Positive semiquantitative cultures have a 15% to 40% concordance with concomitant bacteremia and are strongly associated with inflammation at the insertion site.[12–15,21,24,31]

The more arduous quantitative culture techniques using broth culture of catheter segments (>100–1000 CFU defines true colonization) have proponents.[16–18] However, studies suggest that culture of the external surface of the catheter segment, which reflects the microbiological status of the percutaneous wound and intravascular environment, distinguishes true catheter-related infection from contamination more reliably than the quantitative broth culture method.[13] Culturing catheters semiquantitatively also allows for more rapid identification of clinically significant isolates, because microbial growth usually occurs within 12 to 18 hours, whereas quantitative (broth) culture growth may take 24 to 48 hours. As a practical matter, most centers offer semiquantitative catheter culture rather than quantitative.

For those catheters that cannot be removed and safely replaced, comparison of quantitative peripheral and catheter-drawn blood cultures can make the diagnosis of catheter-associated bacteremia or fungemia (without catheter removal) with sensitivity and specificity of approximately 90%.[36–40] Quantitative cultures of blood drawn from infected central venous catheters are usually 5 to 10 times higher than those from peripheral blood. Similarly, intraluminal brushes[41] and specialized staining of cytospin of lysed blood[42] drawn from infected central lines shows potential in the diagnosis of CRS without removal of the catheter. Another approach currently in development involves using polymerase chain reaction (PCR) to look for bacterial 16S ribosomal DNA in blood samples drawn from the catheter. Concentrations of such DNA above a certain threshold have been shown to have a very high predictive value for CR-BSI in febrile patients.[43]

An intriguing and potentially immediately useful new approach to the noninvasive diagnosis of CRS involves comparison of time to positivity of blood cultures drawn simultaneously from the catheter and peripheral sites.[44,45] Greater than 120 minutes' difference in time to detection of growth from the catheter versus peripheral site appears to be highly suggestive of catheter infection. However, all these techniques make medical and economic sense only in assessment of long-term indwelling catheters in cases where intraluminal colonization is likely, and where the patient's condition makes removal and replacement of the intravascular catheter unacceptably risky.

Safdar and colleagues[46] have recently performed a meta-analysis on the utility of a variety of currently available diagnostic tests for infusion-related sepsis. Overall, paired quantitative peripheral and catheter blood cultures were found to be superior to other techniques for diagnosis when such samples could be obtained, while quantitative segmental cultures appeared to be the most useful catheter culture technique.

A sudden onset of septic symptoms shortly after the start of infusion is suggestive of contamination of the intravenous fluid. If infusate contamination is suspected, the infusion must be immediately terminated. The entire infusate apparatus and infusate bag should be transported to the microbiology laboratory, where the infusate can be aseptically removed and cultured in broth.

A recommended approach to assessment of fever/sepsis in a patient with a central venous catheter is outlined in **Fig. 1**.

MICROORGANISMS ASSOCIATED WITH INFUSION-RELATED SEPSIS

CRS is associated with 2 major groups of organisms, those that are part of the normal skin flora (coagulase-negative staphylococci [CNS], S aureus, Bacillus species, Corynebacterium species) and those organisms that are transferred from the hands of medical staff and equipment (Pseudomonas aeruginosa, Acinetobacter species, Stenotrophomonas maltophila, and Candida species). Certain microorganisms are so prevalent in catheter-related infection that their recovery from blood should substantially raise the suspicion that an intravascular catheter is the source. These organisms include S aureus, S epidermidis, and Candida, the most common microorganisms in sepsis from infected catheters. For example, high-grade candidemia (>25 CFU/mL of peripheral blood) indicates CR-BSI in more than 90% of cases.[47]

Contaminated infusate solutions are strongly suggested by isolation of Enterobacter cloacae, Enterobacter agglomerans, or Pseudomonas cepacia, because these are major pathogens in sepsis from contaminated fluid.[20–22,30,31] The latter gram-negative organisms are able to multiply rapidly in 5% dextrose in water solution.[20–22,30] For this reason, the use of dextrose-containing solutions as irrigants for intravascular monitoring catheters should be discouraged.

S epidermidis is a normal skin inhabitant. For this reason, in the past blood-culture reports of S epidermidis were considered to be the result of skin contamination. Studies of central venous and peripheral venous catheter–related infections indicate that CNS such as S epidermidis are now the most common pathogens in intravenous

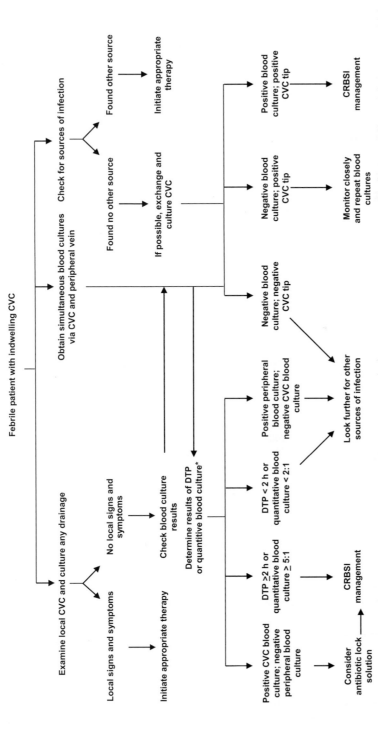

Fig. 1. Diagnosis of acute febrile episode in a patient with a central venous catheter. CVC, central venous catheter; DTP, differential time to positivity. Asterisk indicates that a blood culture is considered positive if the ratio of colony forming units growing from simultaneously drawn central and peripheral blood is at least 5:1 or the DTP is at least 2 hours (central blood culture turns positive before simultaneously drawn peripheral blood culture). (*From* Raad I, Hanna H, Maki D. Intravascular catheter-related infections: advances in diagnosis, prevention, and management. Lancet Infect Dis 2007;7:646; with permission.)

catheter–related sepsis and one of the most important pathogens in infection of all types of percutaneous and implantable devices.[11,12,20–25] CNS are important nosocomial pathogens because of their increasing resistance to many commonly used antibiotic agents, and their ability to adhere to and colonize vascular catheters. Many strains can withstand the application of topical antiseptics, and can grow well on foreign bodies and disrupted epithelium.[20–22]

The approach to therapy with specific pathogens and catheters is described in **Fig. 2**.

RISK FACTORS FOR INFUSION-RELATED SEPSIS

Understanding and consideration of the risk factors and sources of microorganisms predisposing patients to infusion-related infections may guide the development and implementation of control measures for prevention of these potentially lethal complications. The risk factors that predispose the patient to infusion-related sepsis include (1) patient factors, (2) concomitant therapies, and (3) catheter-specific factors (**Box 2**).

Patient Factors

Many patient and therapeutic factors predict an increased risk of health care–associated infection. Prospective studies[22,48–50] have shown that the following factors are associated with an increased risk of infection: age older than 65 years; severe and numerous underlying diseases; sepsis; major trauma, surgery, or burns; invasive devices; underlying immune system dysfunction and/or immunosuppressive drugs; breakdown of anatomic barriers; and confinement in a critical care environment.

Therapy-Related Factors

Overall, patients in ICUs have the highest risk profile for complicating infection. Most of these patients endure prolonged hospitalization and have serious underlying conditions associated with disease-related impairment of the immune system. Virtually all critically ill patients are exposed to multiple invasive procedures and monitoring equipment, and many receive TPN or acute hemodialysis, both of which are associated with an increased risk of IRS.[51] Increased nurse workload also appears to be a substantial risk factor for catheter-related infections.[52]

Catheter-Related Factors

Poor aseptic technique (such as during traumatic vascular catheter insertion) is unquestionably associated with a risk of catheter or infusate infection. This risk is related to not only the technique (Seldinger technique vs surgical cutdown) in catheter insertion, but also the quality of aseptic technique during vascular line maintenance. Catheter introduction using the Seldinger technique (catheter over a guide wire) for percutaneous catheter placement has almost completely replaced the cutdown technique for vascular access. In addition, studies have shown that the use of a trained team for catheter insertion and maintenance can significantly reduce central venous catheter infection rates.[53–55]

The longer the vascular catheter is left in situ, the greater the risk for local and systemic infection. An indwelling time longer than 5 days significantly increases the risk of catheter-related infection.[36,56] The necessity of breaking the closed fluid-filled delivery system and the requirements for catheter manipulation compound any risk factors inherent to the specific type of catheter.

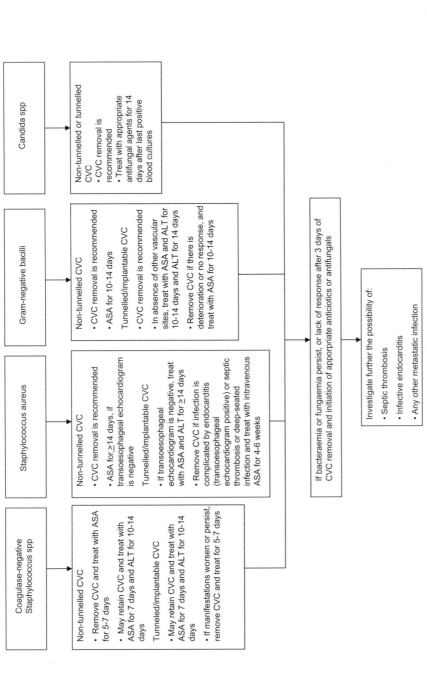

Fig. 2. Management of catheter-related bloodstream infections. ALT, antibiotic-lock therapy; ASA, appropriate systemic antibiotic; CRBSI, catheter-related bloodstream infection; CVC, central venous catheter. (*From* Raad I, Hanna H, Maki D. Intravascular catheter-related infections: advances in diagnosis, prevention, and management. Lancet Infect Dis 2007;7:645–57; with permission.)

Box 2
Risk factors for infusion-related sepsis

Patient-Related Factors

1. Extremes of age (neonates or age greater than 65 years)
2. Critical illness/sepsis
3. Remote active infection with coincident vascular catheter
4. Impaired host defenses
5. Major trauma
6. Major surgery
7. Major burn injury
8. Malnutrition
9. Immunosuppressive diseases (eg, diabetes mellitus, uremia, chronic alcoholism, liver disease, neutropenia)
10. Interruption of anatomic barriers (eg, severe psoriasis or eczema, major burns or wounds, mucositis)

Therapy-Related Factors

1. Catheter insertion or maintenance by other than a dedicated team
2. Multiple invasive devices
3. Hospitalization in intensive care unit
4. Use of immunosuppressive or antibiotic drugs
5. Use of total parenteral nutrition
6. Excessive time intervals (longer than 5 days) between replacements of components of the delivery system
7. Excessive time intervals between dressing changes (longer than 3 days) or failure to change dressings when soiled
8. Faulty decontamination of transducer between patients (reusable transducers)

Catheter-Specific Factors

1. Open surgical placement (cutdown rather than percutaneous)
2. Emergent rather than elective catheter insertion
3. Use of polyvinyl chloride or polyethylene catheters, polyurethane, or Teflon (for peripheral intravenous catheters)
4. Complex closed delivery system with multiple stopcocks and other ports
5. Interruption of closed fluid-filled system or need for catheter manipulation after initial insertion
6. Prolonged intravascular retention (longer than 5 days)
7. Suboptimal skin decontamination (2% chlorhexidine is superior to 10% povidone-iodine or 70% alcohol)
8. Use of multilumen rather than single-lumen catheter (possible)
9. Failure to use antiseptic or antibiotic-bonded catheter
10. Failure to use catheter with silver-impregnated tissue cuff
11. Internal jugular rather than subclavian insertion site (femoral site risk intermediate)

CATHETER MATERIAL

The major infectious risk factor is whether the catheter material provides an attractive surface for adherence by pathogenic microorganisms, such as S epidermidis.[57,58] Most published research linking type of catheter material and infection risk has been done in peripheral intravenous catheters. In vitro studies have shown that Teflon, silicone, and polyurethane are more resistant to adherence by CNS than polyvinyl chloride and polyethylene.[59,60] Although conflicting, current data do not support conclusions linking central venous catheter materials to risk of infection.[10]

The development of intravascular catheters and implantable devices that resist microbial adherence as well as fibrin formation, while retaining desired flexibility characteristics, must receive high priority. This goal remains a major challenge to manufacturers.

SPECIFIC CENTRAL VENOUS CATHETER INSERTION SITES

Studies of pulmonary artery and central venous catheters have revealed that there is an increased risk of CRS with insertion in the jugular vein in comparison with insertion in the subclavian vein.[61-63] This risk may be caused by heavier skin colonization with gram-negative rods and yeasts, owing to the catheter being placed close to the openings of the respiratory tract (tracheostomy tube, nose, mouth).

Placement in the femoral veins is generally not preferred because of the heavy growth of bacteria and yeast in the area, the likelihood of site contamination if the patient is involuntary of stool and/or incontinent of urine, the difficulty in keeping the groin dressing intact and sterile, and the difficulty in immobilizing the patient's leg and the risk of deep venous thrombosis incited by the presence of the catheter. Some data suggest an increased infection risk with femoral venous catheterization in comparison with subclavian and internal jugular sites.[64] Peripherally inserted central catheters (PICCs), despite suggestions to the contrary, appear to be associated with an infection risk comparable with that of standard central venous catheters when assessed in comparable (high-risk) groups of patients.[65,66]

SEPTIC RISK SPECIFIC TO TYPES OF VASCULAR CATHETERS

Catheter-related bacteremia or fungemia is the most frequent serious complication of these devices. In fact, 80% to 90% of intravascular device–related bacteremias and candidemias arise from central venous catheters,[63,67,68] and central venous catheterization is the single greatest risk factor for nosocomial candidemia.[69-71] The rate of catheter-related infection with central venous catheters is far higher than with peripheral venous catheters, which is in the range of 2% to 7%.[12,14,15,23–25,27,28,72–78]

Except for pulmonary artery catheters, central venous catheters generally have either single or triple lumens. Studies have reported inconsistent results regarding the risk of infection with single-lumen versus triple-lumen catheters. For example, one study[74] reported an incidence of catheter-associated bacteremia of 3.1% with triple-lumen catheters; all bacteremias were caused by S epidermidis. However, this study concluded that catheter-related infection occurred with similar frequency between single-lumen and triple-lumen catheters. A meta-analysis/systematic review, however, demonstrated that triple-lumen catheters were associated with an increased incidence of CRS when compared with single-lumen catheters.[79] In this analysis, 1 CR-BSI was prevented for every 20 single-lumen (rather than triple-lumen) catheter inserted. An important factor to consider is that in this latter study, the patients with triple-lumen catheters were more ill, and therefore at greater risk of CRS, than patients with single-lumen catheters. A single trial has suggested that infection risk is unaffected when TPN is delivered by single-, double-, or triple-lumen catheters.[80]

Among the variety of central venous catheters, hemodialysis catheters are associated with the highest risk of CRS, at approximately 10%.[81–83] The lowest risk of infection is with cuffed, tunneled, surgically implanted devices (eg, Hickman, Broviac) with infection risks of 0.2% to 0.5%.[36] PICCs have been reputed to carry an extremely low (<1%) risk of infection,[66] and this is certainly the case in the usual, low-risk outpatient setting. However, in recent years such catheters have become more commonly used in high-risk ICU patients. Safdar and Maki[65] have shown that use of PICCs in such patients is associated in infection rates similar to those for standard central venous catheters.

Pulmonary artery catheters, once a hallmark of critical care management, have substantially declined in usage given a large body of evidence that invasive devices do not decrease mortality. Mermel[61] previously had estimated the rate of CRS to be 0.7%. The investigators concluded that with "reasonable care" the risk of bacteremic infection is low, generally in the range of 1.0%.

Arterial pressure monitoring with arterial catheters, on the other hand, remains an essential component in the management of more than 80% of the 4 to 5 million patients cared for in the ICUs in United States hospitals each year. Maki and Ringer[11] conducted a prospective study of 489 percutaneously inserted arterial catheters in a large medical-surgical ICU, using microbiological methods for identification of all potential sources of infusion-related infection. The septic risk was found to be very low, with local catheter-related infection at 3.1% and infusate-related or hub-related infections at 0.8%. This rate of invasive infection is 3- to 6-fold lower than that encountered with central venous catheters used in similar ICU patients for a comparable period of time in situ.[20,33] Although the rate of infection with arterial catheters was low in this large study, other studies have suggested an equivalent infection risk with arterial catheters when compared with central venous catheters.[84] Flush solutions used for hemodynamic monitoring are vulnerable to contamination, and are the most important cause of epidemic infusion-related gram-negative bacteremia in ICU patients.

MANAGEMENT OF CATHETER-RELATED AND INFUSION-RELATED SEPSIS

A common error seen in management of catheter colonization is the assumption that a colonizing organism does not represent infection or high risk of infection. The question of how to handle catheter asymptomatic colonization of intravascular catheters (semiquantitative count >15 CFU) in the absence of positive blood cultures is difficult, owing to the lack of randomized trials. Certainly routine screening of cultures from extracted catheters frequently yields evidence of colonization with commensals in asymptomatic patients. Most of these do not require therapy. However, catheter tip colony counts of greater than 15 CFU with certain pathogens are clearly associated with increased risk of CR-BSIs.[85,86] As a consequence, catheter colonization with pathogenic noncommensals including S aureus, gram negatives, and Candida species require empiric antimicrobial therapy even in the absence of signs of clinical infection and positive blood cultures.

Without evidence of clinical sepsis or documented bacteremia, most clinicians will not treat patients with antibiotics if catheter colonization with commensal organisms is found following catheter removal. On the other hand, such catheters are sometimes switched over a guide wire. If the original catheter tip grows to greater than 15 CFU, any new catheter placed into the same site over a guide wire should be removed.

In all cases, patients who have experienced high-grade catheter-related bacteremia or candidemia should always be assessed carefully for the development of late complications, including endocarditis or other metastatic complications.[36] This aspect is particularly important for infections with *Candida* species and *S aureus* and for those patients with intravascular prosthetic devices including heart valves.

Recent data suggest that many infected central venous catheters, particularly those infected with coagulase-negative staphylococci, can be effectively treated without catheter removal. However, there is a significant risk of recurrent bacteremia (approximately 20% after 3 weeks vs 3% if the catheter is removed).[87] Because the presence of an infected catheter puts the patient at risk for serious septic complications including septic thrombosis and endocarditis, such an approach should be reserved only for those catheters that cannot be easily and safely replaced. As a general rule, any short-term intravascular catheter suspected of being the source of sepsis (unexplained fever, local inflammation, cryptogenic staphylococcal bacteremia, or candidemia) should be removed and replaced. Exceptions should be limited to those patients with severe coagulopathy/thrombocytopenia or exceptional problems with venous access whereby removal and/or replacement is untenable.

By contrast, CRS associated with surgically implanted catheters (eg, Hickman, Broviac) can be assessed for in situ antibiotic treatment. An attempt at antibiotic treatment with retention of the catheter may be worthwhile if there is no evidence of a persistent exit-site infection, tunnel infection, endocarditis, septic thrombosis, or septic shock; if the infecting organism is other than *Corynebacterium jeikeium*, *S aureus*, *Bacillus* species, *Stenotrophomonas* species, yeast, fungus or mycobacteria; and if bacteremia or candidemia has persisted for less than 3 days.[36] Up to two-thirds of CRS in surgically implanted catheters (apart from those conditions listed here) may be cured with antibiotics administered through the device for 7 to 10 days.[71,88–93] Bacteremia caused by CRS in such devices may be cured even more simply by locking a concentrated antibiotic-containing solution (usually vancomycin or an aminoglycoside) into the lumen of the catheter for 12 hours per day for 2 weeks.[94,95] If this approach is attempted, early initiation of therapy is important to maximize chances of cure.[96]

The role of local thrombolytics in in situ therapy for catheter-related infection is unclear. Some advocate such an approach as part of therapy for retained catheters, because local thrombosis is known to be associated with catheter infections and should theoretically make it more difficult to clear an infection.[93,97] However, to date no randomized trial has been performed to definitively answer this question. For this reason, there are no uniformly accepted recommendations regarding this issue.

PREVENTION OF CATHETER-RELATED AND INFUSION-RELATED SEPSIS

Infection and infectious sequelae, such as sepsis and multiple system organ failure, are the most common causes of death in surgical and trauma ICUs. It has been estimated that the ICU incidence of nosocomial sepsis is 24 times higher than that of general medical-surgical areas.[98] One major reason for this high incidence of health care–associated infection in the ICU is that invasive devices, which are a major risk factor for sepsis, are a standard part of ICU patient care; their use should, therefore, be kept to a minimum. The importance of meticulously following sepsis prophylaxis in all aspects of patient care cannot be overstated. An advisory statement on prevention of intravascular catheter-related infection has been published and is recommended for those requiring a detailed analysis.[8] A simple "golden rule" on this issue is never to insert an intravascular device without a clear indication and never retain that device longer than the minimum period required. Abbreviated suggestions for the prophylaxis and management of infusion-related sepsis are discussed here.

Hand Washing

Infusion-related infections may originate from microorganisms present on the hands of medical personnel inserting or manipulating the devices. The hands of the caregiver are a primary source of antibiotic-resistant bacterial contamination that causes health care–associated infection. Vigorous rubbing together of all lathered hand surfaces for a minimum of 10 seconds (preferably for 30 seconds) is one of the oldest yet most important infection control measures before and after manipulating any invasive device. Wearing gloves may provide an additional measure of patient safety when the closed fluid system requires disruption (changing connecting tubing or stopcocks, and/or aspiration of blood).

Antiseptic hand-washing soaps do not reduce the amount of time, friction, or water required for effective hand degerming. Consistent, careful hand-washing technique and gloving also protects caregivers from acquiring transferable diseases such as hepatitis, acquired immune deficiency diseases, and herpetic infections.

Dedicated Infusion Therapy Team/Training

Many studies have conclusively demonstrated that the use of a dedicated infusion therapy team for intravascular catheter placement and care can substantially reduce the risk of IRS by up to 8-fold.[53,99] If such a team is not possible, rigorous training of nurses and physicians involved in catheter insertion and care, along with meticulous adherence to catheter care protocols, can achieve similar results.[100,101] This latter approach is specifically recommended in an advisory statement by a group of experts in the field.[8]

Skin Disinfection

A strong concordance exists between microorganisms colonizing catheters and the skin at the catheter-insertion site.[11,12,24,25] The data in related studies suggest that the importance of reliable suppression of the skin microflora with an antiseptic solution before catheter insertion and the follow-up care of the insertion site cannot be overemphasized.

The ideal means of skin disinfection (nonirritating and effective in antimicrobial activity) has not yet been identified. In a study by Maki and colleagues,[102] insertion sites were disinfected with 70% alcohol, 10% povidone-iodine, or 2% aqueous chlorhexidine, by random allocation. Alcohol and povidone-iodine were equivalent in protection against infection but significantly less effective than chlorhexidine in preventing catheter-related infection.[102] Although other studies have failed to show such a difference,[103] chlorhexidine has been recommended as the first-line antiseptic for prevention of infection with percutaneously inserted intravascular devices of all types.[103] Other studies demonstrate a decreased risk of CRS with use of a topical polyantibiotic regiment (polymyxin B, neomycin, bacitracin) or mupirocin (an antistaphylococcal agent).[104,105] One study has shown superiority of 5% povidone-iodine in 70% ethanol over the 10% aqueous form.[106] Future studies should examine other agents for cutaneous disinfection to improve the effectiveness and duration of flora suppression at the catheter-insertion site. Even with adequate suppression of skin microflora at the time of insertion, the suppressed microorganisms can rapidly grow back and invade the wound.

SURGICAL ASEPTIC TECHNIQUE FOR INTRAVASCULAR CATHETER INSERTION

For central venous catheter insertion, the operator and assistant should wear gown, gloves, and mask, and the patient should be surgically draped. All those assisting in the room should wear a surgical mask and cap. When possible, the door to the room should be closed during the insertion procedure, and the number of persons entering and leaving the room should be limited. The use of maximal barrier precautions has been shown to result in a highly significant 4- to 6-fold decrease in the risk of catheter-related infections.[33,61,107]

INTRAVASCULAR CATHETER DRESSING PROTOCOL

To prevent contamination of the insertion site, a sterile occlusive dressing should be applied. The dressing and not the tape should cover the wound. The date of catheter insertion should be recorded where it can be easily found, such as in the medical record and, if possible, directly on the dressing or tape.

As discussed earlier, there is a strong correlation between microorganisms present at the catheter-insertion site and microorganisms implicated in CRS. In the past it was believed that frequent dressing changes at the site would reduce the incidence of CRS. Studies regarding dressing material and frequency of dressing changes have produced conflicting results. At this point, the CDC has no recommendation on the frequency of dressing changes or the type of dressing material.[10] However, dressings should be changed also whenever wet, soiled with drainage, or disrupted. Wet dressings particularly favor bacterial growth.

A semipermeable clear membrane dressing has been introduced in recent years. Vasquez and Jarrad[108] studied one such dressing, Opsite, and found an overall CRS rate of 1% for the 100 patients studied. It was concluded that Opsite was both a safe and cost-effective dressing for central venous catheters. Young and colleagues[109] also compared a standard protocol of gauze changed 3 times per week with Opsite changed 3 times per week, or every 7 to 10 days. Sepsis rates were low in all groups. It was concluded by these investigators that Opsite could be safely left in place for up to 7 days. However, 2 studies[110,111] have revealed a much higher incidence of catheter-related infection and sepsis when transparent dressings were used for central venous catheters. Patients were found to have higher rates of colonization of the subcutaneous tract and subsequent bacteremia that coincided with microorganisms found at the catheter-insertion site.[111] Bacterial colonization may actually be enhanced when moisture accumulates under the transparent dressing. Transparent dressings are less bulky and allow for visualization of the site while being vapor-permeable and waterproof. Further studies are required to determine the safety and efficacy of transparent polyurethane dressings. Sterile gauze and an antimicrobial ointment are currently acceptable and economical dressings.

The recent development of a chlorhexidine sponge of about 1-inch (2.5 cm) diameter that can be affixed over the catheter-insertion site has shown promise in at least one study.[112] In another meta-analysis, a trend toward decreased vascular and epidural catheter infection was shown.[113] However, other studies have been contradictory, and guidelines do not support this approach at this time.

Regular maintenance and observation of the intravenous site are important for prevention or early detection of intravenous-related complications.[114] Intravenous sites should be inspected at least every 24 hours. If visual inspection is not possible, the insertion site should be gently palpated to detect pain, tenderness, or swelling. At each dressing change and at catheter removal, the insertion site should be observed for erythema, purulence, swelling, and tenderness.

INFUSION SYSTEM PROTOCOLS

Intraluminal antibiotic locks as part of routine catheter care may be effective in reducing intraluminal colonization and infection rates.[115–117] Antibiotics that can be locked into the infusion ports with a reduction in IRS include aminoglycosides and minocycline.[117] A recent meta-analysis has demonstrated that this vancomycin lock can halve the incidence of CR-BSI.[118] Despite this, vancomycin locking is not currently recommended because of the risk of the development of vancomycin-resistant organisms (especially enterococci).

Most IRS is, in fact, CRS. However, contamination of the infusate may occur, often in the setting of a cluster. Historically, United States hospital practice has been to routinely replace the entire infusion delivery system on a 24- to 48-hour basis to reduce the risk from extrinsically contaminated fluid.[20] This action minimizes the opportunity of any potential organisms in the infusate to grow to numbers large enough to cause adverse effects. However, recent studies suggest that the infusate delivery systems do not require replacement more than every 72 hours.[19,119,120] Exceptions may be made for infusion sets used for delivery of blood products, lipid emulsions, or arterial pressure monitoring, whereby more frequent changes may be prudent.[36]

CATHETER-DESIGN IMPROVEMENTS/ANTISEPTIC-ANTIMICROBIAL BONDING

Improvements in catheter design have been intrinsic to improvement in rates of CRS. Methods to prevent invasion of the transcutaneous tract by skin flora following catheter insertion have been studied. Surgically implanted, tunneled, Dacron-cuffed devices such as Hickman and Broviac catheters used for long-term vascular access are an example. Both tunneling and the cuff limit the migration of cutaneous microorganisms to the bloodstream. An attachable subcutaneous cuff constructed of a biodegradable collagen matrix impregnated with bactericidal silver was studied by Maki and colleagues,[12] who found that the silver-impregnated cuff can confer a 3-fold reduction of catheter-related infection with PICCs. Antiseptic hubs and in-line filters have also been studied.[9,36] In addition, needleless luer-activated devices (ports) are an important source of catheter infection, and improvements in their design and materials can be expected to reduce rates of infusion-related sepsis.[121,122]

Three different commercially available antiseptic-/antibiotic-bonded central venous catheters exist: (1) minocycline-/rifampicin-bonded catheters; (2) chlorhexidine-/silver sulfadiazine–impregnated catheters; and (3) platinum/silver/carbon iontophoretic catheters. Each device is currently available in the United States. A series of studies and meta-analyses have demonstrated that antiseptic and antimicrobial bonded intravascular catheters are effective in reducing the risk of catheter colonization and infection.[123] Recent data suggest that the use of antiseptic (chlorhexidine and silver sulfadiazine)-bonded and antibiotic (minocycline and rifampin)-bonded catheters results in a 3- to 4-fold reduction in the risk of CRS.[124–126] A single head-to-head comparison of the 2 types of catheter has favored the antibiotic-bonded device.[125,127]

Despite data showing a decrease in catheter colonization with the silver/platinum iontophoretic catheter, 2 studies have failed to demonstrate any reduction in CR-BSI with these devices.[9,128,129] Irrespective of these data, no formal recommendation favoring one type of catheter over another has been adopted in formal consensus advisories.[8] Their use in general has been recommended in institutions where catheter infection risk remains high despite implementation of other recommendations in high-risk patients.

New antiseptic and antimicrobial catheters continue to be developed, including catheters coated or bonded with new combinations or formulations of chlorhexidine, silver, vancomycin, and miconazole.[128,130–133]

INSERTION SITE

Because studies of pulmonary artery catheters and central venous catheters have shown that there is an increased risk of CRS with insertion in the jugular vein compared with insertion in the subclavian vein,[61–63] the subclavian venous site is the preferred insertion site as regards the prevention of CRS. Recent data suggest an increased CRS risk using the femoral insertion site.[5,64]

DURATION OF INTRAVASCULAR CATHETERIZATION

Previous studies have indicated that the duration of vascular catheterization[134–137] is related to the incidence of both catheter colonization and CRS. In general, an in situ duration of more than 72 hours significantly increases the risk of catheter-related infection. Consequently, it had been generally recommended that central venous catheters be changed routinely every 3 to 5 days (most clinicians use 5 days). Other studies support the theory that both arterial and pulmonary catheters can remain in place as long as needed, provided there are no signs or symptoms of CRS occurring more than 48 hours after catheter insertion, local signs of infection at the insertion site, or positive blood cultures.[61,64,138–140] The most recent consensus recommendations suggest that in the absence of evidence of colonization/infection, routine replacement of central venous catheters is not required.[8]

INTEGRATIVE, MULTIFACTORIAL PROTOCOLS (BUNDLES)

A series of studies have shown that increasing nursing workload substantially increases the probability of acquiring CR-BSI.[52] The mechanism of this effect is likely to be a multifactorial deterioration in standard infection-prevention techniques. At least 2 major studies have now demonstrated astonishing decreases in incidence of catheter-related infection through an implementation of central-line "bundles" (a broad group of proven standard infection-control methods endorsed by the Institute of Healthcare Improvement [IHI]) as previously discussed.[141,142] Care bundles, in general, are groupings of best practices with respect to a disease process that individually improve care, but when applied together result in substantially greater improvement. The science supporting the bundle components is sufficiently established to be considered standard of care. The key elements of the catheter bundles are hand hygiene, routine use of maximum barrier precautions during insertion, chlorhexidine as the preferred antiseptic, the subclavian vein as the preferred access, and daily assessment for continued retention of intravascular catheters. One simple way to ensure compliance with these elements is to use a standard checklist.[142] Of note, these studies indicated that once these efforts were effectively implemented, the benefits were sustainable if the protocols were incorporated into hospital guidelines.

REFERENCES

1. Maki DG. Infections due to infusion therapy. In: Bennett JV, Brachman PS, editors. Hospital infections. Boston: Little Brown & Co; 1986. p. 849–98.
2. Raad I, Darouiche RO. Catheter-related septicemia: risk reduction. Infect Med 1996;13:807–23.

3. Vincent JL, Bihari DJ, Suter PM, et al. The prevalence of nosocomial infection in intensive care units in Europe. Results of the European Prevalence of Infection in Intensive Care (EPIC) Study. EPIC International Advisory Committee. JAMA 1995;274(8):639–44.
4. Vincent J, Rello J, Marshall J, et al. International study of the prevalence and outcomes of infection in intensive care units. JAMA 2009;302(21):2323–9.
5. Mermel LA. Prevention of intravascular catheter-related infections. Ann Intern Med 2000;132:391–402.
6. Srinivasan A, Wise M, Bel M, et al. Vital signs: central line-associated blood stream infections - United States, 2001, 2008, and 2009. MMWR Morb Mortal Wkly Rep 2011;60(8):243–8.
7. Scott RD. The direct medical cost of healthcare-associated infections in U.S. hospitals and the benefits of prevention. Atlanta (GA): Center for Disease Control; 2010.
8. O'Grady NP, Alexander M, Dellinger EP, et al. Guidelines for the prevention of intravascular catheter-related infections. Infect Control Hosp Epidemiol 2002; 23(12):759–69.
9. Raad I, Hanna H, Maki D, et al. Intravascular catheter-related infections: advances in diagnosis, prevention, and management [166 refs]. Lancet Infect Dis 2007;7(10):645–57.
10. Pearson ML. Hospital Infection Control Practice Advisory Committee: guidelines for prevention of intravascular-device-related infections. Infect Control Hosp Epidemiol 1996;17:438–73.
11. Maki DG, Ringer M. Evaluation of dressing regimens for prevention of infection with peripheral intravenous catheters. JAMA 1987;258:2396–403.
12. Maki DG, Cobb L, Garman JK, et al. An attachable silver-impregnated cuff for prevention of infection with central venous catheters: a prospective randomised multicenter trial. Am J Med 1988;85:307–14.
13. Maki DG, Weise CE, Sarafin HW. A semiquantitative culture method for identifying intravenous catheter-related infection. N Engl J Med 1977;296:1305–9.
14. Snydman DR, Murray SA, Kornfeld SJ. Total parental nutrition-related infections. Prospective epidemiologic study using semiquantitative methods. Am J Med 1982;73:695–9.
15. Collignon PJ, Soni N, Pearson IY. Is semiquantitative culture of central vein catheter tips useful in the diagnosis of catheter-associated bacteremia? J Clin Microbiol 1986;24:532–5.
16. Cleri DJ, Corrado ML, Seligman SJ. Quantitative culture of intravenous catheters and other intravascular inserts. J Infect Dis 1987;141:781–6.
17. Sherertz RJ, Raad I, Belani A, et al. Three-year experience with sonicated vascular catheter cultures in a clinical microbiologic laboratory. J Clin Microbiol 1990;28:76–82.
18. Raad I, Sabbagh MF, Rand KH, et al. Quantitative tip culture methods and the diagnosis of central venous catheter-related infections. Diagn Microbiol Infect Dis 1992;15:13–20.
19. Band JD, Maki DG. Safety of changing intravenous delivery systems at longer than 24-hour intervals. Ann Intern Med 1979;91:173–8.
20. Maki DG, Goldman DA, Rhame FS. Infection control in intravenous therapy. Ann Intern Med 1973;79:867–87.
21. Maki DG. Infections associated with intravascular lines. In: Swartz M, Remington JS, editors. Current topics in clinical infectious disease. New York: McGraw Hill; 1982. p. 309–63.

22. Maki DG. Nosocomial bacteremia: an epidemiologic overview. Am J Med 1981; 70:719–32.
23. McGeer A, Righter J. Improving our ability to diagnose infections associated with central venous catheters: value of Gram's staining and culture of entry site swabs. Can Med Assoc J 1987;137:1009–15.
24. Snydman DR, Pober BR, Murray SA. Predictive values of surveillance skin cultures in total-parenteral-nutrition-related infection. Lancet 1982;2:1385.
25. Bjornson HS, Colley R, Bower RH. Association between microorganism growth at the catheter insertion site and colonization of the catheter in patients receiving total parenteral nutrition. Surgery 1982;92:720–7.
26. Kovacevich DS, Faubion WC, Bender JM, et al. Association of parenteral nutrition catheter sepsis with urinary tract infections. JPEN J Parenter Enteral Nutr 1986;10:639–41.
27. Pettigrew RA, Lang SD, Haydock DA. Catheter-related sepsis in patients on intravenous nutrition: a prospective study of quantitative catheter cultures and guidewire changes for suspected sepsis. Br J Surg 1985;72:52–5.
28. Sitges-Serra A, Linares J, Garau J. Catheter sepsis: the clue is the hub. Surgery 1985;97:355–7.
29. Raad I, Costerton W, Sabharwal U. Ultrastructural analysis of indwelling vascular catheters: a quantitative relationship between luminal colonization and duration of placement. J Infect Dis 1993;168:400–7.
30. Maki DG, Rhame FS. Nationwide epidemic of septicemia caused by contaminated intravenous products. Am J Med 1977;60:471–85.
31. Hamory BH. Nosocomial bloodstream and intravascular device-related infections. In: Wenzel R, editor. Prevention and control of nosocomial infections. Baltimore (MD): Williams and Wilkins; 1987. p. 283.
32. Bennett SN, McNeil MM, Bland LA, et al. Postoperative infections traced to contamination of an intravenous anesthetic, propofol. N Engl J Med 1995;333: 147–54.
33. Goldman DG, Martin WT, Worthington JW. Growth of bacteria and fungi in total parenteral nutrition solutions. Am J Surg 1973;126:314–8.
34. Freeman J, Goldmann DA, Smith NE, et al. Association of intravenous lipid emulsion and coagulase-negative staphylococcal bacteremia in neonatal intensive care units. N Engl J Med 1990;323:301–8.
35. Safdar N, Maki DG. Inflammation at the insertion site is not predictive of catheter-related bloodstream infection with short-term, noncuffed central venous catheters. Crit Care Med 2002;30(12):2632–5.
36. Maki DG. Infections caused by intravascular devices used for infusion therapy: pathogenesis, prevention, and management. In: Bisno AL, Waldvogel FA, editors. Infections associated with indwelling medical devices. Washington, DC: American Society for Microbiology; 1994. p. 155–212.
37. Ascher DP, Shoupe BA, Robb M, et al. Comparison of standard and quantitative blood cultures in the evaluation of children with suspected central venous line sepsis. Diagn Microbiol Infect Dis 1992;15:499–503.
38. Benezra D, Kiehn T, Gold JW, et al. Prospective study of infections in indwelling central venous catheters using quantitative blood cultures. Am J Med 1988;85: 495–8.
39. Vanhuynegem L, Parmentier P, Potvliege C. In situ bacteriologic diagnosis of total parenteral nutrition catheter infection. Surgery 1987;103:174–7.
40. Raad I. Intravascular-catheter-related infections. Lancet 1998;351(9106): 893–8.

41. Kite P, Dobbins BM, Wilcox MH, et al. Evaluation of a novel endoluminal brush method for in situ diagnosis of catheter related sepsis. J Clin Pathol 1997;50: 278–82.

42. Rushforth JA, Hoy CM, Kite P, et al. Rapid diagnosis of central venous catheter sepsis. Lancet 1993;342:402–3.

43. Millar MR, Johnson G, Wilks M, et al. Molecular diagnosis of vascular access device-associated infection in children being treated for cancer or leukaemia. Clin Microbiol Infect 2008;14(3):213–20.

44. Guerti K, Ieven M, Mahieu L. Diagnosis of catheter-related bloodstream infection in neonates: a study on the value of differential time to positivity of paired blood cultures. Pediatr Crit Care Med 2007;8(5):470–5.

45. Raad I, Hanna HA, Alakech B, et al. Differential time to positivity: a useful method for diagnosing catheter-related bloodstream infections. Ann Intern Med 2004;140(1):18–25 [Erratum Ann Intern Med. 2004 Jan 6;140(1):I39; PMID: 14706995].

46. Safdar N, Fine JP, Maki DG. Meta-analysis: methods for diagnosing intravascular device-related bloodstream infection. Ann Intern Med 2005;142(6): 451–66 [Erratum appears in Ann Intern Med. 2005 May 3;142(9):803].

47. Telenti A, Steckelberg JM, Stockman L, et al. Quantitative blood cultures in candidemia. Mayo Clin Proc 1991;66:1120–3.

48. Craven DE, Kunches LM, Lictenberg DA. Nosocomial infections and fatality in medical and surgical intensive care unit patients. Arch Intern Med 1988;148: 1161–8.

49. Freeman J, McGowan JE. Risk factors for nosocomial infection. J Infect Dis 1978;138:811–9.

50. Armstrong CW, Mayhall CG, Miller KB. Prospective study of catheter replacement and other risk factors for infection of hyperalimentation catheters. J Infect Dis 1986;154:808–16.

51. Yilmaz G, Koksal I, Aydin K, et al. Risk factors of catheter-related bloodstream infections in parenteral nutrition catheterization. JPEN J Parenter Enteral Nutr 2007;31(4):284–7.

52. Hugonnet S, Chevrolet JC, Pittet D. The effect of workload on infection risk in critically ill patients. Crit Care Med 2007;35(1):76–81.

53. Faubion WC, Wesley JR, Khalidi N, et al. Total parenteral nutrition catheter sepsis: impact of the team approach. JPEN J Parenter Enteral Nutr 1986;10: 642–5.

54. Nelson DB, Kien CL, Mohr B. Dressing changes by specialized personnel reduced infection rates in patients receiving central venous parenteral nutrition. JPEN J Parenter Enteral Nutr 1986;10:220–2.

55. Tomford JW, Hershey CO, McLaren CE. Intravenous therapy team and peripheral venous catheter-associated complications: a prospective controlled study. Arch Intern Med 1984;144:1191–4.

56. Mermel LA, Maki DG. Infectious complications of Swan-Ganz pulmonary artery catheters. Pathogenesis, epidemiology, prevention and management. Am J Respir Crit Care Med 1994;149:1020–36.

57. Christensen GD, Simpson WA, Beachey EH. Adherence of slime-producing strains of Staphylococcus epidermidis to smooth surfaces. Infect Immun 1982;37:318–26.

58. Peters G, Locci R, Pulverer G. Adherence and growth of coagulase-negative staphylococci on surfaces of intravenous catheters. J Infect Dis 1982;146: 479–82.

59. Sheth NK, Rose HD, Franson TR. In vitro quantitative adherence of bacteria to intravascular catheters. J Surg Res 1983;34:213–8.
60. Sheth NK, Franson TR, Rose HD. Colonization of bacteria on polyvinyl chloride and Teflon intravenous catheters in hospitalized patients. J Clin Microbiol 1983; 18:1061–3.
61. Mermel LA, McCormick RD, Springman SR, et al. The pathogenesis and epidemiology of catheter-related infection with pulmonary artery Swan-Ganz catheters: a prospective study utilizing molecular subtyping. Am J Med 1991;91: 197S–205S.
62. Pinilla JC, Ross DF, Martin T, et al. Study of the incidence of intravascular catheter infection and associated septicemia in critically ill patients. Crit Care Med 1983;11:21–5.
63. Richet H, Hubert B, Netemberg G. Prospective multicenter study of vascular catheter-related complications and risk factors for positive central-catheter cultures in intensive care unit patients. J Clin Microbiol 1990;28:2520–5.
64. Norwood S, Ruby A, Civetta J, et al. Catheter-related infections and associated septicemia. Chest 1988;99:968–75.
65. Safdar N, Maki DG. Risk of catheter-related bloodstream infection with peripherally inserted central venous catheters used in hospitalized patients [54 refs]. Chest 2005;128(2):489–95.
66. Graham DR, Keldermans MM, Klemm LW, et al. Infectious complications among patients receiving home intravenous therapy with peripheral, central, or peripherally placed central venous catheters. Am J Med 1991;91(Suppl 3B): 95S–100S.
67. Maki DG. The epidemiology and prevention of nosocomial bloodstream infections. In: Program and abstracts of the third international conference on nosocomial infections 1990. Atlanta, (GA): Centers for Disease Control. The National Foundation for Infectious Disease and the American Society for Microbiology; 1990. p. 20.
68. Nystrom B, Olesen Larsen S, Daschner F, et al. Bacteraemia in surgical patients with intravenous devices: a European multicentre incidence study. J Hosp Infect 1983;4:338–49.
69. Bross J, Talbot GH, Maislin G, et al. Risk factors for nosocomial candidemia: a case-control study in adults without leukemia. Am J Med 1989;87:614–20.
70. Komshian SV, Uwaydah AK, Sobel JD, et al. Fungemia caused by Candida species and Torulopsis glabrata in the hospitalized patient: frequency, characteristics, and evaluation of factors influencing outcome. Rev Infect Dis 1989;3: 379–90.
71. Wang EE, Prober CG, Ford-Jones L, et al. The management of central intravenous catheter infections. Pediatr Infect Dis 1984;3:110–3.
72. Capell S, Linares J, Sitges-Serra A. Catheter sepsis due to coagulase-negative staphylococci in patients on total parental nutrition. Eur J Clin Microbiol 1985;5: 40–2.
73. Linares J, Sitges-Serra A, Garau J. Pathogenesis of catheter sepsis: a prospective study with quantitative and semiquantitative cultures of catheter and hub segments. J Clin Microbiol 1985;21:357–60.
74. Kelly CS, Ligas JR, Smith CA. Sepsis due to triple lumen central venous catheters. Surg Gynecol Obstet 1986;163:14–6.
75. Pemberton LB, Lyman B, Lander V, et al. Sepsis from triple vs. single-lumen catheters during total parenteral nutrition in surgical or critically ill patients. Arch Surg 1986;121:591–4.

76. Padberg FT, Ruggiero J, Blackburn GL, et al. Central venous catheterization for parenteral nutrition. Ann Surg 1981;193:264–70.

77. Bozzetti F, Terno G, Bonfanti G. Prevention and treatment of central venous catheter sepsis by exchange via a guidewire. A prospective controlled trial. Ann Surg 1983;198:48–52.

78. Sitzmann JV, Townsend TR, Siler MC, et al. Septic and technical complications of central venous catheterization. A prospective study of 200 consecutive patients. Ann Surg 1985;202:766–70.

79. Zurcher M, Tramer MR, Walder B. Colonization and bloodstream infection with single- versus multi-lumen central venous catheters: a quantitative systematic review [58 refs]. Anesth Analg 2004;99(1):177–82.

80. Ma TY, Yoshinaka R, Banaag A, et al. Total parenteral nutrition via multilumen catheters does not increase the risk of catheter-related sepsis: a randomized, prospective study. Clin Infect Dis 1998;27(3):500–3.

81. Cheesbrough JS, Finch RG, Burden RP. A prospective study of the mechanisms of infection associated with hemodialysis catheters. J Infect Dis 1986;154:579–89.

82. Pezzarossi HE, Ponce de Leon S, Calva JJ, et al. High incidence of subclavian dialysis catheter-related bacteremias. Infect Control 1986;7:596–9.

83. Sherertz RJ, Falk RJ, Huffman KA, et al. Infections associated with subclavian Uldall catheters. Arch Intern Med 1983;143:52–6.

84. Traore O, Liotier J, Souweine B, et al. Prospective study of arterial and central venous catheter colonization and of arterial- and central venous catheter-related bacteremia in intensive care units. Crit Care Med 2005;33(6):1276–80.

85. O'Grady NP, Barie PS, Bartlett J, et al. Practice parameters for evaluating new fever in critically ill adult patients. Crit Care Med 1998;26(2):392–408.

86. Ekkelenkamp MB, van der BT, van de Vijver DA, et al. Bacteremic complications of intravascular catheters colonized with *Staphylococcus aureus*. Clin Infect Dis 2008;46(1):114–8.

87. Raad I, Davis S, Khan A, et al. Impact of central venous catheter removal on the recurrence of catheter-related coagulase-negative staphylococcal bacteremia. Infect Control Hosp Epidemiol 1992;13:215–21.

88. Cappello M, De Pauw L, Bastin G, et al. Central venous access for haemodialysis using the Hickman catheter. Nephrol Dial Transplant 1989;4:988–92.

89. Hartman GE, Shochat SJ. Management of septic complications associated with silastic catheters in childhood malignancy. Pediatr Infect Dis 1987;6:1042–7.

90. Johnson PR, Decker MD, Edwards KM, et al. Frequency of Broviac catheter infections in pediatric oncology patients. J Infect Dis 1986;154:570–8.

91. Press OW, Ramsey PG, Larson EB, et al. Hickman catheter infections in patients with malignancies. Medicine 1984;63:189–200.

92. Prince A, Heller B, Jevy J, et al. Management of fever in patients with central vein catheters. Pediatr Infect Dis 1986;5:20–4.

93. Schuman ES, Winters V, Gross GF, et al. Management of Hickman catheter sepsis. Am J Surg 1985;149:627–8.

94. Douard MC, Leverger G, Paulien R, et al. Quantitative blood cultures for diagnosis and management of catheter-related sepsis in pediatric hematology and oncology patients. Intensive Care Med 1991;17:30–5.

95. Messing B, Peitra-Cohen S, Debure A, et al. Antibiotic-lock technique: a new approach to optimal therapy for catheter-related sepsis in home-parenteral nutrition patients. JPEN J Parenter Enteral Nutr 1988;12:185–9.

96. Onder AM, Chandar J, Billings AA, et al. Comparison of early versus late use of antibiotic locks in the treatment of catheter-related bacteremia. Clin J Am Soc Nephrol 2008;3(4):1048–56.

97. Jones GR, Konsler GK, Dunaway RP, et al. Prospective analysis of urokinase in the treatment of catheter sepsis in pediatric hematology-oncology patients. J Pediatr Surg 1993;28:350–8.

98. Wenzel RP, Osterman CA, Donowitz LG, et al. Identification of procedure-related nosocomial infections in high-risk patients. Rev Infect Dis 1981;3:701–7.

99. Maki DG. Yes, Virginia, aseptic technique is very important: maximal barrier precautions during insertion reduce the risk of central venous catheter-related bacteremia. Infect Control Hosp Epidemiol 1994;15:227–30.

100. Puntis JW, Holden CE, Smallman S, et al. Staff training: a key factor in reducing intravascular catheter sepsis. Arch Dis Child 1990;65:335–7.

101. Vanherweghem JL, Dhaene M, Goldman M, et al. Infections associated with subclavian dialysis catheters: the key role of nurse training. Nephron 1986;42:116–9.

102. Maki DG, Alvarado CJ, Ringer M. A prospective, randomized trial of povidone-iodine, alcohol and chlorhexidine for prevention of infection with central venous and arterial catheters. Lancet 1991;338:339–43.

103. Humar A, Ostromecki A, Direnfeld J, et al. Prospective randomized trial of 10% povidone-iodine versus 0.5% tincture of chlorhexidine as cutaneous antisepsis for prevention of central venous catheter infection. Clin Infect Dis 2000;31(4):1001–7.

104. Hill RL, Fisher AP, Ware RJ, et al. Mupirocin for the reduction of colonization of internal jugular cannulae-a randomised controlled trial. J Hosp Infect 1990;15:311–21.

105. Maki DG, Band JD. A comparative study of polyantitotic and iodophor ointments in prevention of vascular catheter-related infection. Am J Med 1981;70:739–44.

106. Parienti JJ, du Cheyron D, Ramakers M, et al. Members of the NSG. Alcoholic povidone-iodine to prevent central venous catheter colonization: a randomized unit-crossover study. Crit Care Med 2004;32(3):708–13.

107. Raad I, Hohn DC, Gilbreath J. Prevention of central venous catheter-related infections using maximal barrier precautions during insertion. Infect Control Hosp Epidemiol 1994;15:231–8.

108. Vasquez RM, Jarrad MM. Care of the central venous catheterization site: the use of a transparent polyurethane film. JPEN J Parenter Enteral Nutr 1984;8:181–6.

109. Young GP, Alexeyeff M, Russell DM, et al. Catheter sepsis during parenteral nutrition: the safety of longterm Opsite dressing. JPEN J Parenter Enteral Nutr 1988;12:365–70.

110. Conly JM, Grieves K, Peters B. A prospective randomized study comparing transparent and dry gauze dressings for central venous catheters. J Infect Dis 1989;159:310–9.

111. Dickerson N, Horton P, Smith S, et al. Clinically significant central venous catheter infections in a community hospital: association with type of dressing. J Infect Dis 1989;160:720–2.

112. Maki DG, Mermel LA, Kluger D, et al. The efficacy of a chlorhexidine-impregnated sponge (Biopatch TM) for the prevention of intravascular catheter-related infection: a prospective, randomized controlled multicenter study. 40th Interscience

Conference on Antimicrobial Agents and Chemotherapy. Toronto (ON), September 17–20, 2000.

113. Ho KM, Litton E. Use of chlorhexidine-impregnated dressing to prevent vascular and epidural catheter colonization and infection: a meta-analysis. J Antimicrob Chemother 2006;58(2):281–7.

114. Simmons BP. CDC guidelines for the prevention and control of nosocomial infections. Guidelines for prevention of intravascular infections. Am J Infect Control 1983;11:183–99.

115. Jaffer Y, Selby NM, Taal MW, et al. A meta-analysis of hemodialysis catheter locking solutions in the prevention of catheter-related infection. Am J Kidney Dis 2008;51(2):233–41.

116. Schwartz C, Henrickson KJ, Roghmann K, et al. Prevention of bacteraemia attributed to luminal colonization of tunnelled central venous catheters with vancomycin-susceptible organisms. J Clin Oncol 1990;80:591–7.

117. Raad I, Buzaid A, Rhyne J, et al. Minocycline and ethylenediaminetetraacetate for the prevention of recurrent vascular catheter infections. Clin Infect Dis 1997; 25:149–51.

118. Safdar N, Maki DG. Use of vancomycin-containing lock or flush solutions for prevention of bloodstream infection associated with central venous access devices: a meta-analysis of prospective, randomized trials. Clin Infect Dis 2006;43(4):474–84.

119. Buxton AE, Highsmith AK, Garner JS. Contamination of intravenous fluid: effects of changing administration sets. Ann Intern Med 1979;90:764–8.

120. Gorbea HF, Snydman DR, Delaney A. Intravenous tubing with burettes can be safely changed at 48-hour intervals. JAMA 1984;251:2112–5.

121. Menyhay SZ, Maki DG. Disinfection of needleless catheter connectors and access ports with alcohol may not prevent microbial entry: the promise of a novel antiseptic-barrier cap. Infect Control Hosp Epidemiol 2006;27(1): 23–7.

122. Maragakis LL, Bradley KL, Song X, et al. Increased catheter-related bloodstream infection rates after the introduction of a new mechanical valve intravenous access port. Infect Control Hosp Epidemiol 2006;27(1):67–70.

123. Falagas ME, Fragoulis K, Bliziotis IA, et al. Rifampicin-impregnated central venous catheters: a meta-analysis of randomized controlled trials. J Antimicrob Chemother 2007;59(3):359–69.

124. Maki DG, Stolz SM, Wheeler S, et al. Prevention of central venous catheter-related bloodstream infection by use of an antiseptic-impregnated catheter: a randomised, controlled trial. Ann Intern Med 1997;127:257–66.

125. Raad I, Darouiche RO, Hachem R, et al. The broad spectrum activity and efficacy of catheters coated with minocycline and rifampicin. J Infect Dis 1996; 173:418–24.

126. Raad I, Darouiche RO, Dupuis J. Central venous catheters coated with minocycline and rifampin for the prevention of catheter-related colonization and bloodstream infection: a randomised, double-blind trial. Ann Intern Med 1997;127: 267–74.

127. Darouiche RO, Raad I, Heard SO, et al. A comparison of two antimicrobial-impregnated central venous catheters. N Engl J Med 1999;340:1–8.

128. Bong JJ, Kite P, Wilco MH, et al. Prevention of catheter related bloodstream infection by silver iontophoretic central venous catheters: a randomised controlled trial. J Clin Pathol 2003;56(10):731–5.

129. Moretti EW, Ofstead CL, Kristy RM, et al. Impact of central venous catheter type and methods on catheter-related colonization and bacteraemia. J Hosp Infect 2005;61(2):139–45.

130. Yucel N, Lefering R, Maegele M, et al. Reduced colonization and infection with miconazole-rifampicin modified central venous catheters: a randomized controlled clinical trial. J Antimicrob Chemother 2004;54(6):1109–15.

131. Brun-Buisson C, Doyon F, Sollet JP, et al. Prevention of intravascular catheter-related infection with newer chlorhexidine-silver sulfadiazine-coated catheters: a randomized controlled trial. Intensive Care Med 2004;30(5):837–43.

132. Rupp ME, Lisco SJ, Lipsett PA, et al. Effect of a second-generation venous catheter impregnated with chlorhexidine and silver sulfadiazine on central catheter-related infections: a randomized, controlled trial. Ann Intern Med 2005;143(8):570–80 [Erratum Ann Intern Med. 2005 Oct 18;143(8):I36; PMID: 16230719].

133. Thornton J, Todd NJ, Webster NR. Central venous line sepsis in the intensive care unit. A study comparing antibiotic coated catheters with plain catheters. Anaesthesia 1996;51(11):1018–20 [Erratum appears in Anaesthesia 1997 Feb;52(2):192].

134. Gil RT, Krause JA, Thill-Baharozian MC. Triple vs single lumen central venous catheters. Arch Intern Med 1989;149:1139–43.

135. Roy O, Billiau V, Beuscart C. Nosocomial infections associated with long-term radial artery cannulation. Intensive Care Med 1989;15:241–6.

136. Band JD, Maki DG. Infections caused by arterial catheters used for hemodynamic monitoring. Am J Med 1979;67:735–41.

137. Applefeld JJ, Caruthers TE, Reno DJ. Assessment of the sterility of long-term cardiac catheterization using thermodilution Swan-Ganz catheter. Chest 1978;74:377–80.

138. Eyer S, Brummitt C, Crossley K. Catheter-related sepsis: prospective randomized study of three methods of long-term catheter maintenance. Crit Care Med 1990;18:1073–9.

139. Snyder RH, Ardrer FJ, Endy T. Catheter infection: comparison of two catheter maintenance techniques. Ann Surg 1988;208:651–3.

140. Mermel LA, Maki DG. Epidemic bloodstream infections from hemodynamic pressure monitoring: signs of the times. Infect Control Hosp Epidemiol 1989;10(2):47–53.

141. Eggimann P, Harbarth S, Constantin MN, et al. Impact of a prevention strategy targeted at vascular-access care on incidence of infections acquired in intensive care. Lancet 2000;355(9218):1864–8.

142. Pronovost P, Needham D, Berenholtz S, et al. An intervention to decrease catheter-related bloodstream infections in the ICU. N Engl J Med 2006;355(26):2725–32.

Abdominal Catastrophes in the Intensive Care Unit Setting

Joao B. Rezende-Neto, MD, Ori D. Rotstein, MD*

KEYWORDS

- Intra-abdominal infection • Abdominal compartment syndrome
- *Clostridium difficile* colitis • Surgical emergencies

KEY POINTS

- In the critically ill patient in the intensive care unit, several intra-abdominal pathologic processes may supervene and cause deterioration of the patient's status.
- Intra-abdominal pathologic processes are difficult to diagnose because of the compromised status of the patient, and advanced imaging is invaluable in establishing a diagnosis.
- Timely intervention is indicated, as delay is invariably associated with poor outcome.

BACKGROUND

Intra-abdominal complications, often requiring surgical intervention, are known to occur in critically ill patients admitted to intensive care for nonsurgical problems. Intensivists and surgeons face significant challenges when managing such patients. Associated comorbidities, particularly respiratory, cardiovascular, and renal dysfunction, result in minimal margin for error in management.[1]

The overall incidence of intra-abdominal complications in this particular group of patients is not well established. Data from large studies also include patients who have a primary surgical diagnosis and are admitted to the medical intensive care unit (MICU) because of clinical comorbidities.[1–3] Moreover, most studies typically focus on intra-abdominal infectious complications in this group of patients.[4–7] Nonetheless, a review of 6000 MICU admissions reported a 1.3% incidence of intra-abdominal catastrophe. Sedation, mechanical ventilation, and altered mental status interfere with physical examination of the abdomen, and can obscure the characteristic signs of peritoneal irritation in these patients.[1] Therefore, diagnosis becomes highly dependent on advanced imaging techniques and laboratory tests. MICU patients diagnosed with an acute

Disclosures: The authors have nothing to disclose.
Department of Surgery, St. Michael's Hospital, 30 Bond Street 16CC-044, Toronto, Ontario M5B1W8, Canada
* Corresponding author.
E-mail address: rotsteino@smh.ca

Crit Care Clin 29 (2013) 1017–1044
http://dx.doi.org/10.1016/j.ccc.2013.06.005   criticalcare.theclinics.com
0749-0704/13/$ – see front matter © 2013 Elsevier Inc. All rights reserved.

surgical abdominal catastrophe showed that delay in surgical intervention, Acute Physiology and Chronic Health Evaluation III (APACHE-III) scores, renal failure, and the diagnosis of bowel ischemia were significant risk factors associated with mortality.[1]

Although it is evident that postponing a surgical intervention can be disastrous in this group of critically ill patients, it is also crucial to avoid unnecessary and premature operations.[1–4,8,9] Surgical teams are often consulted to review a patient in the MICU whose status has deteriorated, with a view to determining whether this is derived from an intra-abdominal source. Deciding whether to surgically intervene, and the most appropriate time to do so, requires sound judgment and expertise.[4,8,10] Operative times and the complexity of the surgical procedures performed are also important, as limited physiologic reserve and perioperative systemic inflammatory derangements increase operative risk in these patients.[9,11,12]

The purpose of this overview is to address the diagnosis and treatment of some of the common abdominal processes arising in patients in the MICU setting. This discussion does not specifically cover abdominal processes that might have led to admission to the MICU, such as postsurgical anastomotic dehiscence, severe necrotizing pancreatitis, or patients with sepsis following surgery for peritonitis (eg, perforated diverticulitis). Rather, it focuses on abdominal catastrophes that may develop in patients in the MICU setting. The following entities are described herein:

- Abdominal compartment syndrome (ACS)
- Ischemic bowel affecting the small or large intestine (or both)
- Cholecystitis
- Fulminant *Clostridium difficile* colitis
- Perforated duodenal ulcer

ABDOMINAL COMPARTMENT SYNDROME
Background

ACS is defined as the development of pressure-induced organ dysfunction or failure caused by a manifestation of the pathophysiologic consequences of raised intra-abdominal pressures. ACS is classified as primary, secondary, or recurrent. Primary ACS denotes a condition originating within the abdomen, whereas secondary ACS occurs without a primary intra-abdominal abnormality or intervention. Recurrent ACS refers to the recurrence of the syndrome after surgical and and/or medical treatment have been implemented.[13,14]

Clinical and experimental research have led to a better understanding of the underlying pathophysiology and management strategies for intra-abdominal hypertension (IAH) and ACS.[14–22] Despite this, IAH and ACS are still important causes of morbidity and mortality, particularly in medical critically ill patients.[15,16]

Epidemiology

The incidence of IAH and ACS in MICU patients is difficult to determine.[23] A study involving a mixed population of patients in the intensive care unit (ICU) showed that the incidence of IAH was 50.5% and that of ACS 8.2%.[24] A more comprehensive study, with a similar patient population, reported lower rates of IAH and ACS on admission: 32.1% and 4.2%, respectively.[25] However, the incidence of ACS increased to 12.9% in the subsequent days of ICU stay.[25]

A few studies have investigated the epidemiology of ACS in primary MICU patients.[26–28] One consistent finding in these studies was that secondary ACS was the most common mechanism in this group of patients.[23,29,30] In addition, it was shown that primary MICU patients present with significant comorbidities, have a higher rate of multiple-organ failure (MOF), and a lower survival rate (34%) compared with their surgical counterparts with ACS (54%), despite the similar severity of illness (APACHE-II and Simplified Acute Physiology Score 2).[23] The incidence of MOF was almost 2.5 times higher in medical patients than in trauma patients, further emphasizing the severity of IAH/ACS in this patient population.[30]

Clinical Presentation

Intra-abdominal hypertension provokes physiologic derangement in practically every organ system, resulting in a multitude of clinical manifestations (**Table 1**).[14,16,18,19,26,29,31]

Table 1
Clinical manifestations of intra-abdominal hypertension and abdominal compartment syndrome

Organ/System	Dysfunction
Central nervous system	Increased ICP
	Decreased CPP
Cardiovascular system	Increased SVR
	Increased CVP, PAP, PCWP
	Decreased venous return
	Decreased CO
	Decreased left ventricle function/compliance
Respiratory system	Increased intrathoracic pressure
	Increased auto-PEEP, hypercarbia
	Increased peak and plateau airway pressure
	Increased intrapulmonary shunt formation
	Increased pulmonary inflammation
	Decreased lung volume
	Decreased Pao_2/Fio_2
Gastrointestinal system	Increased intestinal permeability
	Increased bacterial translocation
	Increased gastrointestinal bleeding
	Increased splanchnic venous compression
	Decreased splanchnic blood flow
	Decreased CO_2-gap
	Decreased intramucosal pH
Liver	Decreased hepatic blood flow
	Decreased lactate clearance
	Decreased glucose metabolism
	Decreased cytochrome P450 function
Kidneys	Increased vascular resistance
	Increased ureter compression
	Increased ADH
	Decreased renal perfusion
	Decreased GFR
Endocrine system	Increased proinflammatory response
Abdominal wall	Increased edema
	Increased wound complications
	Decreased perfusion
	Decreased muscle function and compliance

Abbreviations: ADH, antidiuretic hormone; CO, cardiac output; CPP, cerebral perfusion pressure; CVP, central venous pressure; GFR, glomerular filtration rate; IAH, intra-abdominal hypertension; ICP, intracranial pressure; Pao_2/Fio_2, partial pressure of oxygen/fraction of inspired oxygen ratio; PAP, pulmonary artery pressure; PCWP, pulmonary capillary wedge pressure; PEEP, positive end-expiratory pressure; SVR, systemic vascular resistance.

More importantly, IAH/ACS is a sequential phenomenon that can ultimately lead to irreversible end-organ dysfunction. Hence, early recognition of those clinical manifestations is important in implementing measures to halt the increase in intra-abdominal pressure (IAP).

Diagnosis

Physical examination has poor sensitivity and accuracy for elevated IAP in critically ill patients. Therefore, quantitative measurement of IAP is required to define IAH/ACS.[24]

Normal IAP in an adult is between 0 and 5 mm Hg. IAH is defined as IAP greater than or equal to 12 mm Hg. The diagnosis of ACS requires a sustained elevation of the IAP greater than 20 mm Hg, associated with new organ dysfunction or failure, regardless of the abdominal perfusion pressure (APP); APP is calculated as the mean arterial pressure (MAP) minus the IAP.[13,14]

According to The World Society of the Abdominal Compartment Syndrome (WSACS), IAP should be assessed with the patient in supine position, and the pressure transducer zeroed at the mid-axillary line; the reading should be obtained at the end of expiration. Absence of abdominal muscular contractions should be ensured before reading the IAP.[32]

Intra-abdominal pressure can be assessed through several routes; the WSACS recommends the intravesical approach, which is readily accessible, noninvasive, and closely reproduces direct IAP values. Studies have shown that smaller fluid volumes injected into the bladder result in more accurate estimates of IAP compared with larger volumes; the WSACS recommends infusion of 25 mL of sterile saline at the patient's body temperature.[32,33] In addition, a delay of 30 to 60 seconds should be observed before the actual reading of the intravesicular pressure (IVP), which allows for relaxation of the detrusor muscle. Disregarding these steps can result in values higher than normal.[33]

Critically ill patients often have elevated IAP. IAPs of 15 to 25 mm Hg are common in critically ill patients who are in septic shock for extra-abdominal diseases.[34] However, IAH/ACS in MICU patients is frequently insidious, therefore delayed diagnosis and worse outcome are more frequent than in surgical/trauma patients with this condition. Thus, early recognition of IAH, as per the WSACS criteria, is important in promptly implementing preventive measures of full-blown ACS.

The WSACS grades IAH as follows:

- Grade I: IAP 12 to 15 mm Hg
- Grade II: IAP 16 to 20 mm Hg
- Grade III: IAP 21 to 25 mm Hg
- Grade IV: IAP greater than 25 mm Hg

Awareness of the main risk factors for IAH/ACS in medical patients is also important for appropriate diagnosis. A study of 81 consecutive critically ill patients with septic shock showed an incidence of IAH of 73% among those who were admitted with a primary medical diagnosis.[34] More importantly, 21% of the medical patients who were initially diagnosed with IAH went on to develop ACS.[34] As expected, an intra-abdominal infection was the most common cause of IAH. However, septic shock caused by pneumonia, urinary tract infections, obstetric infections, and oncologic infections were, in that order, also responsible for IAH in this patient population.[34] One of the few studies to investigate ACS specifically in primary MICU patients showed that acute pancreatitis, extra-abdominal sepsis, and cardiac arrest were the most common causes of IAH/ACS.[25] In severe acute pancreatitis, IAH is an early phenomenon.

In general, risk factors for IAH/ACS in primary MICU patients can be classified as:

- Increased intraluminal contents (ileus, colonic pseudo-obstruction, *Clostridium difficile* colitis, bowel obstruction, bowel ischemia)
- Increased intra-abdominal contents (ascites/liver dysfunction, retroperitoneal hematomas in anticoagulated patients)
- Fluid overload (>18 L/24 h) and capillary leak (sepsis from several sources, acute renal failure, metabolic acidosis)
- Decreased abdominal wall compliance (mechanical ventilation resulting in elevated intrathoracic pressure, morbid obesity)

The ideal frequency of IAP assessment is controversial. Nonetheless, when IAH is suspected or at least 2 risk factors are present, IAP should be measured.[35] If an intermittent measurement strategy is selected, IAP should be assessed every 4 hours, or every hour in high-risk patients.[35] Continuous measurement of the IAP in a mixed population of medical and surgical critically ill patients showed similar results in comparison with intermittent assessment.[27] Therefore, the use of special urinary catheters designed for continuous measurement of the IAP still require further investigation.

ISCHEMIA OF THE SMALL INTESTINE AND COLON
Acute Intestinal Ischemia

Background
Acute intestinal ischemia can be mechanical, vascular nonocclusive, or vascular occlusive, with the last of these either arterial or venous in origin. Acute mechanical strangulation of the mesentery or the bowel is the most common cause of acute intestinal ischemia, usually a result of strangulated hernias or bowel obstruction, with a closed intestinal loop.

Nonocclusive intestinal ischemia occurs as a complication of "low-flow states" whereby vasoconstriction of the splanchnomesenteric vasculature decreases blood flow to the bowel. In severe cases, prolonged decrease in blood flow can lead to bowel infarction. The presence of shock and frequent use of vasopressors render critically ill ICU patients prone to this type of complication.[28,36,37] Acute intestinal ischemia is considered nonocclusive in roughly 3% of patients.[37]

Acute arterial intestinal ischemia can be embolic or thrombotic. Approximately 65% of all vascular-related cases are embolic phenomena, arterial thrombosis accounts for 27%, while mesenteric venous thrombosis is the cause of acute intestinal ischemia in 3% to 5% of patients.[37] Intestinal ischemia in venous mesenteric thrombosis results from prolonged vasospasm caused by venous congestion of the bowel wall.

Acute intestinal ischemia in the intensive care setting carries a grave prognosis. Despite advances in diagnostic imaging, intensive care support, and surgical treatment, the average mortality rate from all causes of acute intestinal ischemia has not changed significantly in the past 30 years, and is still around 60% to 80%.[38–40] Principal determinants of poor outcome in acute intestinal ischemia are:

- Acute arterial thrombosis
- Significant preexisting disease
- Poor collateral circulation
- Age older than 60 years (relative risk of mortality is 3 compared with younger patients)
- Duration of ischemia
- Delay in diagnosis and treatment[36,40–42]

Timely intervention is critical for a favorable outcome.[40,41,43] A retrospective study on patients operated on for acute intestinal ischemia showed 100% intestinal viability in patients who were symptomatic for less than 12 hours, whereas only 18% if symptoms were present for more than 24 hours before diagnosis.[44] In a more recent study, patients who were treated before developing multiple organ failure, increased blood lactate level, and pneumoperitoneum on computed tomography (CT) required a shorter length of bowel resection and ICU stay.[38]

Unfortunately, early diagnosis of acute mesenteric ischemia may be challenging in the ICU, where clinical assessment is often limited by sedation and mechanical ventilation, and patients often present as unstable for several other reasons.

Epidemiology

Acute intestinal ischemia is an uncommon abdominal emergency, less than 1% of all acute laparotomies being performed for acute mesenteric ischemia. The reported incidence is approximately 0.1% of all hospital admissions.[37,41] Embolism is the most common cause of vascular-related mesenteric ischemia, and is frequently a result of embolism from cardiac origin. The main risk factors are:

- Atrial fibrillation
- Impaired heart-wall motion after myocardial infarction
- Right to left shunts
- Valvular vegetation (endocarditis) and mycotic aneurysms
- Fragments of a ruptured atheromatous plaque
- Thrombus formed/dislodged from prosthetic grafts

Embolic intestinal ischemia is an acute event, therefore impeding arterial collateralization or ischemic adaptation, and mortality rates are as high as 70%.[40] By contrast, thrombotic intestinal ischemia is usually a long-term complication of severe arteriosclerotic disease. Approximately 50% to 75% of these patients have preexisting chronic mesenteric ischemia, as well as comorbid atherosclerotic disease in other organs. This feature is important in ICU patients with low physiologic reserve, whereby hemodynamic events that lead to a low-flow state can ultimately occlude a stenotic arterial segment or hinder collateral blood flow, thus provoking intestinal ischemia. It is the most deadly of all causes of acute intestinal ischemia, with mortality rates as high as 90%.[40]

Arterial vascular occlusion in thrombotic intestinal ischemia is frequently close to the origin of the superior mesenteric artery (SMA). Therefore, infarction usually affects long segments of the small bowel, including part of the duodenum and the transverse colon. However, blood vessel collateralization and the chronic nature of this type of bowel ischemia can result in less extensive infarction despite proximal vascular occlusion.[45]

Mesenteric venous thrombosis is associated with preexisting prothrombotic conditions in 80% of cases. A medical history of deep venous thrombosis is reported in up to 40% of the patients.[46] At present, less than 1 in 1000 laparotomies for acute abdomens are for the treatment of mesenteric venous thrombosis.[46,47]

Patients with mesenteric venous thrombosis are generally younger than those with other types of acute intestinal ischemia, the mean age being between 45 and 60 years.[46,47] The initial location of the thrombus is an important pathophysiologic element. Distal thromboses, particularly within intramural vessels, tend to progress more rapidly to infarction than proximal ones, and have shorter duration of symptoms.[48] With respect to the major veins, isolated thrombosis of the superior mesenteric vein is more frequently associated with peritonitis and the need for surgical intervention than is thrombosis of the portal or splenic veins.[48] In addition, isolated thrombosis of this vessel is frequently linked to preexisting prothrombotic medical conditions.[48]

MICU patients are at significant risk for nonocclusive intestinal ischemia, particularly those in shock, those receiving high-dose vasoactive agents, and patients who have been treated with digoxin for congestive heart failure. Another high-risk group is long-term dialysis patients, who develop hypotension caused by rapid fluid shifts. Nonocclusive intestinal ischemia was also reported in ICU patients receiving enteral feeding. The incidence in this group is 0.3% to 8%, and is believed to be caused by an imbalance between oxygen demand and supply (blood flow) precipitated by the enteral feeding.[37,38,40,49]

Clinical presentation and diagnosis

Severe abdominal pain unaccompanied by correlative physical signs is the hallmark symptom of embolic and thrombotic acute mesenteric ischemia. Unfortunately, in the ICU setting the presentation is not that straightforward, and mesenteric ischemia may not be perceived until bowel infarction occurs and the patient rapidly deteriorates.[37,38,41,50]

There are no specific laboratory tests for intestinal ischemia, and in many cases the diagnosis of mesenteric ischemia is one of exclusion.[51] The most common findings are:

- Leukocytosis
- High serum L-lactate and D-lactate
- Hyperamylasemia
- High level of aspartate aminotransferase
- High level of lactate dehydrogenase
- Anion-gap metabolic acidosis

Hyperphosphatemia and hyperkalemia are often present in late stages. Elevated serum L-lactate is frequently considered a marker of mesenteric ischemia. However, this finding has a very low specificity of approximately 50%.[51–53] A systematic review of all diagnostic markers of intestinal ischemia showed that high levels of serum D-lactate, the stereoisomer of L-lactate, were the most accurate.[51] Nonetheless, an elevated level of serum L-lactate is considered a reliable predictor of mortality. A retrospective study on 121 patients demonstrated that 81% of those with an L-lactate level higher than 5.2 mEq/L died.[52]

The lack of specific laboratory markers for acute intestinal ischemia has made imaging the key to diagnosis. Plain radiographs of the abdomen and the chest provide unspecific findings until late phases when pneumatosis and pneumoperitoneum are detected. Abdominal CT findings provide earlier evidence of intestinal ischemia, and are also important in ruling out other diagnoses.[54] The diagnostic capability of CT scanning has significantly improved for all types of acute intestinal ischemia with the use of new multidetector angiography scans, for which a pooled sensitivity of 93% and a pooled specificity of 94% were described in a systematic review and meta-analysis.[55] Air in the SMA or the portal vein seen on CT represents advanced, and frequently lethal, intestinal ischemia. Pneumatosis intestinalis, pneumoperitoneum, and solid-organ infarction are linked to greater than 75% mortality.[56] Other important CT features of acute intestinal ischemia demonstrated on the bowel wall and the mesentery are:

- Bowel-wall thickening, particularly after reperfusion in arterial and nonocclusive types
- Diminished bowel-wall enhancement on contrast CT, which increases with reperfusion in arterial occlusive type ischemia

- Bowel dilatation in acute mechanical strangulation and venous types
- Vascular defects in mesentery vessels in acute arterial or venous types of intestinal ischemia
- Hazy infiltration of the mesentery

Mesenteric angiography is traditionally considered the gold standard for the diagnosis of mesenteric arterial occlusion, with sensitivity of 75% to 100% and specificity of 100% having been reported. It is also useful for the diagnosis of nonocclusive intestinal ischemia, whereby vasospasm and multiple narrowing, and "string of sausage" sign of the SMA are demonstrated. Furthermore, if the diagnosis of acute intestinal ischemia is obtained at a potentially reversible stage by arteriography, endovascular therapeutic procedures and papaverine infusion can be performed during the same intervention.[36] To a significant extent, the use of angiography has been challenged and supplanted by less invasive and readily available multidetector CT angiography, particularly in the acutely ill ICU patient.[54,55]

Magnetic resonance imaging (MRI) angiography was shown to have sensitivity and specificity comparable with those of angiography in the diagnosis of intestinal ischemia, particularly in severe stenosis at the origins of the SMA and the celiac axis. However, this method is not reliable for more peripheral occlusions and nonocclusive intestinal ischemia.[36] These reasons, in addition to long acquisition times, constitute important limitations for the use of MRI angiography in the diagnosis of acute intestinal ischemia in ICU patients.[36–38] Endoscopy and tonometry have not been thoroughly investigated in this patient population.

Several studies have investigated the use of diagnostic laparoscopy (DL) in critically ill patients with suspected intra-abdominal complications. The 2 most common conditions for which this method was used were acalculous cholecystitis and acute intestinal ischemia.[57–63]

Bedside DL in the ICU has been shown to be safe and reliable. The diagnostic accuracy of the procedure depends on the primary disease and local factors, with accuracy rates ranging from 90% to 100%.[57–64] Acalculous cholecystitis and acute intestinal ischemia yield the highest diagnostic accuracies when the procedure is performed in the ICU.[58,59,61,64] The presence of intra-abdominal adhesions and retroperitoneal location of the disease are the main limiting factors to the use of DL.[64] Reported complication rates with the procedure are low, between 0% and 8%, and no mortalities have been described.[58,59,61,64,65] Although data from specialized centers suggest that bedside DL is a valuable adjunct in the management of critically ill patients, its use requires specialized equipment as well as surgical expertise and experience. In many ICUs, it is simply not feasible to perform DL at bedside, therefore a preferred approach might be to transport the patient to the operating room, perform laparoscopy under more favorable conditions, and make decisions in a setting where laparotomy for definitive treatment is feasible.

Ischemic Colitis

Background

Ischemic colitis (IC) is a disease that affects predominantly the elderly. Patients with IC commonly have significant coexisting health disorders, particularly cardiovascular and pulmonary disease, and therefore are usually managed in a MICU setting.[66] Even though many cases are mistakenly diagnosed as other types of colitis or inflammatory bowel disease, IC is the most common cause of gastrointestinal tract ischemia and the second most common cause of lower gastrointestinal bleeding.[67] Inadequate regional colonic perfusion is considered the triggering process for IC.

Clinically, IC can be self-limited or have a catastrophic presentation with a high mortality rate. Severity of clinical presentation depends on the primary cause of the ischemic event, extensiveness and degree of the ischemia, and the patient's comorbidities. Although significant improvement has been achieved in reaching prompt diagnosis and in the surgical treatment of severe IC, mortality rates are still very high, between 60% and 80%.[68]

Epidemiology

The incidence of IC in the general population varies from 4.5 to 44 cases per 100,000 people per year.[66] There are no specific data on the incidence of IC in MICU patients. However, given the similarities between the epidemiologic aspects of IC and those of critically ill ICU patients, a high incidence is probable in this patient population, particularly the elderly.

A systematic review of the epidemiology of IC showed that approximately 90% of the cases occur in patients older than 65 years (median age 70.6 years), with patients having chronic obstructive pulmonary disease and irritable bowel syndrome (IBS) at higher risk.[66]

Constipation is another problem that has been linked to IC.[66,69,70] It is believed that high intraluminal pressure in the colon interferes with mucosal blood flow and induces IC. Constipation is a common problem in the critically ill. A study in a medical/surgical ICU patient population showed an 85% incidence of constipation in medical patients; a sequential survey among several ICUs in the United Kingdom produced similar findings.[70]

Gender is an important epidemiologic aspect of IC. Several studies have shown that female gender is an important risk factor for the disease.[66,69,70] The incidence in females is 1.5 to 2 times higher than in males. Only spontaneous IC is more frequent in women, whereas postoperative IC is more frequent in men. Risk factors for IC in the MICU patient population are listed in **Table 2**.

Clinical presentation and diagnosis

There are 2 basic clinical presentations of IC, acute nongangrenous and gangrenous. Nongangrenous IC accounts for 85% of the cases and responds well to nonoperative management; it is frequently a reversible condition (50%). However, patients with comorbidities such as those in the ICU or with associated colonic diseases are at risk for progression to more severe forms of IC, and may require surgical intervention.[71–73] The nongangrenous type can also evolve to chronic colitis (20%–25%) or segmental strictures of the colon (10%–15%).

Gangrenous IC represents a transmural involvement of the colon and accounts for 15% of the cases. Progression to perforation and multiple-organ failure, and mortality rates of greater than 60% are common in this group of patients.[74–76] Approximately 20% of patients with IC will require acute surgical treatment, and practically all patients have gangrenous-type IC.[71,72,74] Unfortunately, there are no reliable factors capable of predicting gangrenous-type IC in ICU patients. However, in a non-ICU setting, age older than 90 years, hypertension, and a history of cancer predicted gangrenous IC in 85% of the cases.[75] Furthermore, rectal bleeding and diarrhea were significantly less frequent in gangrenous IC than in the nongangrenous type.[75]

The left colon is affected in 75% of the patients with IC. "Watershed" areas of the left colon, such as the splenic flexure and the rectal sigmoid transition (Sudek point), are often involved in regional nonocclusive type ischemia, whereas watershed segments of the ascending colon, where the marginal vessels are scarce, are particularly vulnerable to low-flow states.[73] It has been shown that mortality rates are doubled in IC

Table 2
Risk factors for ischemic colitis in medical ICU patient population

Patient-Related Risk Factors	Medication-Related Risk Factors[9]
Vascular: surgical (1%–7%) or endovascular repair of ruptured AAA; peripheral artery occlusive disease	Agents with constipation as a side effect: clonidine, morphine, nifedipine, digitalis, amiodarone, piperacillin, propafenone
Cardiologic: congestive heart failure, myocardial infarction	Antibiotics
Respiratory: COPD (RR* = 3.88)	Vasopressor agents (vasopressin, glypressin)
Metabolic: diabetes, dyslipidemia, hypercoagulability (factor V Leiden), thrombophilia. Hypoalbuminemia (<3.5 g/dL)	Chemotherapeutic agents: vinca alkaloid, taxane
Oncologic comorbidity, radiation vasculitis	NSAIDs (aspirin RR* = 1.97)
History of abdominal surgery during the preceding 6 mo	Diuretics (ethacrynic acid, furosemide)
Age >65 y	Glycerin, cleansing enemas
Infections: cytomegalovirus Escherichia coli O157:H7, hepatitis C with cryoglobulinemia	Immunosuppressive agents
Gastrointestinal: constipation, IBS (RR* = 3.1), mesenteric thrombosis, portal hypertension, acute pancreatitis, Ogilvie syndrome, bowel obstruction, colon neoplasm	
Low-flow state: hemodialysis, hypotension, septic shock, dehydration	

Abbreviations: AAA, abdominal aortic aneurysm; COPD, chronic obstructive pulmonary disease; IBS, irritable bowel syndrome; NSAIDs, nonsteroidal anti-inflammatory drugs; RR*, relative risk for ischemic colitis versus general population.

involving the right colon in comparison with the left colon, and the need for surgical treatment increases 5 times compared with other regions of the colon.

Diagnosis of IC is based on patients' risk factors, clinical findings, and diagnostic tests. Patients who develop IC while in the ICU for other medical conditions present a significant diagnostic challenge, because important clinical findings and diagnostic tests contributive to the diagnosis are often inaccessible or discouraged. For example, abdominal pain is a symptom in approximately two-thirds of the patients with IC. Obviously this cannot be readily detected in the sedated or intubated ICU patient. When present, abdominal pain starts abruptly and is associated with abdominal distension; urge to defecate and mild rectal bleeding usually follow.[71–73]

Regarding small intestinal ischemia, routine laboratory test results are nonspecific. Furthermore, no biochemical marker of ischemia has demonstrated legitimate diagnostic value in IC. Imaging and colonoscopy together create the cornerstone of the diagnosis.[66,71,72]

Plain radiographs of the abdomen provide nonspecific findings in approximately 20% of cases during the initial phases. Pneumatosis, free air, thumbprinting, and air in the portal system are late radiographic signs that indicate severe IC. CT is widely used as the initial imaging method for assessing intestinal ischemia in general.[67,72] Although CT lacks specificity for the diagnosis of IC, it is useful in ruling out other intra-abdominal conditions. Certain CT findings correlate with the severity of IC. Thumbprinting, pericolonic stranding, and bowel-wall thickening indicate IC with partial wall involvement.[16] Severe ischemia provoked by total vascular occlusion results in colonic dilatation and thin, unenhanced wall.[75] High-quality thin-slice CT can detect vascular occlusion. Other signs of severe IC on CT are pneumatosis coli, air in the portal system, and pneumoperitoneum with or without free intra-abdominal fluid. These findings, coupled with risk factors for IC, indicate a poor prognosis.

Colonoscopy is the most specific and sensitive test for IC. Visible mucosal changes determine the severity of the disease. Sharp demarcation of the ischemic area, particularly preserving the rectum, is suggestive of IC. Areas of pale mucosa intercalated by areas of erythema occur during early phases. If unequivocal signs of necrosis are detected (gray, green, or black mucosa) the procedure should be aborted, owing to the risk of colonic perforation. As the ischemia advances, submucosal edema, hemorrhage, and mucosal nodules are detected in the lumen, corresponding to thumbprinting on radiographic tests.[66,67,72,73] These findings recede as submucosal hemorrhage is reabsorbed or evacuated into the lumen.[67,72]

Colonoscopy is an invasive procedure and has some inherent drawbacks for the diagnosis of IC. There is a need to exercise prudence when inflating the colon, and intraluminal pressure should be kept below 30 mm Hg. Alternatively colonoscopy can be performed with CO_2, which is more rapidly absorbed than room air. In addition, CO_2 also provokes vasodilatation, improving colonic-wall perfusion.[67,72]

Severe Clostridium difficile Colitis

Background

Clostridium difficile is a gram-positive anaerobic bacillus. It is a normal component of the intestinal flora of children younger than 2 years, and of 3% to 5% of the adult population. *C difficile* infection (CDI) is an important cause of death among critically ill ICU patients.[77] Prior antibiotic treatment, including prophylactic use, is reported in approximately 95% of the patients who develop CDI (relative risk 5.9).[78] Even the 2 most common antibiotics used in the treatment of CDI, metronidazole and vancomycin, can actually cause the disease. However, clindamycin, ampicillin, fluoroquinolones, and cephalosporins (particularly ceftriaxone) are the most frequent.[77,78] More than 30% of hospitalized patients who receive antibiotics, for any reason, become colonized with *C difficile*, approximately 55% of whom develop CDI.[79]

The period between antibiotics and colonization with *C difficile* and the actual symptoms of CDI is short (median of 2–3 days). However, the risk of CDI persists for several weeks after the cessation of antimicrobial therapy because of prolonged modification of the colonic flora.[77]

In addition to preceding antibiotic therapy, there are several other risk factors for CDI:

- Cancer
- Proton-pump inhibitors
- Low levels of antitoxin
- Low levels of B antibodies
- ICU admission
- Inflammatory bowel disease
- Burns
- Prolonged hospitalization (1% colonization if less than 1 week, up to 50% colonization if more than 4 weeks)[80]
- Long-term care facilities (up to 50% of the patients can be colonized)[81]
- Immunosuppression (chemotherapy, human immunodeficiency virus)
- Organ transplantation (lung transplant patients 8 times more likely to have severe CDI)[77]

- Advanced age (patients older than 65 years have a 20-fold higher risk for CDI than younger patients)[80]
- Enteral feedings (elemental diets)
- Gastrointestinal surgery

Epidemiology

There is substantial evidence showing an increase in prevalence, severity, and mortality from CDI.[79,81–86] Possible reasons are the outbreak of more virulent strains (BI/NAP1/027 strain produces 15–20 times more toxin than less virulent ones) and inadequate immune response (low levels of immunoglobulin G antitoxin).[77,87] Furthermore, recurrent CDI is also becoming more common, particularly in patients older than 65 years, in whom the incidence of more severe forms of the disease is considerably higher.[87]

Approximately 3% to 8% of the patients with CDI will develop fulminant *C difficile* colitis.[88,89] The mortality rate caused by this form of CDI ranges from 30% to 90%, and approximately 50% of the deaths occur within 48 hours of ICU admission.[89–91]

The main risk factors linked to 30-day mortality in fulminant CDI are:

- Age older than 74 years
- White blood cell count (WBC) greater than $50 \times 10^9/L$
- Lactate greater than 5 mmol/L
- Immunosuppression
- Vasopressor therapy for hypotension.

Among these risk factors, high WBC and lactate each had adjusted odds ratios of greater than 10 for fulminant CDI; 18.6 (95% confidence interval [CI], 3.7–94.7) and 12.4 (95% CI, 2.4–63.7), respectively.[90] The need for vasopressor therapy for shock and multiple-organ failure in fulminant CDI was associated with greater than 65% mortality.[92,93]

Studies have shown that early surgical consultation contributes to more timely diagnosis and treatment of patients who present with fulminant CDI.[89,90] However, the lack of validated clinical predictors and management strategy create a significant challenge for those who treat such patients.[89–92]

Diagnosis

Several testing strategies can be used to diagnose CDI. Stool culture is important for epidemiologic studies, while the cytotoxicity cell assay is the gold standard for detection of *C difficile* toxins. However, both methods are clinically impractical because of long turnaround times.[77,78] Furthermore, when stool culture is used as the sole diagnostic method, there is at least a 10% chance of a false-positive result because of nontoxigenic strains of *C difficile*.[78] Enzyme-linked immunosorbent assay and polymerase chain reaction tests are rapid, but can be less reliable than the cytotoxicity cell assay.[77,78,94] Therefore, diagnosis should be based on a combination of history, risk factors, laboratory results, clinical manifestation, imaging tests, and sometimes an endoscopic procedure.

Common clinical manifestations of CDI are watery foul-smelling diarrhea and mild abdominal pain.[77–79,81,82] However, diarrhea can be absent in approximately 20% of critically ill patients who have severe CDI or develop the disease in the postoperative period; opiate use is also a contributing factor.[95]

Clinical manifestations of severe CDI include:

- Ileus
- Abdominal distension with minimal diarrhea

- Toxic megacolon (0.4%–3%)[89]
- Significant dehydration
- Changes in mental status
- Evidence of end-organ failure

With respect to laboratory results, a WBC greater than 20×10^9/L, hypoalbuminemia less than 20 g/L, and creatinine greater than 2.3 mg/L have all been associated with severe CDI.[90–92]

In severe CDI, imaging studies are commonly used to rule out other causes of acute abdomen. Reliability of these studies is variable, and this should be considered when interpreting the findings. A retrospective study showed that plain radiographs of the abdomen were read as normal in 36% of patients who had a confirmed diagnosis of fulminant *C difficile* colitis, and another 18% showed only nonspecific changes.[90] In the same study, abdominal ultrasonographic findings were considered normal in 46% of the cases with confirmed diagnosis.[90] A CT scan, with or without contrast, is more reliable than other imaging methods for the diagnosis of CDI. Common CT findings are:

- Segmental colonic-wall thickening greater than 4 mm (most sensitive finding)
- Colonic-wall nodularity
- Ascites (42%)
- Pericolonic stranding (62%)[96]

Less common findings are:

- Nodular thickening of the haustral folds
- Colonic distension (13% of the patients with fulminant colitis)
- Colonic-fold effacement[96]

Endoscopic methods for the diagnosis of *C difficile* colitis are used inconsistently (3%–31% of the cases), even though pseudomembranes demonstrated by colonoscopy/sigmoidoscopy are pathognomonic of severe *C difficile* colitis.[78,90,91,97–99] Less specific findings are rectal sparing (25%–70% of the patients), mucosal edema, erythema, and ulcerations.[77,91] False-negative rates for endoscopic methods in fulminant *C difficile* colitis range from 10% to 25%.[89,97]

Patients with fulminant *C difficile* colitis who undergo endoscopic diagnosis have a higher risk of colonic perforation.[91,99] Therefore, colonoscopy/sigmoidoscopy should be reserved for situations when laboratory tests are persistently negative despite a high suspicion for *C difficile* colitis, or when treatment for *C difficile* colitis is ineffective, bringing forth the need to elucidate a diagnosis.[89,99]

Acute Acalculous Cholecystitis

Background
Acute acalculous cholecystitis (AAC) accounts for approximately 2% to 15% of all causes of acute cholecystitis, and is a significant problem in critically ill patients.[100–103] In the ICU approximately 50% of all cases of acute cholecystitis in postoperative patients are acalculous.[100–103]

The incidence of gallbladder gangrene in ICU patients with AAC is greater than 50%, and that of perforation greater than 10%.[100,101,103,104] Conversely, in the non-ICU outpatient population the reported incidence of gallbladder gangrene is 36%, with no reports of perforations.[105] A higher incidence of complicated AAC in ICU patients can be attributed, in part, to the delay in treatment as a result of a difficult diagnosis. In combination with significant premorbid conditions, this results in mortality rates of between 30% and 45%.[100,102,103]

There are several factors involved in the pathogenesis of ACC. However, an ischemic process of the gallbladder wall provoked by impaired splanchnic circulation is pivotal, and is a common condition among critically ill patients. Microangiopathy with arterial occlusion and reduced venous filling was demonstrated in patients with ACC, whereas calculous cholecystitis is characterized by vasodilatation.[106]

Moreover, interventions frequently performed in the ICU, such as mechanical ventilation, total parenteral nutrition (TPN), and use of opioids, cause cholestasis and modification of bile composition (increasing lysophosphatidylcholine and β-glucuronidase), thereby inducing AAC.[102,104,107] A study showed that biliary sludge was detected via ultrasonography in approximately 6% of the patients who were on TPN for 3 weeks, which increased to 100% by the sixth week.[108] It is postulated that the combination of bile stasis/altered bile composition and gallbladder ischemia contributes to mucosal injury and secondary bacterial infection.

Epidemiology

Demographically, AAC is more common in men than in women (3:1). This preference is even more striking among patients who undergo surgical procedures unrelated to trauma, of whom approximately 80% are men.[100] Non–trauma-related and burn-related AAC are more common in postoperative older patients (>60 years), particularly those who undergo complicated cardiovascular surgical procedures.[100,109] Approximately 42% of the cases of acute cholecystitis after cardiac surgery are acalculous.[100] Other common predisposing factors to AAC in older patients are:

- Severe atherosclerosis
- Congestive heart failure
- Cardiac arrest and cardiopulmonary resuscitation
- Diabetes
- Hemodialysis

An interesting study showed that de novo presentation of AAC in previously healthy patients was unrelated to advanced age.[105] Patients as young as 30 years developed the condition (mean age 52.4 years).[105] Other general risk factors for AAC are:

- Trauma
- Burns[110]
- Multiple blood transfusions[110]
- Hypotension
- Childbirth
- Acute myeloid leukemia
- Bone marrow transplantation
- Immunosuppression
- Vasculitis
- Cholesterol embolization
- Medications (vasopressors, sunitinib)[111]

Sepsis from various sources is also an important risk factor for AAC in ICU patients. A report from a mixed ICU population showed that an admission diagnosis of sepsis and pneumonia accounted for 54% of cases of AAC.[103]

Diagnosis

In general, the diagnosis of acute cholecystitis is essentially linked to clinical impression and physical examination.[112] The Murphy sign and right upper quadrant tenderness have high positive and negative likelihood ratios (LR), respectively, for the diagnosis of acute cholecystitis (positive LR 2.8; 95% CI, 0.8–8.6; negative LR 0.4; 95% CI, 0.2–1.1); Of note, the CI for both findings included 1.[112] Unfortunately, physical examination of the intubated and sedated critically ill ICU patient is unreliable.[112] Older patients frequently have acute cholecystitis without any findings on physical examination, even if not sedated. Furthermore, clinical signs of cholestasis are common in critically ill patients for conditions other than AAC, complicating the diagnosis even more.[100,103,112]

Laboratory tests are nonspecific for AAC, particularly in patients who are critically ill from other conditions.[103,112] Among 39 ICU patients with a confirmed diagnosis of AAC, only 13% had fever (38.5°C), 54% had leukocytosis, and liver enzymes were abnormal in only 59% to 79%.[103] Therefore, AAC should be suspected in ICU patients with unexplained fever and leukocytosis, and an undefined source of sepsis.

Imaging studies are important adjuncts in the diagnosis of AAC. Although abdominal ultrasonography is considered the most accurate diagnostic imaging technique for acute cholecystitis, the absence of gallstones in AAC decreases the sensitivity of this method from 88% to approximately 67%.[112,113] A study involving 62 critically ill trauma patients showed an even worse performance of abdominal ultrasonography in the diagnosis of AAC, with 30% sensitivity and 93% specificity.[114] Nonetheless, bedside abdominal ultrasonography is the most widely used imaging study in the diagnosis of AAC in ICU patients.[100,103,112,114] The most common abnormal ultrasonographic findings in AAC are:

- Gallbladder-wall thickening (>3.5 mm)
- Pericholecystic fluid or perforation of the gallbladder
- Subserosal edema (halo)
- Emphysematous gallbladder
- Gallbladder distension (>5 mm transversely)
- Positive Murphy sign with ultrasound probe

Gallbladder sludge, abdominal ascites, hypoalbuminemia, and cholesterolosis are associated with false-positive results.[100]

CT scanning is helpful when other conditions need to be investigated. Although CT is inferior to ultrasonography in the evaluation of acute biliary conditions, the pathologic findings are similar to those detected with abdominal ultrasonography.[100,112,114] A cholescintigraphy (hepatobiliary iminodiacetic acid) scan and bedside laparoscopy are of limited value in the critically ill ICU patient.

Perforated Duodenal Ulcer

Background

Perforation occurs in approximately 5% to 10% of patients with peptic ulcer disease, being 7 times more common in duodenal ulcers than in gastric ulcers. In both organs, the perforations are usually located on the anterior wall.[115–118] Effective treatment against *Helicobacter pylori* has drastically decreased the need for elective surgical treatment in peptic ulcer disease. At present, approximately 80% of the operations in patients with peptic ulcer disease are performed for acute complications.[115–118] Nonetheless, *H pylori* is still the principal cause of perforated duodenal ulcers, while nonsteroidal anti-inflammatory drugs (NSAIDs) are responsible for approximately 40% to 50% of cases.[115–119]

Epidemiology

Although the frequency of perforated peptic ulcer is decreasing in the general population, it is becoming more frequent among elderly patients and those with comorbidities.[115,116,120] The mean age for this complication is currently between 60 and 70 years,[120] a fact that can be explained by a frequently positive (50%–60%) medical history for peptic ulcer and an increase in the use of NSAIDs among these patients. Perforation is more common in men (male/female ratio 2:1). However, the incidence in women has increased significantly in the last 45 years, as the previous male/female ratio was almost 7:1.[120] Women with perforated duodenal ulcers tend to be 10 years older than men.[120]

In addition to *H pylori* and NSAIDs, other risk factors for perforated peptic ulcers that commonly present in ICU patients are chronic obstructive lung disease, shock, major burns, steroid therapy, and multiple-organ failure.[116,118–120]

Diagnosis

Similarly to other intra-abdominal catastrophes, early diagnosis of perforated duodenal ulcer and timely intervention result in better outcomes. The classic presentation of sudden epigastric pain becoming generalized is rarely observed in critically ill ICU patients, who are frequently debilitated, under sedation and steroids, and consequently present minimal or no symptoms related to perforated ulcers. Therefore, the diagnosis is frequently delayed until patients become hypotensive and febrile and bacterial peritonitis ensues.[116–118,121]

Mortality rate increases significantly (3–5 times) when the diagnosis and treatment of perforated ulcers are delayed for more than 24 hours, particularly if systolic blood pressure is less than 100 mm Hg.[116,117] In the elderly patient with comorbidities, these findings are associated with a 42% mortality.[117,120]

Differential diagnosis should include mesenteric infarction, acute pancreatitis, and ruptured aortic aneurysm. Early hypotension increases the likelihood of a diagnosis of ruptured abdominal aortic aneurysm. Although pneumoperitoneum can be detected on supine chest radiograph in approximately 70% to 80% of cases, the absence of this finding may lead to a misdiagnosis of acute appendicitis, acute pancreatitis, or cholecystitis.[116–118,121] Therefore, CT is the most frequently used diagnostic imaging method. Bedside ultrasonography is of limited value in the diagnosis of perforated duodenal ulcer, and the use of bedside DL requires further research.

TREATMENT OF ABDOMINAL CATASTROPHES IN THE ICU

Patients in the ICU are invariably receiving both hemodynamic and ventilator support. Clearly, overlay of an acute intra-abdominal process may affect these parameters, and requires an adjustment in the management. In addition to supportive care, antimicrobial therapy and source control of the underlying pathologic processes represent the mainstay of treatment. This section addresses these issues for each of the main pathologic processes discussed in the prior sections.

Antimicrobial Therapy

Most pathologic processes discussed in the prior sections are infectious in nature and therefore represent an indication for the administration of antimicrobial therapy. The major exception is ACS, which results from the pathophysiologic consequences of elevated IAP. There is therefore no indication for initiation of antimicrobial therapy specifically for this entity.

C difficile–associated disease (CDAD) is infectious in nature, but differs from the other diseases in that the offending microorganism remains in the colon and the toxins elaborated by the microbe lead to its manifestation. Antimicrobial therapy is therefore directed at the responsible colonic microbe, namely *C difficile*. Much of the discussion regarding treatment of this microbe centers on how to achieve therapeutic concentrations in the colon. Recent clinical practice guidelines published by the Society for Healthcare Epidemiology of America and the Infectious Diseases Society of America have developed a classification of disease severity, and have aligned treatment with the severity of disease (**Table 3**).[77]

The vast majority of patients with CDAD fall into the first category of mild to moderate disease, and invariably respond well to oral therapy with metronidazole for mild disease, or with vancomycin if patients are considered to have more severe disease as evidenced by leukocytosis and mild renal dysfunction in the setting of the older patient.[122] These patients are rarely in the ICU setting, and if so their CDAD usually presents as a bystander in their illness rather than as an abdominal catastrophe. For patients described as having complicated CDAD with abdominal ileus and hemodynamic instability, the recommendation suggests that oral vancomycin plus intravenous metronidazole are given together. In the patient with profound ileus, instillation of vancomycin via a nasogastric tube and via enema is recommended.

The other pathologic processes discussed, namely ischemic small and large intestine, cholecystitis, and perforated duodenal ulcer disease, are associated with loss of the integrity of the wall of the viscera affected, and therefore warrant initiation of antimicrobial therapy. As a general approach to antimicrobial therapy in intra-abdominal infection, treatment should be directed against the most common microbes causing infection related to the diseased organ. The ICU patient population is unique in that the typical microbial flora associated with various parts of the gastrointestinal tract may be modified by several factors including prior antibiotic use, the use of gastric acid–reducing therapy, intestinal ileus and obstruction, and immunosuppressive therapies. For example, the upper small bowel is usually populated by gram-positive cocci such as *Streptococcus viridans* and staphylococci, whereas in the setting of obstruction/ileus the flora look more like colonic flora, with a shift of microbes to include

Table 3
Classification schema for *Clostridium difficile* infection and recommended antibiotic treatment strategy as outlined in Society for Healthcare Epidemiology of America/Infectious Diseases Society of America Treatment Guidelines

Category	Criteria	Treatment	Strength/Quality of Evidence
Mild or moderate	Diarrhea	Metronidazole 500 mg per os tid	A-I
Severe	WBC >15 × 10^9/µL or creatinine level increased 1.5-fold greater than baseline level	Vancomycin 125 mg per os qid	B-I
Severe, complicated	Ileus, megacolon, hypotension, or shock	Metronidazole 500 mg intravenously tid + vancomycin 500 mg by mouth qid (+ vancomycin enemas in ileus)	C-III

This scoring system is not yet validated.

Abbreviation: WBC, white blood cell count.

Adapted from Cohen SH, Gerding DN, Johnson S, et al. Clinical practice guidelines for *Clostridium difficile* infection in adults: 2010 update by the Society for Healthcare Epidemiology of America (SHEA) and the Infectious Diseases Society of America (IDSA). Infect Control Hosp Epidemiol 2010;31:447; with permission.

gram-negative enteric bacteria and *Bacteroides* species.[123] The picture is further complicated by the facts that the intra-abdominal infection is hospital-acquired and that patients have frequently been on antimicrobial therapy. This situation leads to a shift such that the gastrointestinal tract is colonized by hospital-acquired, multidrug-resistant, gram-negative bacteria.[8,124]

Consensus guidelines recently published by the Surgical Infection Society and the Infectious Diseases Society of America address the management of intra-abdominal infections. The guidelines separate patients into 2 groups: (1) those with community-acquired infection and (2) those with health care–associated infection. The community-acquired infection group is further subdivided into "mild to moderate severity" and "high severity," where high risk defines patients who are at increased risk for treatment failure. The high-risk patients are identified by several factors, almost all of which are applicable to the ICU patient:

- High severity of illness (ie, physiologic derangement as defined by APACHE II)
- Advanced age
- Comorbidity and degree of organ dysfunction
- Immunologic suppression (including malnutrition, malignancy, immunosuppressive agents)
- Diffuse peritonitis
- Poor control of underlying pathologic process
- Prolonged preoperative hospital stay
- Prior use of antimicrobial agents

In this high-risk patient group, the microbial flora are characterized by the presence of multiresistant microbes, and according to the guidelines, broad-spectrum antimicrobial agents are indicated. Several of these agents are recommended:

- Single-agent therapy with carbapenem agents such as piperacillin/tazobactam, imipenem/cilastatin, meropenem, doripenem
- Combination therapy with ceftazidime plus metronidazole

In the health care–associated setting, the presence of multiresistant microbes is even more likely, including methicillin-resistant *Staphylococcus aureus*, vancomycin-resistant enterococci, *Candida* species, and multiresistant gram-negative enteric bacilli. This likelihood underscores the importance of taking cultures at the time of surgery. In addition, decisions regarding coverage should take into account the antibiotic susceptibility pattern of the individual institution. In essence, antibiotic selection should be similar to those for high-severity community-acquired infections plus addition/replacement based on institutional patterns. Furthermore, the regimen should be tailored to the culture and sensitivity data derived from the infection. This regimen would include the addition of antifungal therapy should fungi be cultured from infection.

Surgery and Other Interventions

Clostridium difficile–associated disease

C difficile manifests as a range of disease ranging from mild diarrhea to a very severe illness characterized by diffuse abdominal tenderness, hypotension requiring inotrope support, and multiple-organ failure. Up to 8% of MICU patients are more likely to exhibit a spectrum of more severe disease, which presents itself as a fulminant colitis.[125] At this point in the patient's care, surgical consultation occurs for consideration of surgical intervention. Unfortunately, the preferred surgical intervention of a total abdominal colectomy with ileostomy is associated with a mortality rate of 34% to 80%.[125] Advanced age, preoperative shock, preoperative dialysis dependence, postoperative cardiac arrest, and Wound Classification III predicted mortality in a recent study using an administrative database.[126] Elevated lactate (>5 mmol/L), more than 50×10^9/L leukocytes, immunosuppression, and vasopressor therapy also predicted poor outcome. Delay in surgery from the time of diagnosis was also associated an increased mortality. Clearly, the key to optimizing outcomes in this group of patients is to be able to predict progression of disease soon after it is obvious that the patient is not responding to medical therapy. Unfortunately this is a problem, because no single parameter or constellation of parameters is able to do so. Therefore, the surgical and MICU team is left with recommending total colectomy and ileostomy, a procedure that itself is fairly morbid, in a patient who may yet respond to medical treatment.

The University of Pittsburgh group has recently reported on an alternative approach to the management of fulminant CDAD.[89,127,128] These investigators hypothesized that failure of medical therapy was due to excessive toxin accumulation in the colon and the failure of vancomycin to reach this site. The group established a protocol wherein a laparoscopic loop ileostomy is created, this stoma then being used to both flush the colon with polyethylene glycol and instill vancomycin enemas in an antegrade direction into the colon. In their comparison of this treatment group (42 patients) with a matched group of 42 patients treated with colectomy at the same institution, they reported a reduction in mortality rate to 19% from 50%. The investigators further suggested that initiation of this protocol at an early stage of complicated disease might further improve outcome, through preventing progression of disease and minimizing the need for colectomy.

Abdominal compartment syndrome

The main goal in the treatment of IAH is to decrease the abdominal pressure. The WSACS guidelines recommend surgical decompression of the abdomen when noninvasive measures are incapable of achieving that goal. However, surgeons are well aware of the ensuing morbidity created by the "open abdomen." Therefore, determining the actual failure of nonsurgical management and the best time to perform decompressive laparotomy in IAH/ACS is a matter of debate.[23,26,30,34,35]

Approximately 8% to 16% of the patients who undergo decompressive laparotomy for ACS will never achieve primary closure of the fascia.[129,130] This aspect becomes a significant problem in the ICU, often leading to complications such as enterocutaneous and enteroatmospheric fistulas, fluid and electrolyte imbalance, malnutrition, surgical-site infection, and difficult ventilatory management. The incidence of small-bowel fistula ranged from zero to 26% in an extensive review of more than 150 articles on the management of open abdomens; the mortality rate ranged from zero to 42%.[131]

Delayed abdominal closure is also associated with significant long-term problems. In a recent study, almost 25% of the patients who underwent delayed closure of the abdominal wall did not return to work, 65% screened positive for depression, and 23% were found to have symptoms of posttraumatic stress disorder.[132] Therefore, nonsurgical management of IAH should be implemented early in the ICU patient **(Table 4)**.[13,35]

Cholecystitis

Gajic and colleagues[1] reported that cholecystitis accounted for 14% of the patients presenting with acute abdominal complications in the MICU. The recent Tokyo Guidelines reviewed the various approaches to treatment.[133] While noting that early cholecystectomy represented definitive therapy, the investigators observed that this procedure was associated with increased perioperative mortality in high-risk critically

Table 4
Nonsurgical management of intra-abdominal hypertension and abdominal compartment syndrome

General Management Strategy[a]	Procedures
Decrease abdominal content	Decompress stomach and rectum (tubes) Paracentesis (ascites) Percutaneous drainage (fluid collections) Enemas and prokinetic agents GI endoscopic decompression Reduce GI feeding
Improve abdominal wall compliance	Remove tight dressings Avoid head of bed >30° Neuromuscular blockade
Decrease excess fluid balance	Diuretics Colloids/hypertonic fluids/vasoactive medications Hemodialysis/hemofiltration
Improve end-organ perfusion	Maintain APP ≥60 mm Hg Optimize alveolar recruitment Goal-directed fluid resuscitation Use vasoactive medications

Abbreviations: APP, abdominal perfusion pressure; GI, gastrointestinal.
[a] General management strategy should be initiated if intra-abdominal pressure is 12 mm Hg or higher.

ill patients, and recommended that percutaneous transhepatic gallbladder drainage is a safe alternative that effectively leads to resolution of the cholecystitis. The literature specifically addressing these questions is generally poor, and multicenter, randomized trials comparing percutaneous cholecystostomy with early cholecystectomy are required to definitively answer the question of superior therapy.[134] The analysis will have to take into account the fact that following percutaneous cholecystostomy, approximately 50% of patients develop gallstone-related symptoms, one-fifth of which are due to complex biliary disease.[135]

Ischemic bowel disease

At the time of laparotomy gangrenous intestine is obvious, and the bowel should be resected. When the cause of infarction is a mesenteric vascular embolus or volvulus of the intestine, the demarcation sites between live and dead bowel are usually obvious, and the decision regarding the extent of bowel resection is straightforward. In this setting a primary anastomosis may be feasible, depending on local factors in the peritoneal cavity and systemic factors such as patient hemodynamic stability and medical comorbidities. In nonocclusive mesenteric ischemia, perforation may occur at 1 or more sites, with some areas of obvious gangrene but other areas where the bowel looks dusky (ie, ischemic but not necrotic). In this setting, the surgeon usually resects the clearly gangrenous parts of intestine (which presumably include the sites of perforation) and plans for a second-look laparotomy at 24 to 48 hours after the initial surgery. At the second stage, any residual ischemic/infarcted bowel should be resected. This second operation usually consists of a repeat laparotomy, although the use of a second-look laparoscopy has been reported.[63] The surgeon must again decide at this juncture whether primary anastomosis is feasible and/or desirable. A similar general approach is used following resection of colon for IC, although there is far less enthusiasm for primary anastomosis involving colon in this setting.

The use of a second-look laparotomy is conceptually now encompassed more broadly under the title of "damage control laparotomy."[136] In essence, the first operation is performed under emergent circumstances with a view to resecting obviously gangrenous bowel, managing any hemorrhage, and lavaging and debriding infected or necrotic material from the peritoneal cavity. Intestinal ends are stapled and left in the peritoneal cavity. The abdomen is then closed temporarily and the patient returned to the ICU for stabilization, warming, and correlation of acidosis and coagulopathy. Patients return to the operating room 48 hours later for the second look and surgical management. The literature is not robust, but suggests that this approach leads to a higher probability of intestinal anastomosis at the second procedure and, in addition, improved outcome. Negative-pressure wound therapy has been suggested for temporary closure, although a recent systematic review does not support its superiority over other techniques.[137]

Perforated duodenal ulcer disease

Perforation results in spread of gastrointestinal contents throughout the peritoneal cavity, and is manifested by diffuse peritoneal findings, fluid in the peritoneum, and, usually, a pneumoperitoneum. In this setting, surgical intervention is indicated. In general, the defect is managed by direct closure when the defect is small with easily opposable edges, reinforced by patching of the defect with vascularized omentum. Intraoperative lavage of gastrointestinal content and particulate matter should be performed. The role of drainage in this setting has not been critically studied, and may be influenced by the surgeon's preference and opinion regarding the quality of the patch/closure. A systematic review comparing a laparoscopic approach with this procedure has been shown to be comparable with open surgery in terms of overall outcome.[138] As previously noted, the decision to perform this approach should be made based on the skill and experience of the operating surgeon. Given that the intra-abdominal process is occurring against the backdrop of a critically ill patient, a laparotomy with expeditious definitive therapy and washout may be preferable. In addition, pneumoperitoneum in the hemodynamically unstable patient may preclude a laparoscopic approach.[139] Occasionally the perforation is well walled off, and can be managed conservatively with antibiotics with or without percutaneous drainage if an abscess is present.

SUMMARY

In the critically ill patient in the ICU, several intra-abdominal pathologic processes may supervene and cause deterioration of the patient's status. These processes are difficult to diagnose because of the compromised status of the patient, and advanced imaging, in particular CT scanning, is invaluable in establishing a diagnosis. Timely intervention is indicated, because delay is invariably associated with poor outcome.

REFERENCES

1. Gajic O, Urrutia LE, Sewani H, et al. Acute abdomen in the medical intensive care unit. Crit Care Med 2002;30:1187–90.
2. Liolios A, Oropello JM, Benjamin E. Gastrointestinal complications in the intensive care unit. Clin Chest Med 1999;20:329–45.
3. Rozycki G, Tremblay L, Feliciano DV, et al. Three hundred consecutive emergent celiotomies in general surgery patients: influence of advanced diagnostic imaging techniques and procedure diagnosis. Ann Surg 2002;235:681–9.

4. Marshall JC, Innes M. Intensive care unit management of intra-abdominal infection. Crit Care Med 2003;31:2228–37.
5. McLauchlan GJ, Anderson ID, Grant IS, et al. Outcome of patients with abdominal sepsis treated in an intensive care unit. Br J Surg 1995;82:524–9.
6. Moore LJ, McKinley BA, Turner KL, et al. The epidemiology of sepsis in general surgery patients. J Trauma 2011;70:673–80.
7. Sartelli M. A focus on intra-abdominal infections. World J Emerg Surg 2010;5:9.
8. Solomkin JS, Mazuski JE, Bradley JS, et al. Diagnosis and management of complicated intra-abdominal infection in adults and children: guidelines by the Surgical Infection Society and the Infectious Diseases Society of America. Clin Infect Dis 2010;50:133–64.
9. Becher RD, Hoth JJ, Miller PR, et al. Systemic inflammation worsens outcomes in emergency surgical patients. J Trauma 2012;72:1140–9.
10. Marshall JC, Maier RV, Jimenez M, et al. Source control in the management of severe sepsis and septic shock: an evidence-based review. Crit Care Med 2004;32:S513–26.
11. Diaz JJ, Bokhari F, Mowery NT, et al. Guidelines for management of small bowel obstruction. J Trauma 2008;64:1651–64.
12. Yazdi SS, Shapiro ML. Small bowel obstruction: the eternal dilemma of when to intervene. Scand J Surg 2010;99:78–80.
13. Malbrain ML, Cheatham ML, Kirkpatrick A, et al. Results from the International Conference of Experts on Intra-abdominal Hypertension and Abdominal Compartment Syndrome. Intensive Care Med 2006;32:1722–32.
14. Malbrain ML, Cheatham ML. Definitions and pathophysiological implications of intra-abdominal hypertension and abdominal compartment syndrome. Am Surg 2011;77(Suppl 1):S7–11.
15. Balogh ZJ, van Wessem K, Yoshino O, et al. Postinjury abdominal compartment syndrome: are we winning the battle? World J Surg 2009;33:1134–41.
16. Cheatham ML, Safcsak K. Intra-abdominal hypertension and abdominal compartment syndrome: the journey forward. Am Surg 2011;77(Suppl):S1–5.
17. Citerio G, Vascotto E, Villa F, et al. Induced abdominal compartment syndrome increases intracranial pressure in neurotrauma patients: a prospective study. Crit Care Med 2001;29:1466–71.
18. Diebel LN, Dulchavsky SA, Brown WJ. Splanchnic ischemia and bacterial translocation in the abdominal compartment syndrome. J Trauma 1997;43:852–5.
19. Malbrain ML, Deeren D, De Potter TJ. Intra-abdominal hypertension in the critically ill: it is time to pay attention. Curr Opin Crit Care 2005;11:156–71.
20. Kirkpatrick AW, Brenneman FD, McLean RF, et al. Is clinical examination an accurate indicator of raised intra-abdominal pressure in critically injured patients? Can J Surg 2000;43:207–11.
21. Rezende-Neto J, Moore EE, Masuno T, et al. The abdominal compartment syndrome as a second insult during systemic inflammatory neutrophil priming provokes multiple organ injury. Shock 2003;20:303–8.
22. Schachtrupp A, Wauters J, Wilmer A. What is the best animal model for ACS? Acta Clin Belg Suppl 2007;(1):225–32.
23. Cheatham ML, Safcsak K, Fiscina C, et al. Advanced age may limit the survival benefit of open abdominal decompression. Am Surg 2011;77:856–61.
24. Malbrain ML, Chiumello D, Pelosi P, et al. Prevalence of intra-abdominal hypertension in critically ill patients: a multicentre epidemiological study. Intensive Care Med 2004;30:822–9.

25. Malbrain ML, Chiumello D, Pelosi P, et al. Incidence and prognosis of intraabdominal hypertension in a mixed population of critically ill patients: a multiple-center epidemiological study. Crit Care Med 2005;33:315–22.
26. Smith C, Cheatham ML. Intra-abdominal hypertension and abdominal compartment syndrome in the medical patient. Am Surg 2011;77(Suppl):S67–71.
27. Zengerink I, McBeth PB, Zygun DA, et al. Validation and experience with a simple continuous intra-abdominal pressure measurement in a multidisciplinary medical/surgical critical care unit. J Trauma 2008;64:1159–64.
28. Bailey RW, Bulkley GB, Hamilton SR, et al. Protection of the small intestine from nonocclusive mesenteric ischemic injury due to cardiogenic shock. Am J Surg 1987;153:108–16.
29. Balogh Z, Moore FA, Moore EE, et al. Secondary abdominal compartment syndrome: a potential threat for all trauma clinicians. Injury 2007;38:272–9.
30. Cothren CC, Moore EE, Johnson JL, et al. Outcomes in surgical in surgical versus medical patients with the secondary abdominal compartment syndrome. Am J Surg 2007;194:804–7.
31. Sugrue M, Jones F, Deane SA, et al. Intra-abdominal hypertension is an independent cause of postoperative renal impairment. Arch Surg 1999;134:1082–5.
32. Keulenaer BL, Regli A, Malbrain ML. Intra-abdominal measurement techniques: is there anything new? Am Surg 2011;77(Suppl):S17–22.
33. DeWaele J, Pletinckx P, Blot S, et al. Saline volume in transvesical intra-abdominal pressure measurement: enough is enough. Intensive Care Med 2006;32:455–9.
34. Regueira T, Bruhn A, Hasbun P, et al. Intra-abdominal hypertension: incidence and association with organ dysfunction during early septic shock. J Crit Care 2008;23:461–7.
35. Cheatham ML, Malbrain ML, Kirkpatrick A, et al. Results from the conference of experts on intra-abdominal hypertension and abdominal compartment syndrome. Part II. Recommendations. Intensive Care Med 2007;33:951–62.
36. Brandt LJ, Boley SJ. AGA technical review on intestinal ischemia. American Gastrointestinal Association. Gastroenterology 2000;118:954–68.
37. Herbert GS, Steele SR. Acute and chronic mesenteric ischemia. Surg Clin North Am 2007;87:1115–34.
38. Corcos O, Castier Y, Sibert A, et al. Effects of a multimodal management strategy for acute mesenteric ischemia on survival and intestinal failure. Clin Gastroenterol Hepatol 2013;11:158–65.
39. Kassahun WT, Schulz T, Richter O, et al. Unchanged high mortality rates from acute occlusive intestinal ischemia: six year review. Langenbecks Arch Surg 2008;393:163–71.
40. Schoots IG, Kofeman GI, Legemate DA, et al. Systematic review of survival after acute mesenteric ischaemia according to disease aetiology. Br J Surg 2004;91:17–27.
41. Dorudi S, Lamont PM. Intestinal ischaemia in the unconscious intensive care unit patient. Ann R Coll Surg Engl 1992;74:356–9.
42. Schoots IG, Levi MM, Reekers JA, et al. Thrombolytic therapy for acute superior mesenteric occlusion. J Vasc Interv Radiol 2005;16:317–29.
43. Wadman M, Syk I, Elmstahl S. Survival after operations for ischaemic bowel disease. Eur J Surg 2000;166:872–7.
44. Lobo Martinez E, Carvajosa E, Sacco O, et al. Embolectomy in mesenteric ischemia. Rev Esp Enferm Dig 1993;83:351–4.

45. Ottinger LW. The surgical management of acute occlusion of the superior mesenteric artery. Ann Surg 1978;188:721–31.

46. Harnik IG, Brandt LJ. Mesenteric venous thrombosis. Vasc Med 2010;15: 407–18.

47. Acosta S, Alhadad A, Svensson P. Epidemiology, risk and prognostic factors in mesenteric venous thrombosis. Br J Surg 2008;95:1245–51.

48. Kumar S, Kamath PS. Acute mesenteric venous thrombosis: one disease or two? Am J Gastroenterol 2003;98:1299–304.

49. Taylor CT, Colgan SP. Hypoxia and gastrointestinal disease. J Mol Med 2007;85: 1295–300.

50. Abu-Daff S, Abu-Daff N, Al-Shahed M. Mesenteric venous thrombosis and factors associated with mortality: a statistical analysis with five-year follow-up. J Gastrointest Surg 2009;13:1245–50.

51. Evennett NJ, Petrov MS, Mittal A, et al. Systematic review and pooled estimates for the diagnostic accuracy of serological markers for intestinal ischemia. World J Surg 2009;33:1374–83.

52. Newman TS, Magnuson TH, Ahrendt SA, et al. The changing face of mesenteric infarction. Am Surg 1998;64:611–6.

53. Demir IE, Ceyhan GO, Friess H. Beyond lactate: is there a role for serum lactate measurement in diagnosing acute mesenteric ischemia? Dig Surg 2012;29: 226–35.

54. Furukawa A, Kanasaki S, Kono N, et al. CT diagnosis of acute mesenteric ischemia from various causes. AJR Am J Roentgenol 2009;192:408–16.

55. Menke J. Diagnostic accuracy of multidetector CT in acute mesenteric ischemia: systematic review and meta-analysis. Radiology 2010;256:93–101.

56. Kirkpatrick ID, Kroeker MA, Greenberg HM. Biphasic CT with mesenteric angiography in the evaluation of acute mesenteric ischemia: initial experience. Radiology 2003;229:91–8.

57. Brandt CP, Priebe PP, Eckhauser ML. Diagnostic laparoscopy in the intensive care patient: avoiding the nontherapeutic laparotomy. Surg Endosc 1993;7:168–72.

58. Brandt CP, Priebe PP, Jacobs DG. Value of laparoscopy in trauma ICU patients with suspected acalculous cholecystitis. Surg Endosc 1994;8:361–4.

59. Jaramillo EJ, Trevino JM, Berghoff KR, et al. Bedside diagnostic laparoscopy in the intensive care unit: a 13-year experience. JSLS 2006;10:155–9.

60. Orlando R 3rd, Crowell KL. Laparoscopy in the critically ill. Surg Endosc 1997; 11:1072–4.

61. Seshadri PA, Poulin EC, Mamazza J, et al. Simplified laparoscopic approach to second look laparotomy: a review. Surg Laparosc Endosc Percutan Tech 1999; 9:286–9.

62. Wang YZ. Staged second-look laparoscopy to evaluate ischemic bowel. JSLS 2009;13:560–3.

63. Yanar H, Taviloglu K, Ertekin C, et al. Planned second-look laparoscopy in the management of acute mesenteric ischemia. World J Gastroenterol 2007; 13(24):3350–3.

64. Hackert T, Kienle P, Weitz J, et al. Accuracy of diagnostic laparoscopy for early diagnosis of abdominal complications after cardiac surgery. Surg Endosc 2003; 17:1671–4.

65. Persi A, Matano S, Manca G, et al. Bedside diagnostic laparoscopy to diagnose intraabdominal pathology in the intensive care unit. Crit Care 2009;13:R25.

66. Higgins PD, Davis KJ, Laine L. Systematic review: the epidemiology of ischemic colitis. Aliment Pharmacol Ther 2004;19:729–38.

67. Greenwald DA, Brandt LJ. Colonic ischemia. J Clin Gastroenterol 1998;27: 122–8.
68. Ritz JP, Germer CT, Buhr HJ. Prognostic factors for mesenteric infarction: multi-variate analysis of 187 patients with regard to patient age. Ann Vasc Surg 2005; 19:328–34.
69. Nassar AP, da Silva FM, de Cleva R. Constipation in intensive care unit: inci-dence and risk factors. J Crit Care 2009;24:630.e9–12.
70. Mostafa SM, Bhandari S, Ritchie G, et al. Constipation and its implications in the critically ill patient. Br J Anaesth 2003;91:815–9.
71. Theodoropoulou A, Koutroubakis IE. Ischemic colitis: clinical practice in diag-nosis and treatment. World J Gastroenterol 2008;14:7302–8.
72. Sun MY, Maykel JA. Ischemic colitis. Clin Colon Rectal Surg 2007;20:5–12.
73. Baixauli J, Kiran RP, Delaney CP. Investigation and management of ischemic co-litis. Cleve Clin J Med 2003;70:920–34.
74. Anon R, Bosca MM, Sanchiz V, et al. Factors predicting poor prognosis in ischemic colitis. World J Gastroenterol 2006;12:4875–8.
75. Barouk J, Gournay J, Bernard P, et al. Ischemic colitis in the elderly: predictive factors of gangrenous outcome. Gastroenterol Clin Biol 1999;23:470–4.
76. Thoeni RF, Cello JP. CT imaging of colitis. Radiology 2006;240:623–38.
77. Cohen SH, Gerding DN, Johnson S, et al. Clinical practice guidelines for *Clos-tridium difficile* infection in adults: 2010 update by the Society for Healthcare Epidemiology of America (SHEA) and the Infectious Diseases Society of Amer-ica (IDSA). Infect Control Hosp Epidemiol 2010;31:431–55.
78. Riddle DJ, Dubberke ER. *Clostridium difficile* infection in the intensive care unit. Infect Dis Clin North Am 2009;23:727–43.
79. US Department of Health and Human Services. HCUPnet 2010. Available at: http://hcupnet.ahrq.gov. Accessed May 23, 2013.
80. Garey KW, Dao-Tran TK, Jiang ZD, et al. A clinical risk index for *Clostridium diffi-cile* infection in hospitalized patients receiving broad-spectrum antibiotics. J Hosp Infect 2008;70:142–7.
81. Riggs MM, Sethi AK, Zabarsky TF, et al. Asymptomatic carriers are a poten-tial source for transmission of epidemic and nonepidemic *Clostridium diffi-cile* strains among long-term care facility residents. Clin Infect Dis 2007; 45:992–8.
82. Jaber MR, Olafsson S, Fung WL, et al. Clinical review of the management of fulminant *Clostridium difficile* infection. Am J Gastroenterol 2008;103: 195–203.
83. Loo VG, Poirier L, Miller MA, et al. A predominately clonal multi-institutional outbreak of *Clostridium difficile*-associated diarrhea with high morbidity and mortality. N Engl J Med 2005;353:2442–9.
84. Morris AM, Jobe BA, Stoney M, et al. *Clostridium difficile* colitis: an increasingly aggressive iatrogenic disease? Arch Surg 2002;137:1096–100.
85. Ricciardi R, Rothenberger DA, Madoff RD, et al. Increasing prevalence and severity of *Clostridium difficile* colitis in hospitalized patients in the United States. Arch Surg 2007;142:624–31.
86. Zilberberg MD, Shorr AF, Kollef MH. Increase in adult *Clostridium difficile*-related hospitalizations and case-fatality rate, United States 2000-2005. Emerg Infect Dis 2008;14:929–31.
87. Pepin J, Saheb N, Coulombe MA, et al. Emergence of fluoroquinolones as the predominant risk factor for *Clostridium difficile*-associated diarrhea: a cohort study during an epidemic in Quebec. Clin Infect Dis 2005;41:1254–60.

88. Dial S, Alrasadi K, Manoukian C, et al. Risk of *Clostridium difficile* diarrhea among hospitals inpatients prescribed proton pump inhibitors: cohort and case-control studies. CMAJ 2004;171:33–8.

89. Carchman EH, Peitzman AB, Simmons RL, et al. The role of acute care surgery in the treatment of severe complicated *Clostridium difficile*-associated disease. J Trauma Acute Care Surg 2012;73:789–800.

90. Lamontagne F, Labbe AC, Haeck O, et al. Impact of emergency colectomy on survival of patients with fulminant *Clostridium difficile* colitis during an epidemic caused by a hypervirulent strain. Ann Surg 2007;245:267–72.

91. Adams SD, Mercer DW. Fulminant *Clostridium difficile* colitis. Curr Opin Crit Care 2007;13:450–5.

92. Koss K, Clark MA, Sanders DS, et al. The outcome of surgery in fulminant *Clostridium difficile* colitis. Colorectal Dis 2006;8:149–54.

93. Swindells J, Brenwald N, Nathan R, et al. Evaluation of diagnostic tests for *Clostridium difficile* infection. J Clin Microbiol 2010;48:606–8.

94. Hurley BW, Nguyen CC. The spectrum of pseudomembranous enterocolitis and antibiotic-associated diarrhea. Arch Intern Med 2002;162:2177–84.

95. Longo WE, Mazuki JE, Virgo KS, et al. Outcome after colectomy for *Clostridium difficile* colitis. Dis Colon Rectum 2004;47:1620–6.

96. Ash L, Baker ME, O'Malley CM Jr, et al. Colonic abnormalities on CT in adult hospitalized patients with *Clostridium difficile* colitis: prevalence and significance of findings. Am J Roentgenol 2006;186:1393–400.

97. Dallal RM, Harbrecht BG, Boujoukas AJ, et al. Fulminant *Clostridium difficile*: an underappreciated and increasing cause of death and complications. Ann Surg 2002;235:363–72.

98. Marra AR, Edmond MB, Wenzel RP, et al. Hospital-acquired *Clostridium difficile*-associated disease in the intensive care unit setting: epidemiology clinical course and outcome. BMC Infect Dis 2007;7:42.

99. Hookman P, Barkin JS. *Clostridium difficile* associated infection, diarrhea and colitis. World J Gastroenterol 2009;15:1554–80.

100. Barie PS, Eachempati SR. Acute acalculous cholecystitis. Curr Gastroenterol Rep 2003;5:302–9.

101. Barie PS, Fischer E. Acute acalculous cholecystitis. J Am Coll Surg 1995;180: 232–44.

102. Kalliafas S, Ziegler DW, Flancbaum L, et al. Acute acalculous cholecystitis: incidence, risk factors, diagnosis, and outcome. Am Surg 1998;64:471–5.

103. Laurila J, Syrjala H, Laurila PA, et al. Acute acalculous cholecystitis in critically ill patients. Acta Anaesthesiol Scand 2004;48:986–91.

104. Wang AJ, Wang TE, Lin CC, et al. Clinical predictors of severe gallbladder complications in acute acalculous cholecystitis. World J Gastroenterol 2003;9: 2821–3.

105. Ganpathi IS, Diddapur RK, Eugene H, et al. Acute acalculous cholecystitis: challenging the myths. HPB (Oxford) 2007;9:131–4.

106. Hakala T, Nuuiten PJ, Ruokonen ET, et al. Microangiopathy in acute acalculous cholecystitis. Br J Surg 1997;84:1249–52.

107. Johnson EE, Hedley-White J. Continuous positive-pressure ventilation and choledochoduodenal flow resistance. J Appl Physiol 1995;39:937–42.

108. Messing B, Bories C, Kuntslinger F, et al. Does total parenteral nutrition induce gallbladder sludge formation and lithiasis? Gastroenterology 1983;84:1012–9.

109. Ryu JK, Ryu KH, Kim KH. Clinical features of acute acalculous cholecystitis. J Clin Gastroenterol 2003;36:166–9.

110. Theodorou P, Maurer CA, Spanholtz TA, et al. Acalculous cholecystitis in severely burned patients: incidence and predisposing factors. Burns 2009;35:405–11.
111. Nakano K, Suzuki K, Morita T. Life-threatening acute acalculous cholecystitis in a patient with renal cell carcinoma treated by sunitinib: a case report. J Med Case Rep 2012;6:69.
112. Trowbridge RL, Rutkowski NK, Shojania KG. Does this patient have acute cholecystitis? JAMA 2003;289:80–6.
113. Cooperberg PL, Gibney RG. Imaging of the gallbladder. Radiology 1987;163: 605–13.
114. Puc MM, Trans HS, Wry PW, et al. Ultrasound is not a useful screening tool for acute acalculous cholecystitis in critically ill trauma patients. Am Surg 2002;68: 65–9.
115. Canoy DS, Hart AR, Todd CJ. Epidemiology of duodenal ulcer perforation: a study on hospital admissions in Norfolk, United Kingdom. Digestive and Liver Disease. Can J Gastroenterol 2009;23:604–8.
116. Boey J, Choi SK, Poon A, et al. Risk stratification in perforated duodenal ulcers. A prospective validation of predictive factors. Ann Surg 1987;205:22–6.
117. Lohsiriwat V, Prapasrivorakul S, Lohsiriwat D. Perforated peptic ulcer: clinical presentation, surgical outcomes, and the accuracy of the Boey scoring system in predicting postoperative morbidity and mortality. World J Surg 2009;33:80–5.
118. Noguiera C, Silva AS, Santos JN, et al. Perforated peptic ulcer: main factors of morbidity and mortality. World J Surg 2003;27:782–7.
119. Gutthann SP, Garcia RL, Raiford DS. Individual nonsteroidal anti-inflammatory drugs and other risk factors for upper gastrointestinal bleeding and perforation. Epidemiology 1997;8:18–24.
120. Uccheddu A, Floris G, Altana ML, et al. Surgery for perforated peptic ulcer in the elderly. Evaluation of factors influencing prognosis. Hepatogastroenterology 2003;50:1956–8.
121. Wysocki A, Budzynski P, Kulawik J, et al. Changes in the localization of perforated peptic ulcer and its relation to gender and age of the patients throughout the last 45 years. World J Surg 2011;35:811–6.
122. Zar FA, Bakkanagari SR, Moorthi KM, et al. A comparison of vancomycin and metronidazole for the treatment of *Clostridium difficile*-associated diarrhea, stratified by disease severity. Clin Infect Dis 2007;45:302–7.
123. Cohn I Jr, Burnside GH. Imbalance of the normal microbial flora: influence of strangulation obstruction upon the bacterial ecology of the small intestine. Am J Dig Dis 1965;10(10):873–82.
124. Roehrborn A, Thomas L, Potreck O, et al. The microbiology of postoperative peritonitis. Clin Infect Dis 2001;33:1513–9.
125. Osman KA, Ahmed MH, Hamad MA, et al. Emergency colectomy for fulminant *Clostridium difficile* colitis: striking the right balance. Scand J Gastroenterol 2011;46(10):1222–7.
126. Lee DY, Chung EL, Guend H, et al. Predictors of mortality after emergency colectomy for *Clostridium difficile* colitis: an analysis of ACS-NSQIP. Ann Surg 2013. [Epub ahead of print].
127. Neal MD, Alverdy JC, Hall DE, et al. Diverting loop ileostomy and colonic lavage: an alternative to total abdominal colectomy for the treatment of severe, complicated *Clostridium difficile* associated disease. Ann Surg 2011;254(3):423–7.
128. Olivas AD, Umanskiy K, Zuckerbraun B, et al. Avoiding colectomy during surgical management of fulminant *Clostridium difficile* colitis. Surg Infect (Larchmt) 2010;11(3):299–305.

129. Ball CG, Kirkpatrick AW, McBeth P. The secondary abdominal compartment syndrome: not just another post-traumatic complication. Can J Surg 2008;51: 399–405.

130. Miller PR, Thompson JT, Faler BJ, et al. Late fascial closure in lieu of ventral hernia: the next step in open abdomen management. J Trauma 2002;53:843–9.

131. Becker HP, Willms A, Schwab R. Small bowel fistulas and the open abdomen. Scand J Surg 2007;96:263–71.

132. Zarzaur BL, DiCocco JM, Shahan CP, et al. Quality of life after abdominal wall reconstruction following open abdomen. J Trauma 2011;70:285–91.

133. Tsuyuguchi T, Itoi T, Takada T, et al. TG13 indications and techniques for gallbladder drainage in acute cholecystitis (with videos). J Hepatobiliary Pancreat Sci 2013;20(1):81–8.

134. Winbladh A, Gullstrand P, Svanvik J, et al. Systematic review of cholecystostomy as a treatment option in acute cholecystitis. HPB (Oxford) 2009;11(3):183–93.

135. deMestral C, Gomez D, Haas B, et al. Cholecystostomy: a bridge to hospital discharge but not delayed cholecystectomy. J Trauma Acute Care Surg 2013; 74(1):175–9.

136. Finlay IG, Edwards TJ, Lambert AW. Damage control laparotomy. Br J Surg 2004;90(Suppl 1):83–5.

137. Roberts DJ, Zygun DA, Grendar J, et al. Negative-pressure wound therapy for critically ill adults with open abdominal wounds: a systematic review. J Trauma Acute Care Surg 2012;73(3):629–39.

138. Sanabria AE, Villegas MI, Morales Uribe CH. Laparoscopic repair for perforated peptic ulcer disease. Cochrane Database Syst Rev 2013;2:CD004778.

139. Egresta F, Ansaloni L, Baiocchi GL, et al. Laparoscopic approach to the acute abdomen from the Consensus Development Conference. Surg Endosc 2012; 26:2134–64.

Other Viral Pneumonias
Coronavirus, Respiratory Syncytial Virus, Adenovirus, Hantavirus

Nelson Lee, MD, FRCP (Lond. Edin.)[a], Salman T. Qureshi, MD, FRCPC[b],*

KEYWORDS

- SARS • Coronavirus • RSV • Adenovirus • Hantavirus • Acute respiratory failure
- Immunocompromised host

KEY POINTS

- Severe acute respiratory syndrome–associated coronavirus and the Middle East respiratory syndrome coronavirus are novel pathogens that can cause severe respiratory infections and acute respiratory distress syndrome, which is associated with high mortality.
- Sustained human-to-human transmission of coronavirus can occur; thus, early case recognition, laboratory diagnosis, isolation, and implementation of appropriate infection control measures in the health care setting are important to prevent disease transmission.
- The diagnosis of respiratory syncytial virus in adults can be challenging and there are no vaccines or antivirals available; these unmet needs should be urgently addressed.
- The diagnosis and surveillance of adenovirus infection has been greatly improved by the development of highly sensitive and quantitative polymerase chain reaction assays of mucosal samples or plasma.
- The diagnosis of hantavirus pulmonary syndrome is primarily based on a history of exposure to potentially infected rodents in endemic areas such as the rural southwestern United States and may be confirmed by polymerase chain reaction or serologic testing.
- Clinical management of hantavirus pulmonary syndrome includes excellent supportive care with particular attention to careful management of fluid status.

Contributors: N. Lee drafted the sections on coronavirus and RSV; S.T. Qureshi drafted the sections on adenovirus and hantavirus, edited, and assembled the final content of the article.
Potential Conflicts of Interest: The authors declare that they do not have any conflicts of interest.
S.T. Qureshi holds a Tier II Canada Research Chair in Respiratory Infection and receives research funding from the Canadian Institutes of Health Research.
[a] Division of Infectious Diseases, Department of Medicine and Therapeutics, Faculty of Medicine, Prince of Wales Hospital, The Chinese University of Hong Kong, 30-32 Ngan Shing Street, Shatin, New Territories, Hong Kong, China; [b] Division of Respirology, Department of Critical Care Medicine, McGill University Health Centre, Room L11-403, 1650 Cedar Avenue, Montréal, Québec, H3G 1A4 Canada
* Corresponding author.
E-mail address: salman.qureshi@mcgill.ca

Crit Care Clin 29 (2013) 1045–1068
http://dx.doi.org/10.1016/j.ccc.2013.07.003
0749-0704/13/$ – see front matter © 2013 Elsevier Inc. All rights reserved.

HUMAN CORONAVIRUS INFECTIONS
Virology

Most human coronaviruses (eg, hCoV 229E, OC43, NL63) cause mild upper respiratory tract diseases, except occasionally in immunocompromised hosts. However, 2 novel coronaviruses, the severe acute respiratory syndrome–associated coronavirus (SARS-CoV), and a recently identified Middle East respiratory syndrome coronavirus (MERS-CoV) may cause serious viral pneumonitis, leading to hospitalization and death.[1,2] Coronaviruses are large, lipid-enveloped, positive-sense, single-stranded RNA viruses. Viral genome analyses revealed that SARS-CoV and MERS-CoV are Group B and Group C betacoronavirus, respectively, and are closely related to coronaviruses found in bats.[1–4] Intermediate mammalian hosts such as civet cats have been implicated for SARS-CoV before its adaptation for human transmission,[1,3] but no such host has been identified for MERS-CoV. These coronaviruses encode a surface spike glycoprotein (S protein) that attaches the virus to host cells, determining its host range and tropism, and is the target for neutralizing antibodies.[1,3] It has been shown that SARS-CoV uses human angiotensin-converting enzyme 2 (ACE-II) as the primary cellular receptor; the human C-type lectin (DC/L-SIGN) has also been implicated as an alternative receptor.[1,3,5] MERS-CoV has been shown to bind to dipeptidyl peptidase 4 (DPP4; also called CD26), an interspecies-conserved protein found on the surface of several cell types including the nonciliated cells in human airways,[4–6] and this interaction may explain its broad host range and its ability to cause cross-species zoonotic transmission.[4] There is no vaccine available at present for coronaviruses.[7]

Epidemiology and Disease Transmission

SARS-CoV emerged in Southern China (Guangdong Province) in February 2003; the first victims were those who had direct contact with live animals, either in the wet markets or in restaurants selling these animals as winter food.[1,3] The disease quickly spread to Hong Kong; and within a few weeks, through international air travel, it had reached Vietnam, Singapore, Taiwan, and Canada.[1,3,8] By July 2003, more than 30 countries were affected, resulting in 8096 confirmed infections and 774 deaths (9.6%).[8] Mathematical modeling of the early phase of the outbreak estimated that the basic reproductive number (R_0) of SARS-CoV was in the range of 2.2 to 3.7; the primary mode of transmission was via respiratory droplets.[9] Two key epidemiologic features of SARS were frequent nosocomial outbreaks and superspreading events, which exacerbated its transmission. Notably, 1706 of 8096 (21%) of SARS victims were health care workers.[8] It has been suggested that viral replication was at its peak in SARS patients at the time of hospitalization when symptoms worsen (see later discussion). Transmission was facilitated by close bed proximity and the application of aerosol-generating procedures (eg, intubation, resuscitation) and devices (eg, continuous positive airway pressure and biphasic positive airway pressure [BiPAP] treatments).[10] In 1 example, nebulization from a bronchodilator in a SARS patient resulted in a major hospital outbreak involving 138 inpatients, doctors, nurses, allied health workers, and medical students who had worked in the same medical ward.[11] Subsequent studies indicated that the attack rates were between 10% and 60% in the hospital settings.[10] An example of a community superspreading event that involved more than 300 residents occurred in a private housing estate (Amoy Gardens) in Hong Kong. Drying up of the U-shaped bathroom floor drain and backflow of contaminated sewage (from a SARS patient with diarrhea), coupled with the toilet's exhaust fan, might have created infectious aerosols that moved upward through the warm air shaft of the building. Computational fluid-dynamics modeling suggested possible dispersion by wind flow, causing long-range transmission to nearby buildings.[1] This and other evidence suggested that SARS could be opportunistically airborne.[3,12] Appropriate precautions to prevent airborne transmission should be implemented in the health care setting, particularly when respiratory procedures and devices are used.[12] Notably, laboratory-related SARS cases have occurred since the epidemic,[13] which highlights the importance of laboratory safety in handling these contagious viral pathogens.

In 2012, MERS-CoV emerged in the Middle East, and by June 2013, a total of 68 people in Saudi Arabia, Qatar, Jordan, the United Arab Emirates, and the United Kingdom were confirmed to have infections caused by the virus.[14] Epidemiologic investigations so far have revealed sporadic transmission of the disease. Zoonotic transmission has also been implicated even though most of these cases did not report a history of direct animal contact. It is unknown whether there is a low level of virus circulation in asymptomatic human carriers or if there is an animal reservoir that allows multiple introductions into humans.[15] Based on the reports of family and hospital clusters, it is thought that human-to-human transmission is possible.[3,14]

Pathogenesis

Humans have no preexisting immunity to these novel coronaviruses. SARS-CoV and MERS-CoV were shown to have the ability to evade innate host defenses (eg, type I interferon responses and related mechanisms), and replicate efficiently in host tissues (SARS-CoV, respiratory and intestinal tract cells; MERS-CoV, respiratory, intestinal, and kidney cells).[15–17] Besides lytic cell damage, uncontrolled replication of SARS-CoV leads to unabated inflammatory cytokine activation (eg, interleukin [IL]-6, IL-8, monocyte chemotactic protein-1, interferon-inducible protein-10, monokine induced by interferon-γ–inducible protein; commonly known as a cytokine storm), which is implicated in the development of progressive pneumonitis, diffuse alveolar damage/acute respiratory distress syndrome (ARDS), and hemophagocytic syndrome.[17,18] Clinically, the respiratory tract viral load peaked around 7 to 11 days and subsequently decreased[19]; a high viral load and slow viral clearance were associated with progressive disease and fatal outcomes.[4] High-level viremia and intestinal tract involvement also predicted adverse outcomes.[6,20] Little is known about the pathogenesis of MERS-CoV. A macaque model has shown active viral replication in lung tissues causing localized to widespread lesions and clinical illness, which starts to decrease after 1 week.[21]

Clinical Manifestations and Disease Course

SARS was described as a triphasic illness[11,22] with a typical incubation period of 4 to 6 days (range 2–16 days). In the viremic phase, patients experienced fever, chills, and rigor, which partially subsided in a few days; however, in about 90% of cases, this was followed by a resurgence of fever, cough, and shortness of breath (hyperimmune or pneumonia phase). Chest radiographs first showed patchy consolidation and ground-glass changes that rapidly progressed in the next few days to involve multiple lobes (**Fig. 1**).[12] In certain cases, findings on computed tomography scans of the thorax closely resembled bronchiolitis obliterans organizing pneumonia (eg, peripheral air-space consolidation).[23] Laboratory features included lymphopenia, thrombocytopenia, increased transaminases, creatinine kinase and lactate dehydrogenase. By the end of the second week (around day 10–14), 15% to 25% of patients deteriorated further and developed refractory respiratory failure and ARDS (pulmonary destruction phase).[3,11,22] About 20% of patients developed profuse diarrhea containing highly

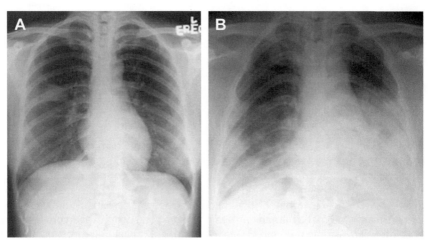

Fig. 1. (*A*) Subtle right middle zone infiltration in a patient with SARS about 3 days after illness onset; (*B*) bilateral, peripheral distributed ground-glass opacities about 7 days after illness onset.

infectious virus particles; nevertheless, renal failure was rare.[6] A substantial proportion of intubated and mechanically ventilated patients developed bacterial superinfection (eg, methicillin-resistant *Staphylococcus aureus*), and some developed complications such as pneumothorax and pneumomediastinum.[22,24] Children typically had a mild disease course that was rarely fatal.[1,3] The overall death rate was 6% to 16%; however, the age-stratified case fatality rate was as follows: less than 25 years, less than 1%; 25 to 44 years, 6%; 45 to 64 years, 15%; and greater than 65 years, greater than 50%.[1,3,8,22]

Preliminary data indicate that the clinical manifestations of MERS-CoV infection closely mimic those of SARS. Patients developed shortness of breath and progressive pneumonia about 1 week after symptom onset; the symptoms were associated with multiple, patchy, consolidation and ground-glass changes on chest imaging, laboratory evidence of lymphopenia, and increased liver enzyme levels. Most strikingly, many patients developed acute renal failure for which there was no clear explanation.[2,5,14] Most patients with confirmed MERS-CoV infection developed critical illness requiring admission to an intensive care unit (ICU) and, thus far, 38 (55.9%) patients have died despite maximal supportive treatment.[14]

Diagnosis

Early case recognition of these novel infections requires a high index of suspicion and a combination of detailed clinical and epidemiologic assessments. Based on the experience with SARS, the World Health Organization recommends that laboratory testing for MERS-CoV is indicated if a patient's pneumonia is otherwise unexplained and there is a history of travel to affected areas.[14] Testing should also be considered if there is direct contact with another sick individual, in case clusters of unexplained pneumonia, and if health care workers are involved. Prompt isolation of suspicious cases may greatly assist infection control and prevent hospital outbreaks.

Reverse transcriptase polymerase chain reaction (RT-PCR) is the test of choice for coronavirus infections. For SARS-CoV, a combination of upper respiratory (nasal, pharyngeal, nasopharyngeal), lower respiratory (higher yield because of higher viral levels, eg, sputum, tracheal aspirate, bronchial alveolar lavage), blood, and fecal specimens were required to maximize the chance of detection.[1,3,20,25] Plasma RT-PCR may detect viremia as early as 2 to 3 days after symptom onset, and has been shown to have prognostic value.[20] A single negative test in an upper respiratory specimen may be insufficient to rule out the diagnosis. Virus culture may provide further confirmation, but it is too slow to assist clinical management and needs to be performed in biosafety level 3 facilities. Serologic diagnosis is largely retrospective but may be useful for epidemiologic surveillance purposes.[1,25] The optimal clinical specimen for MERS-CoV testing is uncertain, but evidence has suggested a better yield with lower respiratory specimens. Given the diversity and periodic emergence of novel coronaviruses that may be extremely challenging to detect, clinicians should consult their local guidelines to determine when to refer cases for coronavirus testing to specialized reference laboratories (eg, pan-coronavirus RT-PCR, specific SARS-CoV and MERS-CoV RT-PCR).[3,14]

Treatment

There is no established therapy for coronavirus infection. During the SARS outbreak in 2003, a range of agents was used in patients but their efficacy is questionable. Ribavirin, although shown to be active in vitro, did not seem to provide clinical benefit (>90% of cases progressed despite treatment).[3,7,11,22,26] Lopinavir-ritonavir, a protease inhibitor used to treat human immunodeficiency virus (HIV)/AIDS with evidence of in vitro activity against SARS-CoV, was given to 41 patients in Hong Kong and was associated with viral load reduction and fewer cases of ARDS and fewer deaths; however, the study was uncontrolled.[7,26,27] Convalescent plasma obtained from recovering individuals that contained neutralizing antibodies had also been used. In 1 study, 19 patients who received such therapy had better survival (100% vs 66.2%) and discharge rates (77.8% vs 23.0%) compared with 21 controls.[28] This form of treatment has also been used in fulminant cases of H5N1 and 2009 H1N1 influenza with apparent success.[3] Subsequent in vitro and animal (ferrets, hamsters, macaques) studies have shown that monoclonal antibodies targeting the S protein may provide neutralizing activity against SARS-CoV, resulting in viral load reduction and resolution of lung lesions[29–33]; however, no clinical data are available. Several in vitro and animal (mice, macaques) studies have consistently shown that type I interferons, if given prophylactically or shortly after exposure, may protect against SARS.[34,35] In humans, it has been shown that interferon-α given within 5 days of illness may result in lower rates of intubation (11.1% vs 23.1%) and death (0.0% vs 7.7%); however, the study was small (9 vs 13 patients) and confounded by corticosteroid use.[7] Preliminary data have shown that type I and type III interferons have in vitro activity against MERS-CoV and these observations may deserve further investigation.[5,15,36] There are no published data on antibody therapies but this approach may also be useful.[6] Other potential treatments that have been tested in animal models include short interfering RNA (siRNA),[37] proteasome inhibitors,[38] prophylactic toll-like receptor agonist administration,[39] and immunomodulants.[3]

Systemic corticosteroid therapy is perhaps the most controversial area in SARS management (**Table 1**). Although favorable clinical and radiological responses have been reported, controlled data were lacking.[1,3,22,40] In the only randomized placebo-controlled study performed, early corticosteroid treatment within the first few days was shown to delay viral clearance.[41] Metabolic side effects, bacterial and fungal superinfections, avascular osteonecrosis, and even acute psychosis had been reported.[22,24,26,42] A systematic review concluded that corticosteroid treatment is not associated with definite benefits and is potentially harmful.[26] Similar adverse

Table 1
Controversies around the use of corticosteroid therapy in SARS

Pros	Cons
Clinical and radiological responses have been observed	Metabolic complications: hyperglycemia, hypertension, hypokalemia
Suppression of inflammatory cytokines	Increased bacterial superinfections
	Avascular osteonecrosis; but incidence was low (0.6%) if total prednisolone dose was <3 g
	Reduced viral clearance
	Others (eg, acute psychosis)

Data from Refs.[1,12,14,16–18,22,24,26,40,42–44,149]

effects have been reported in severe influenza; notably, an increase in mortality was also found.[43] It is unclear whether a lower dose or delayed treatment after viral replication has begun to subside can reduce harm.[44] Currently, it is recommended that corticosteroids be limited to SARS cases with refractory septic shock, and given at a low dose (eg, hydrocortisone 50 mg every 8 hours); a similar recommendation has been made for MERS-CoV infections.[8,14]

RESPIRATORY SYNCYTIAL VIRUS INFECTIONS IN ADULTS
Virology

Respiratory syncytial virus (RSV) is an enveloped, single-stranded RNA paramyxovirus that includes 2 major groups, A and B, each of which consists of 5 to 6 genotypes. The RSV genome encodes 2 nonstructural (NS1 and NS2) and 9 structural proteins, including the F (fusion) and G (attachment) glycoproteins on the viral envelope. Antibodies against the F and G proteins are neutralizing, and have been shown to confer protection against RSV infection in animal models[45]; these targets are likely important for the development of antiviral agents and vaccines. Immunity after primary infection (which generally occurs by 2 years of age) is partial and short-lived; thus, reinfections can occur throughout life.[45,46] Low serum neutralizing antibody levels in adults predicts infection risk and disease severity.[46] Although immunologic mechanisms (eg, cytokine responses) have been implicated in the pathogenesis, emerging evidence suggests that uncontrolled viral replication (indicated by high viral load) drives disease manifestations and leads to severe outcomes.[47–49] Such findings provide an important rationale for the approach to antiviral drug development against RSV.

Epidemiology

RSV is known to be an important cause of lower respiratory tract infection in infants and young children (eg, acute bronchiolitis, wheezy attacks), resulting in hospitalizations and deaths,[50] yet its impact in adults has only been appreciated in recent years. It has been estimated that RSV infects 3% to 10% of adults annually; although most infections are mild, increasing evidence suggest that severe lower respiratory tract infections can occur, especially among older adults (eg, >65 years) and those with underlying conditions (eg, chronic lung diseases, chronic cardiovascular diseases).[45,46] RSV may have accounted for 5% to 15% of community-acquired pneumonia, 9% to 10% of hospital admissions for acute cardiorespiratory diseases, and excessive deaths among adults during seasonal peaks.[45,50–55] Outbreaks among nursing home residents are likely common, but under-recognized.[56,57] The disease burden of RSV has been shown to approach that of seasonal influenza.[51] Patients who are profoundly immunosuppressed, such as hematopoietic stem cell transplant (HSCT) recipients, are at particularly high risk for severe RSV infection (2%–17%), which can be rapidly fatal.[58]

Clinical Manifestations and Outcomes

The clinical manifestations of RSV infection in adults are diverse and mainly determined by host factors such as the underlying chronic medical conditions and degree of immunosuppression. In healthy young adults, RSV may cause self-limiting upper respiratory illnesses; in the profoundly immunosuppressed, progressive lower respiratory tract disease can occur (17%–84%), resulting in fulminant pneumonitis and high mortality (7%–83%).[58] Older adults hospitalized for RSV infection may present with fever, cough, sputum production, wheezing, and dyspnea. Although wheezing and dyspnea may be more common with RSV, and the magnitude of fever sometimes lower, such findings could not reliably differentiate it from influenza.[51,59] Radiographically, about 50% to 60% of cases show active pneumonic changes such as consolidations and ground-glass opacities; the remainder may show evidence of congestive heart failure and features of underlying chronic lung conditions.[59,60] Typically, the pneumonic changes are small, patchy, and unilateral and disproportional to the degree of hypoxemia detected in these patients; a diffuse interstitial infiltration pattern is rare.[59,60] Overall, more than 70% of patients hospitalized with RSV develop severe lower respiratory complications, including pneumonia, acute bronchitis, and exacerbations of chronic obstructive pulmonary disease (COPD)/asthma; 10% to 15% have cardiovascular complications such as congestive heart failure or acute coronary syndrome.[45,46,51,59,60] Bacterial superinfection occurred in 12% to 17% of cases,[59] 10% to 18% of patients required ventilatory support (invasive/noninvasive), and the overall mortality was approximately 8% to 10%.[45,59,60] Late death might occur as a result of multiple cardiorespiratory complications or exacerbations of underlying medical conditions. Studies have shown that the morbidity and mortality from RSV infection in adults are actually similar to that of seasonal influenza.[51,60]

Diagnosis

RSV infection is clinically indistinguishable from other viral respiratory infections and diagnosis requires laboratory testing. Commonly, nasopharyngeal specimens are used; if the patient requires intubation, a lower respiratory tract specimen such as a tracheal aspirate should be obtained. The gold standard for diagnosis is by RT-PCR because of its relative ease and speed; other types of tests such as antigen assays (eg, enzyme immunoassays) and culture have lower sensitivities, which might be related to the lower viral load in adults.[45,61] A negative antigen assay result cannot be used to rule out RSV infection. Serology to detect RSV-specific IgG antibodies may also assist with the diagnosis and, if available, can be used in combination with RT-PCR to maximize the yield.[45]

Treatment and Prevention

At present, there is no established antiviral therapy or vaccine available for RSV. In immunocompromised adults, ribavirin (aerosolized or systemic administration) and palivizumab (an RSV-specific monoclonal antibody directed against the F glycoprotein) have been used to treat RSV infection with the aim of reducing progression to lower respiratory disease and death[58,62,63]; however, controlled data are lacking. In animal models, palivizumab has been shown to reduce viral titers and replication in pulmonary tissues, and in randomized clinical trials, palivizumab given prophylactically to very young high-risk children was shown to reduce hospitalizations related to RSV infections.[45,58] Currently, it is not known whether these approaches can be applied to older adults. New antiviral agents (eg, fusion protein inhibitors, siRNA) and newer generation antibody therapies are under active research.[45,64,65]

Systemic corticosteroids are commonly used to treat wheezing and exacerbations of COPD/asthma in adults, including those triggered by viral infections. Conversely, randomized controlled trials of corticosteroid therapy in young children with RSV infections have revealed a lack of clinical benefit and inconsistent control of inflammatory cytokine responses.[66,67] A recent study of corticosteroids in adults reported that virus control seemed to be unaffected but humoral immunity against RSV was diminished.[68] It is suggested that the decision to treat RSV patients with corticosteroids should be weighed against the potential risks (eg, bacterial superinfections), and be limited to a short course if used.[60,68] Because of the high rates of secondary infections, it is prudent to test and treat bacterial pathogens according to local resistance profiles. In addition to *Streptococcus pneumoniae* and *Hemophilia influenzae*, *Pseudomonas aeruginosa* and other gram-negative bacilli may need to be considered in patients with underlying chronic lung diseases.

In the hospital setting, RSV may spread via contact (eg, hands or via fomites) and droplets, and appropriate infection control measures such as hand washing and use of surgical masks (for both health care workers and infected patients) should be implemented. RSV particles have been detected in air samples from health care facilities, suggesting airborne transmission.[69] Nelson Lee has experienced an RSV outbreak related to the use of BiPAP ventilation (unpublished), and suggests appropriate isolation precautions when aerosol-generating procedures or devices are being used.

ADENOVIRUS INFECTION
Microbiology

Adenoviruses are medium-sized DNA viruses that attach to host cells through the coxsackie B virus-adenovirus receptor.[70] The variation in tissue tropism of individual adenovirus species or serotypes may be attributable to differential receptor expression or binding to alternative receptors. Following endocytosis and nuclear localization, early gene expression inhibits various host immune responses and initiates viral replication, whereas late gene expression directs viral assembly and release through host cell lysis. Human adenoviruses have no animal reservoir and do not infect other species; nonhuman adenoviruses that infect other species do not cause zoonotic disease. The traditional classification of human adenoviruses is complex and includes at least 52 serotypes. Adenoviruses have also been divided into 7 species (A–G) based on various biological and biochemical characteristics; each species includes more than 1 serotype and each serotype includes multiple genotypes. Although there is no strict correlation between species or serotype and disease manifestation, it is possible to make certain generalizations; for example, respiratory disease is caused by species B, C, and E, whereas species F causes gastroenteritis. A comprehensive review of serotype associations with disease has recently been published.[71]

Adenoviruses lack an outer envelope and are relatively resistant to dessication, low pH, and gastric or biliary secretions. The predominant routes of transmission include direct contact with aerosolized droplets in military settings, fecal-oral spread among children or those with prolonged shedding in the stool, and exposure to infected fomites, blood, or tissues. After an incubation period that varies from 2 days to 2 weeks, adenoviruses may be cleared or may cause long-standing asymptomatic infection of lymphoid or other mucosal cells, particularly in children.[72,73] In some cases, adenoviruses may become latent while retaining the potential to undergo endogenous reactivation at a later time point in a highly immune-suppressed host. A combination of innate and adaptive immune responses is required for control or prevention of adenovirus infection in vivo.[74] Innate antiviral immunity is mediated by natural killer (NK) cells, neutrophils, and monocytes/macrophages that are capable of directly killing infected cells or secreting inflammatory cytokines and chemokines that recruit additional effector cell types.[75] Optimal adaptive immunity includes neutralizing antibody production by antigen-specific B cells as well as generation and expansion of CD4+ and CD8+ T lymphocytes that are capable of eliminating infected host cells. Adenoviruses dedicate a significant portion of their genome to subversion of these host defense mechanisms to ensure infected cell survival and facilitate virus transmission in vivo.[76,77]

Epidemiology

In almost all cases, adenoviral infections are mild and self-limiting episodes that occur during childhood and are estimated to cause 5% to 10% of all febrile illnesses in pediatric populations.[72,73,78,79] Compared with children, severe adenoviral disease is much less common in adults and makes timely diagnosis in the critically ill patient quite challenging. Possible epidemiologic clues for adenovirus infection include a cluster of febrile pharyngitis, conjunctivitis, or respiratory disease in individuals living in close quarters, including day-care centers, chronic care facilities, or military barracks. Another clue is the simultaneous presence of circulating adenoviral isolates in the community, particularly during the summer or autumn months when influenza is less common. Several reports from military training centers have shown that serotype 3, 4, or 7 may be associated with severe disease as a result of greater virulence or transmissibility. Prompted by frequent outbreaks beginning in the 1950s that affected up to 10% of all military recruits, enteric-coated live oral vaccines against serotypes 4 and 7 were introduced in 1971 and were successful in diminishing acute respiratory disease. Immunization was progressively stopped from 1996 to 1999 and was followed by a resurgence of epidemic disease caused by the vaccine serotypes 3 and 7.[80] The global epidemiology of adenovirus infections in healthy populations includes 2 novel Ad7 genome types that have been shown to cause severe or fatal disease during several civilian and military outbreaks in North America and are closely related to endemic strains in China and South America.[81] Similarly, a virulent serotype 14 adenovirus strain that had not previously been observed in the United States was recently shown to cause severe and fatal adenovirus disease in children and adult military recruits.[82] Adenovirus infection is also an important emerging pathogen among HSCT recipients; the incidence varies from 4.9% to 29% according to the transplant regimen, age of the study population, and diagnostic testing strategy.[83,84] Relatively little is known about the incidence of adenovirus infection among adult solid-organ transplant recipients; however, plasma DNA was detected in 7.2% of cases during a 1-year prospective surveillance study.[85] Most transplant recipients were asymptomatic at the time of adenovirus detection and all recovered spontaneously. The incidence of adenovirus in patients with HIV infection, undergoing cancer chemotherapy, or with congenital immunodeficiency has been comprehensively reviewed.[86]

Severe Clinical Manifestations in the Healthy Host

In the civilian setting, severe adenoviral disease is extremely unusual in healthy adults with intact immunity. For example, only 18 cases of potentially life-threatening adenoviral pneumonia were published between 1974 and 1998,[87] and since then

14 additional cases have been reported and analyzed.[88] In the more recent series, two-thirds of the patients were male, the mean age was 32.75 years, and the overall mortality rate was 57%. The clinical and radiological features of severe adenoviral disease were generally nonspecific and could mimic bacterial sepsis, although the presence of conjunctivitis or diarrhea served as potential diagnostic clues. A variety of serotypes have been documented to cause sporadic cases of severe civilian[89,90] or fatal military adenoviral pneumonia[91,92] in healthy adults, although the relationship between genotype and virulence has not been comprehensively investigated.[89] The largest reported outbreak occurred in a mental health center and was caused by an unusual adenovirus (serotype 35) that had been associated with disease only among immunocompromised patients.[93] In that outbreak, affected individuals presented with fever and cough associated with diffuse interstitial or dense unilateral pulmonary infiltrates. No other distinguishing clinical features were evident; however, in several instances, the development of mild leukopenia was observed. Six of 18 infected cases required ICU admission, 5 required intubation, and 4 developed ARDS with septic shock; all patients recovered except for 1 individual with chronic renal insufficiency who required prolonged intubation and died 2 months after admission. Typical pathologic findings in fatal cases of adenoviral pneumonia include severe necrotizing bronchiolitis with fibrinous obstruction, interstitial inflammation, and hyaline membranes lined by characteristic alveolar smudge cells that have a large rounded nucleus containing basophilic inclusions with a surrounding halo.[94]

Severe Clinical Manifestations in the Immunocompromised Host

Highly immune-suppressed hosts are susceptible to adenovirus infection of various organ systems (brain, heart, lung, liver, intestine, kidney, pancreas, bladder) (**Box 1**) and may go on to exhibit a spectrum of disease severity that is influenced by their age, underlying disease, clinical interventions, and virus serotype.[86,95] Asymptomatic or clinically evident disease occurs mainly via de novo virus acquisition or through reactivation of latent infection from the host; a minority of cases are attributed to donor-derived infection during stem cell transplantation.[84] In most cases, it is not possible to determine the exact mechanism of adenovirus infection. Clinical illness associated with coinfection by multiple viral serotypes is also more frequent in the immune-suppressed host compared with other susceptible individuals.[96]

Box 1
Severe adenovirus disease manifestations

Interstitial pneumonitis

Meningoencephalitis

Hemorrhagic cystitis

Nephritis

Gastroenteritis

Hepatitis

Myocarditis

Colitis

Adapted from Kojaoghlanian T, Flomenberg P, Horwitz MS. The impact of adenovirus infection on the immunocompromised host. Rev Med Virol 2003;13(3):155–71.

HSCT

The development of extremely sensitive molecular techniques such as quantitative real-time PCR and systematic screening protocols have led to greater recognition of adenovirus infection in HSCT recipients. The infection rates reported in the literature vary widely and are likely due to different diagnostic approaches, host factors, and conditioning regimens; thus, standardization of detection methods is required to definitively quantify the incidence of disease in this patient population.[97] In general, pediatric stem cell transplant recipients are much more likely to develop adenovirus infection (20%–26%) compared with adults (9%) because they have limited natural exposure before transplant and lack species cross-reactive T cells.[98,99] Most adenoviral infections are detected during the first 100 days after transplantation although the median time to detection is much shorter in children (<30 days) compared with adults (>90 days).[97] Several risk factors for adenoviral infection (**Box 2**) and disease (**Box 3**) after transplant that reflect a state of profound host immune deficiency have been identified. Adenoviral infection may cause subclinical viremia, single organ system dysfunction (interstitial pneumonitis, cholangiohepatitis, hemorrhagic cystitis, or colitis, and so forth) or may disseminate to involve 2 or more organ systems and cause a significantly higher mortality (8%–26%).[98] Detection of adenovirus in the blood may precede symptomatic disease by 2 to 3 weeks and provides an opportunity for preemptive intervention[95,98]; however, identification of patients who might benefit most from therapy remains challenging. For example, a retrospective study of 26 pediatric HSCT recipients showed that 7 of the 11 patients diagnosed with adenovirus infection cleared the virus without antiviral therapy.[100] Coinfection or sequential infection with multiple serotypes has been demonstrated in pediatric HSCT recipients and these individuals may have prolonged viral excretion.

Solid-Organ Transplantation

Adenovirus infection typically occurs within the first 3 months of solid-organ transplantation and has a predilection to involve the allograft.[101] Clinical manifestations of liver infection include jaundice and hepatitis, lung infection presents as obliterative bronchiolitis or respiratory failure, cardiac infection leads to coronary vasculopathy, renal infection presents mainly with hemorrhagic cystitis that may be complicated by pneumonia, and intestinal infection presents with diarrhea. In all these situations, severe adenovirus infection may lead to premature graft loss or death. Risk factors for adenoviral infection include younger age (particularly children <5 years old), intestinal transplantation, augmented immune suppression including antilymphocyte antibodies, and transplantation of a seropositive organ into a seronegative recipient.[102] In addition to

---

Box 2
Risk factors for adenovirus infection in hematopoietic stem cell transplantation
Younger age
Mismatched or unrelated grafts
Total body irradiation
Presence of adenovirus antibody in the donor
Use of antithymocyte globulin or anti-CD52 (alemtuzumab)
T-cell depleted or stem cell (CD34+) selected graft
Data from Refs.[83,84,101,117]

Box 3
Risk factors for development of adenovirus disease in HSCTx

High dose immunosuppression

Severe or prolonged lymphopenia

Moderate to severe GVHD

Detection of adenovirus in peripheral blood

Rising viral load in peripheral blood

Rising viral load in stool

Data from Refs.[83,84,101,117]

---

exogenous acquisition or possible transmission via the allograft,[103] organ transplant recipients may reactivate endogenous adenoviral infection after receiving immune suppression. In an older series, the incidence in adult liver transplant patients was 5.8% and most patients had symptomatic disease of varying severity.[104] More recent studies using PCR detection have also shown that asymptomatic infection in the blood of adult solid-organ transplant recipients is common (6.5%–22.5%); however, most cases have not been associated with progressive disease or acute graft rejection and for this reason routine screening is not recommended.[85,101,102] Molecular detection of adenovirus in blood or affected tissue samples is indicated for adult solid-organ transplant recipients with compatible disease manifestations. Conversely, in pediatric solid-organ recipients, serial monitoring of viral load in the blood may precede the development of symptomatic disease and serve as a useful guide for the initiation of antiviral therapy.[105] Currently there are no specific measures for prevention of adenovirus infection in the transplant recipient.

Congenital Immune Deficiency

Patients with congenital immune deficiency are prone to infection with a wide array of microbes (bacterial, fungal, viral, and so forth) including adenovirus.[86] Because of the exceedingly rare nature of these inherited disorders, the true incidence of adenoviral disease is not known. Adenovirus infection is most commonly described in severe congenital immune deficiency (SCID), a condition in which both cellular and humoral immunity is defective. Adenoviral disease in SCID may involve 1 or more organ systems and be rapidly fatal; in addition, there is a higher incidence of unusual serotypes in these patients compared with immunocompetent children.[106]

AIDS

Before the development of highly active antiretroviral therapy (HAART) for patients infected with HIV, adenovirus infection was frequently detected and was associated with several other opportunistic pathogens. Despite this potential confounding effect of multiple coinfections, various case reports have described severe pneumonia, hepatitis, meningoencephalitis, nephritis, gastrointestinal, and potentially fatal disseminated disease caused by adenovirus.[107,108] A comprehensive review estimated that 12% of patients with clinical AIDS develop active adenovirus infection. In these studies, the mean age of patients was 31 years and within 2 months of first detection of adenovirus, the associated mortality was 45%. The most remarkable aspects of adenovirus infection in AIDS were the diversity of serotypes and frequency of antigenically intermediate isolates that are presumed to arise through spontaneous mutation within a strain or recombination between coinfecting serotypes during long-term infection. To clarify the epidemiology of adenovirus infection in patients infected with HIV, a prospective longitudinal study was subsequently performed and determined that the 1-year actuarial incidence of adenovirus infection was 17% with a CD4 count greater than 200 mm^3 and 38% with a CD4 count less than 200 mm^3. Prolonged and generally asymptomatic shedding from the gastrointestinal tract, and to a lesser degree the urinary tract, was documented in most patients. These data suggest that the mortality rate of adenovirus infection in AIDS may be lower than previously stated; however, differences in patient populations and adenovirus detection methods preclude a definitive conclusion of the true attributable mortality. Nonetheless, in the absence of another plausible explanation, adenovirus infection should be considered as a potential causative agent in the critically ill patient infected with HIV who has severe pneumonia, encephalitis, or hepatitis and a high retroviral load and/or a CD4 cell count less than 200 mm^3.

Diagnosis

In addition to exclusion of bacterial and atypical organisms, the main differential diagnosis of severe viral pneumonia in the immunocompetent host includes influenza, parainfluenza, and RSV, followed by several less common agents such as measles, varicella, rhinovirus, and others.[109,110] In the immunocompromised host, reactivation of members of the herpesvirus family (cytomegalovirus [CMV], Epstein-Barr virus [EBV], and human herpesvirus 6 [HHV-6]) as well as adenovirus should also be considered in the differential diagnosis of life-threatening pneumonia, meningoencephalitis, or cases of disseminated organ dysfunction. In such cases, adequate sample procurement from all potentially infected sites is required for further analysis. For severe respiratory failure, a nasopharyngeal aspirate, endotracheal secretions, or bronchoalveolar lavage are all suitable and relatively easy to obtain for viral and other microbiological studies. Comprehensive analysis of lung tissue is also extremely valuable if a transbronchial or surgical biopsy has been performed. When disseminated disease is suspected, a blood sample should also be obtained for detection of circulating adenovirus. Until recently, the gold standard for diagnosis of adenoviral disease from clinical samples was identification of a characteristic cytopathic effect using tissue culture–based methods; however, this approach is slow, costly, technically challenging, and may lack sensitivity. Direct antigen detection in respiratory specimens by immunofluorescence or related techniques is a rapid but less sensitive alternative to viral isolation.[111,112] Serology for determination of antibody responses and viral serotyping or genotyping methods are impractical for use in clinical decision making and are mainly used for epidemiologic investigations. All these techniques have now been supplanted by molecular detection methods that can be applied to blood, stool, sputum, or biopsy specimens.[113] Qualitative PCR and quantitative real-time PCR are rapid and highly sensitive techniques; however, both are critically dependent on the design of primers and probes that are able to amplify and detect the genomes of all clinically relevant adenoviruses.[114,115] Amplification of 1 or more highly conserved adenovirus hexon gene sequence or the use of multiple primer/probe combinations in a single assay have been successfully used by several investigators to identify all disease-associated serotypes. Medical centers may choose to establish their own local PCR protocols for adenovirus detection or refer their samples to commercial laboratories or other service providers. Regardless of where adenovirus PCR testing is done, it is essential to know the sensitivity and specificity of the testing protocol for each type of clinical sample that is analyzed.

In addition to confirming a diagnosis of severe clinical disease, many bone marrow transplant centers now use weekly quantitative PCR to monitor the DNA load of adenovirus (as well as CMV, EBV, and HHV-6) at mucosal sites or in the blood before and after stem cell transplantation.[98] Positive viral identification at a mucosal site in the absence of clinical or laboratory abnormality is consistent with infection but does not necessarily signify disease. On the other hand, adenovirus detection from the same site on multiple occasions or from multiple sites is predictive of disease risk and death.[116] It has been suggested that detection of adenovirus in the blood of stem cell transplant patients should be defined as probable disseminated disease and may signify a window of opportunity for early intervention.[117] One such approach using serial analysis of viral load for therapeutic decision making in pediatric stem cell transplant patients was recently published; however, it is not known whether this strategy is applicable to adults.[98,118] A decreasing viral copy number may be used as a surrogate for a response to therapy; conversely, a titer greater than 10^6/mL is associated with a greater likelihood of death.[116] The usefulness of early intervention after stem cell transplantation is supported by another series in which delayed initiation of cidofovir seemed to be associated with a poor outcome.[119]

Management

The management options for severe adenoviral disease are limited because there are no formally approved antiviral agents with proven efficacy and no prospective randomized trials of antiadenoviral therapy. Several studies have correlated clinical recovery with the return of T cells; therefore, a reduction of immune suppression is generally recommended as soon as a diagnosis of adenovirus infection has been established.[120] A variety of different antiviral agents including ribavirin, ganciclovir, and cidofovir have been used to treat adenovirus infection; however, none of these compounds have been shown to be particularly efficacious for established disease.[102] Cidofovir is an acyclic analogue of deoxycytidine monophosphate, which has in vitro activity against several DNA viruses and is approved for treatment of CMV retinitis. Because of its poor bioavailability, cidofovir must be given intravenously and is converted by host enzymes to an active diphosphate form with a prolonged intracellular half-life. Cidofovir diphosphate exhibits higher binding affinity for viral DNA polymerase compared with the host cell enzyme and inhibits viral replication by competing with host nucleotides for incorporation to viral DNA.[121,122] The most common dosing regimens are 5 mg/kg intravenously weekly for 2 weeks then once every other week until an appropriate clinical response is observed. Cidofovir is filtered and actively secreted by the proximal tubule of the kidney with 90% of the drug excreted unchanged in the urine. Dose-dependent nephrotoxicity is the major adverse effect of cidofovir; it presents as proteinuria, azotemia, glycosuria, metabolic acidosis, and, uncommonly, Fanconi syndrome. Saline prehydration and administration of probenecid are recommended to mitigate cidofovir toxicity; a dose adjustment or discontinuation of cidofovir is recommended in the case of an increasing creatinine level or proteinuria. Lipid analogues such as hexadecyloxypropyl-cidofovir exhibit much better cellular penetration and greater in vitro activity against adenovirus and have shown promising results in an immune-suppressed animal model of disseminated disease.[123] Ribavirin, a guanosine analogue used to treat severe RSV pneumonia, has not shown consistent clinical benefits or efficacy for a variety of severe adenovirus infections and is not recommended.[124] Similarly, ganciclovir shows in vitro activity against some adenovirus isolates and was reported to reduce the incidence of infection in stem cell transplantation[125]; however, there is insufficient clinical experience to support its usefulness.

Various strategies for immune reconstitution of the host are currently being investigated but are not yet widely available. For example, donor lymphocyte infusion has been associated with temporary clearance of adenovirus; however, this approach is currently limited by the risk of exacerbation of graft-versus-host disease (GVHD). Another approach that has been effective in preventing and treating diseases related to EBV and CMV reactivations in HSCT recipients is reconstitution of the host with in vitro expanded virus-specific cytotoxic T lymphocytes (CTLs).[126] Widespread application of this strategy for definitive cure of adenovirus infection is limited by incomplete knowledge of antigen-specific T-cell immunity as well as the practical, technical, regulatory, and financial barriers to generation of sufficient subgroup cross-reactive, adenovirus-specific, cytotoxic T lymphocytes ex vivo.[90,97] Novel CD4 and CD8 T-cell epitopes of the hexon protein have been recently identified and may lead to improved adoptive immunotherapy strategies in the future. Intravenous immunoglobulin has been used to treat severe adenovirus infection; however, its role is currently undefined.[102]

HANTAVIRUS PULMONARY SYNDROME
Introduction

The genus *Hantavirus* includes a diverse group of spherical enveloped viruses that all have a trisegmented negative-sense single-strand RNA genome.[127] Individual viral strains are maintained through prolonged asymptomatic infection of specific rodent hosts and the distribution of human disease depends on local ecological circumstances. Outside North America, a variety of hantaviruses such as the Hantaan virus are known to cause a serious and fatal acute disease termed hemorrhagic fever with renal syndrome. In North America, the related Sin Nombre virus (SNV) is the most common cause of hantavirus cardiopulmonary syndrome, an acute condition characterized by severe respiratory failure, shock, and mild renal dysfunction. In South America, the Andes virus causes a similar condition and is the only hantavirus to be associated with person to person transmission.[128–130] Zoonotic transmission of SNV and related strains occurs by domestic or occupational exposure to aerosols of infected rodent excreta and is more likely when rodent populations are abundant and enter buildings in search of food or cover. The first outbreak of North American hantavirus pulmonary syndrome was described in the Four Corners region of the United States in 1993 with a subsequent outbreak in 1998; both episodes were attributed to higher rodent densities and greater human exposure as a result of increased precipitation.[131,132]

Clinical and Pathologic Features

The clinical manifestations of hantavirus infection follow a long incubation period (7–25 days) and are characterized by a prodrome of fever, chills, myalgia, and gastrointestinal symptoms.[131,133] A mild cough and dyspnea develop after several days and are associated with mild pulmonary disease in one-third of cases.[134] On the other hand, most patients rapidly develop severe respiratory distress and profound oxygen desaturation with progressive radiographic evidence of non-cardiogenic pulmonary edema.[135] The physical findings at the time of presentation are usually nonspecific and include fever, tachypnea, tachycardia, inspiratory crackles, and mild hypotension. Laboratory studies reveal hemoconcentration, mild thrombocytopenia, left shift with circulating myeloblasts and circulating immunoblasts, and mildly abnormal liver function tests. Dizziness, nausea or vomiting, and absence of cough at presentation as well as thrombocytopenia, an increased hematocrit, and a decreased serum bicarbonate level help distinguish hantavirus pulmonary syndrome (HPS) from other common causes of acute respiratory distress such as pneumococcal pneumonia and influenza.[136] In severe cases, hemodynamic analysis is consistent with a shock state that is attributable to a combination of fluid redistribution and myocardial depression.[137,138] The outcome of HPS is unpredictable and varies widely; in some series, all patients with a mild clinical course survived whereas the mortality of those with fulminant disease was as high as 46%.[139,140]

In 40 of 44 fatal cases of HPS, histopathologic analysis showed interstitial pneumonitis with a variable mononuclear cell infiltrate, edema, and focal hyaline membranes; the remainder had diffuse alveolar damage with variable degrees of severe air-space disorganization.[141] Immunohistochemistry and electron microscopy demonstrated the widespread presence of hantavirus antigens and viral inclusions in pulmonary microvascular endothelial cells as well as dendritic cells, macrophages, and lymphocytes. In severe clinical disease, an immunopathologic response has been implicated in the pathogenesis of the capillary leak syndrome that results in severe pulmonary edema.

Diagnosis

HPS is an extremely rare disease in North America; less than 500 cases have been reported in the United States. Historical information such as recent travel to rural areas with endemic hantavirus infection and/or exposure to potentially infected rodents that may have entered human dwellings is crucial to its initial consideration. Patients presenting with severe hantavirus infection invariably have a detectable humoral immune response and positive serologic testing for IgM or IgG is diagnostic of disease in low-prevalence geographic areas.[142] Viremia occurs during the first 10 days of illness and may be detected by RT-PCR of blood[143]; however, isolation of hantavirus requires appropriate containment facilities and is not practical for diagnostic purposes.

Treatment and Prevention

The mainstay of clinical management of HPS is excellent supportive care with particular attention to careful management of fluid status to minimize alveolar edema while maintaining overall organ perfusion.[144] The use of rescue therapies such as steroids and extracorporeal life support are of potential benefit[127,145,146]; however, administration of ribavirin was not shown to be efficacious against SNV despite its in vitro activity against hantavirus.[147] Prevention of human hantavirus infection includes environmental and ecological measures to control or reduce exposure to rodent reservoirs.[148]

ACKNOWLEDGMENTS

The authors thank Adam Flaczyk for assistance with article preparation and Dr Cedric P. Yansouni for critical review of the article content.

REFERENCES

1. Peiris JS, Yuen KY, Osterhaus AD, et al. The severe acute respiratory syndrome. N Engl J Med 2003;349(25):2431–41.
2. Kojaoghlanian T, Flomenberg P, Horwitz MS. The impact of adenovirus infection on the immunocompromised host. Rev Med Virol 2003;13(3):155–71.
3. Chan PK, Tang JW, Hui DS. SARS: clinical presentation, transmission, pathogenesis and treatment options. Clin Sci (Lond) 2006;110(2):193–204.
4. Raj VS, Mou H, Smits SL, et al. Dipeptidyl peptidase 4 is a functional receptor for the emerging human coronavirus-EMC. Nature 2013;495(7440):251–4.

5. Cohen JM, Cooper N, Chakrabarti S, et al. EBV-related disease following hae-matopoietic stem cell transplantation with reduced intensity conditioning. Leuk Lymphoma 2007;48(2):256–69.
6. Gierer S, Bertram S, Kaup F, et al. The spike protein of the emerging betacoro-navirus EMC uses a novel coronavirus receptor for entry, can be activated by TMPRSS2, and is targeted by neutralizing antibodies. J Virol 2013;87(10): 5502–11.
7. Groneberg DA, Poutanen SM, Low DE, et al. Treatment and vaccines for severe acute respiratory syndrome. Lancet Infect Dis 2005;5(3):147–55.
8. World Health Organization (WHO). Severe acute respiratory syndrome (SARS). Available at: http://www.who.int/csr/sars/en/. Accessed May 15, 2013.
9. Zaki AM, van Boheemen S, Bestebroer TM, et al. Isolation of a novel coronavirus from a man with pneumonia in Saudi Arabia. N Engl J Med 2012;367(19): 1814–20.
10. Yu IT, Xie ZH, Tsoi KK, et al. Why did outbreaks of severe acute respiratory syn-drome occur in some hospital wards but not in others? Clin Infect Dis 2007; 44(8):1017–25.
11. Lee N, Hui D, Wu A, et al. A major outbreak of severe acute respiratory syn-drome in Hong Kong. N Engl J Med 2003;348(20):1986–94.
12. Hui DS, Chow BK, Chu LC, et al. Exhaled air and aerosolized droplet dispersion during application of a jet nebulizer. Chest 2009;135(3):648–54.
13. Lim PL, Kurup A, Gopalakrishna G, et al. Laboratory-acquired severe acute res-piratory syndrome. N Engl J Med 2004;350(17):1740–5.
14. World Health Organization (WHO). Coronavirus infections. Available at: http://www.who.int/csr/disease/coronavirus_infections/en/. Accessed June 15, 2013.
15. Kindler E, Jonsdottir HR, Muth D, et al. Efficient replication of the novel human betacoronavirus EMC on primary human epithelium highlights its zoonotic potential. MBio 2013;4(1):e00611–2.
16. Chen J, Subbarao K. The immunobiology of SARS*. Annu Rev Immunol 2007;25: 443–72.
17. Frieman M, Heise M, Baric R. SARS coronavirus and innate immunity. Virus Res 2008;133(1):101–12.
18. Wong CK, Lam CW, Wu AK, et al. Plasma inflammatory cytokines and chemo-kines in severe acute respiratory syndrome. Clin Exp Immunol 2004;136(1): 95–103.
19. Zielecki F, Weber M, Eickmann M, et al. Human cell tropism and innate im-mune system interactions of human respiratory coronavirus EMC compared to those of severe acute respiratory syndrome coronavirus. J Virol 2013; 87(9):5300–4.
20. Ng EK, Hui DS, Chan KC, et al. Quantitative analysis and prognostic implication of SARS coronavirus RNA in the plasma and serum of patients with severe acute respiratory syndrome. Clin Chem 2003;49(12):1976–80.
21. Munster VJ, de Wit E, Feldmann H. Pneumonia from human coronavirus in a ma-caque model. N Engl J Med 2013;368(16):1560–2.
22. Sung JJ, Wu A, Joynt GM, et al. Severe acute respiratory syndrome: report of treatment and outcome after a major outbreak. Thorax 2004;59(5):414–20.
23. Wong KT, Antonio GE, Hui DS, et al. Thin-section CT of severe acute respiratory syndrome: evaluation of 73 patients exposed to or with the disease. Radiology 2003;228(2):395–400.
24. Yap FH, Gomersall CD, Fung KS, et al. Increase in methicillin-resistant Staphy-lococcus aureus acquisition rate and change in pathogen pattern associated

with an outbreak of severe acute respiratory syndrome. Clin Infect Dis 2004; 39(4):511–6.

25. Chan PK, To WK, Ng KC, et al. Laboratory diagnosis of SARS. Emerg Infect Dis 2004;10(5):825–31.

26. Stockman LJ, Bellamy R, Garner P. SARS: systematic review of treatment effects. PLoS Med 2006;3(9):e343.

27. Chu CM, Cheng VC, Hung IF, et al. Role of lopinavir/ritonavir in the treatment of SARS: initial virological and clinical findings. Thorax 2004;59(3):252–6.

28. Soo YO, Cheng Y, Wong R, et al. Retrospective comparison of convalescent plasma with continuing high-dose methylprednisolone treatment in SARS patients. Clin Microbiol Infect 2004;10(7):676–8.

29. Roberts A, Thomas WD, Guarner J, et al. Therapy with a severe acute respiratory syndrome-associated coronavirus-neutralizing human monoclonal antibody reduces disease severity and viral burden in golden Syrian hamsters. J Infect Dis 2006;193(5):685–92.

30. Miyoshi-Akiyama T, Ishida I, Fukushi M, et al. Fully human monoclonal antibody directed to proteolytic cleavage site in severe acute respiratory syndrome (SARS) coronavirus S protein neutralizes the virus in a rhesus macaque SARS model. J Infect Dis 2011;203(11):1574–81.

31. ter Meulen J, Bakker AB, van den Brink EN, et al. Human monoclonal antibody as prophylaxis for SARS coronavirus infection in ferrets. Lancet 2004;363(9427): 2139–41.

32. Sui J, Li W, Murakami A, et al. Potent neutralization of severe acute respiratory syndrome (SARS) coronavirus by a human mAb to S1 protein that blocks receptor association. Proc Natl Acad Sci U S A 2004;101(8):2536–41.

33. Zhu Z, Chakraborti S, He Y, et al. Potent cross-reactive neutralization of SARS coronavirus isolates by human monoclonal antibodies. Proc Natl Acad Sci U S A 2007;104(29):12123–8.

34. Cinatl J, Morgenstern B, Bauer G, et al. Treatment of SARS with human interferons. Lancet 2003;362(9380):293–4.

35. Haagmans BL, Kuiken T, Martina BE, et al. Pegylated interferon-alpha protects type 1 pneumocytes against SARS coronavirus infection in macaques. Nat Med 2004;10(3):290–3.

36. Chan RW, Chan MC, Agnihothram S, et al. Tropism of and innate immune responses to the novel human betacoronavirus lineage C virus in human ex vivo respiratory organ cultures. J Virol 2013;87(12):6604–14.

37. Li BJ, Tang Q, Cheng D, et al. Using siRNA in prophylactic and therapeutic regimens against SARS coronavirus in Rhesus macaque. Nat Med 2005;11(9): 944–51.

38. Ma XZ, Bartczak A, Zhang J, et al. Proteasome inhibition in vivo promotes survival in a lethal murine model of severe acute respiratory syndrome. J Virol 2010; 84(23):12419–28.

39. Zhao J, Wohlford-Lenane C, Zhao J, et al. Intranasal treatment with poly(I*C) protects aged mice from lethal respiratory virus infections. J Virol 2012;86(21): 11416–24.

40. Ho JC, Ooi GC, Mok TY, et al. High-dose pulse versus nonpulse corticosteroid regimens in severe acute respiratory syndrome. Am J Respir Crit Care Med 2003;168(12):1449–56.

41. Lee N, Allen Chan KC, Hui DS, et al. Effects of early corticosteroid treatment on plasma SARS-associated Coronavirus RNA concentrations in adult patients. J Clin Virol 2004;31(4):304–9.

42. Griffith JF, Antonio GE, Kumta SM, et al. Osteonecrosis of hip and knee in patients with severe acute respiratory syndrome treated with steroids. Radiology 2005;235(1):168–75.
43. Lee N, Hui DS. Dexamethasone in community-acquired pneumonia. Lancet 2011;378(9795):979–80 [author reply: 981].
44. Chen RC, Tang XP, Tan SY, et al. Treatment of severe acute respiratory syndrome with glucosteroids: the Guangzhou experience. Chest 2006;129(6):1441–52.
45. Walsh EE. Respiratory syncytial virus infection in adults. Semin Respir Crit Care Med 2011;32(4):423–32.
46. Walsh EE, Peterson DR, Falsey AR. Risk factors for severe respiratory syncytial virus infection in elderly persons. J Infect Dis 2004;189(2):233–8.
47. Duncan CB, Walsh EE, Peterson DR, et al. Risk factors for respiratory failure associated with respiratory syncytial virus infection in adults. J Infect Dis 2009;200(8):1242–6.
48. Walsh EE, Peterson DR, Kalkanoglu AE, et al. Viral shedding and immune responses to respiratory syncytial virus infection in older adults. J Infect Dis 2013;207(9):1424–32.
49. DeVincenzo JP, Wilkinson T, Vaishnaw A, et al. Viral load drives disease in humans experimentally infected with respiratory syncytial virus. Am J Respir Crit Care Med 2010;182(10):1305–14.
50. Nair H, Nokes DJ, Gessner BD, et al. Global burden of acute lower respiratory infections due to respiratory syncytial virus in young children: a systematic review and meta-analysis. Lancet 2010;375(9725):1545–55.
51. Falsey AR, Hennessey PA, Formica MA, et al. Respiratory syncytial virus infection in elderly and high-risk adults. N Engl J Med 2005;352(17):1749–59.
52. Widmer K, Zhu Y, Williams JV, et al. Rates of hospitalizations for respiratory syncytial virus, human metapneumovirus, and influenza virus in older adults. J Infect Dis 2012;206(1):56–62.
53. Jansen AG, Sanders EA, Hoes AW, et al. Influenza- and respiratory syncytial virus-associated mortality and hospitalisations. Eur Respir J 2007;30(6):1158–66.
54. van Asten L, van den Wijngaard C, van Pelt W, et al. Mortality attributable to 9 common infections: significant effect of influenza A, respiratory syncytial virus, influenza B, norovirus, and parainfluenza in elderly persons. J Infect Dis 2012;206(5):628–39.
55. Choi SH, Hong SB, Ko GB, et al. Viral infection in patients with severe pneumonia requiring intensive care unit admission. Am J Respir Crit Care Med 2012;186(4):325–32.
56. Caram LB, Chen J, Taggart EW, et al. Respiratory syncytial virus outbreak in a long-term care facility detected using reverse transcriptase polymerase chain reaction: an argument for real-time detection methods. J Am Geriatr Soc 2009;57(3):482–5.
57. Ellis SE, Coffey CS, Mitchel EF Jr, et al. Influenza- and respiratory syncytial virus-associated morbidity and mortality in the nursing home population. J Am Geriatr Soc 2003;51(6):761–7.
58. Shah JN, Chemaly RF. Management of RSV infections in adult recipients of hematopoietic stem cell transplantation. Blood 2011;117(10):2755–63.
59. Walsh EE, Peterson DR, Falsey AR. Is clinical recognition of respiratory syncytial virus infection in hospitalized elderly and high-risk adults possible? J Infect Dis 2007;195(7):1046–51.

60. Lee N, Lui GC, Wong KT, et al. High morbidity and mortality in adults hospitalized for respiratory syncytial virus infections. Clin Infect Dis 2013. [Epub ahead of print].

61. de-Paris F, Beck C, Machado AB, et al. Optimization of one-step duplex real-time RT-PCR for detection of influenza and respiratory syncytial virus in nasopharyngeal aspirates. J Virol Methods 2012;186(1–2):189–92.

62. Park SY, Baek S, Lee SO, et al. Efficacy of oral ribavirin in hematologic disease patients with paramyxovirus infection: analytic strategy using propensity scores. Antimicrob Agents Chemother 2013;57(2):983–9.

63. Hynicka LM, Ensor CR. Prophylaxis and treatment of respiratory syncytial virus in adult immunocompromised patients. Ann Pharmacother 2012;46(4):558–66.

64. Bonavia A, Franti M, Pusateri Keaney E, et al. Identification of broad-spectrum antiviral compounds and assessment of the druggability of their target for efficacy against respiratory syncytial virus (RSV). Proc Natl Acad Sci U S A 2011;108(17):6739–44.

65. DeVincenzo J, Lambkin-Williams R, Wilkinson T, et al. A randomized, double-blind, placebo-controlled study of an RNAi-based therapy directed against respiratory syncytial virus. Proc Natl Acad Sci U S A 2010;107(19):8800–5.

66. van Woensel JB, Vyas H, Group ST. Dexamethasone in children mechanically ventilated for lower respiratory tract infection caused by respiratory syncytial virus: a randomized controlled trial. Crit Care Med 2011;39(7):1779–83.

67. Fernandes RM, Bialy LM, Vandermeer B, et al. Glucocorticoids for acute viral bronchiolitis in infants and young children. Cochrane Database Syst Rev 2010;(10):CD004878.

68. Lee FE, Walsh EE, Falsey AR. The effect of steroid use in hospitalized adults with respiratory syncytial virus-related illness. Chest 2011;140(5):1155–61.

69. Lindsley WG, Blachere FM, Davis KA, et al. Distribution of airborne influenza virus and respiratory syncytial virus in an urgent care medical clinic. Clin Infect Dis 2010;50(5):693–8.

70. Roelvink PW, Lizonova A, Lee JG, et al. The coxsackievirus-adenovirus receptor protein can function as a cellular attachment protein for adenovirus serotypes from subgroups A, C, D, E, and F. J Virol 1998;72(10):7909–15.

71. Lynch JP 3rd, Fishbein M, Echavarria M. Adenovirus. Semin Respir Crit Care Med 2011;32(4):494–511.

72. Fox JP, Brandt CD, Wassermann FE, et al. The virus watch program: a continuing surveillance of viral infections in metropolitan New York families. VI. Observations of adenovirus infections: virus excretion patterns, antibody response, efficiency of surveillance, patterns of infections, and relation to illness. Am J Epidemiol 1969;89(1):25–50.

73. Fox JP, Hall CE, Cooney MK. The Seattle virus watch. VII. Observations of adenovirus infections. Am J Epidemiol 1977;105(4):362–86.

74. Sumida SM, Truitt DM, Kishko MG, et al. Neutralizing antibodies and CD8+ T lymphocytes both contribute to immunity to adenovirus serotype 5 vaccine vectors. J Virol 2004;78(6):2666–73.

75. Ginsberg HS, Moldawer LL, Sehgal PB, et al. A mouse model for investigating the molecular pathogenesis of adenovirus pneumonia. Proc Natl Acad Sci U S A 1991;88(5):1651–5.

76. Mahr JA, Gooding LR. Immune evasion by adenoviruses. Immunol Rev 1999;168:121–30.

77. Burgert HG, Ruzsics Z, Obermeier S, et al. Subversion of host defense mechanisms by adenoviruses. Curr Top Microbiol Immunol 2002;269:273–318.

78. Cooper RJ, Hallett R, Tullo AB, et al. The epidemiology of adenovirus infections in Greater Manchester, UK 1982-96. Epidemiol Infect 2000;125(2):333–45.
79. Brandt CD, Kim HW, Vargosko AJ, et al. Infections in 18,000 infants and children in a controlled study of respiratory tract disease. I. Adenovirus pathogenicity in relation to serologic type and illness syndrome. Am J Epidemiol 1969;90(6): 484–500.
80. Ryan MA, Gray GC, Smith B, et al. Large epidemic of respiratory illness due to adenovirus types 7 and 3 in healthy young adults. Clin Infect Dis 2002;34(5): 577–82.
81. Erdman DD, Xu W, Gerber SI, et al. Molecular epidemiology of adenovirus type 7 in the United States, 1966-2000. Emerg Infect Dis 2002;8(3):269–77.
82. Binn LN, Sanchez JL, Gaydos JC. Emergence of adenovirus type 14 in US military recruits–a new challenge. J Infect Dis 2007;196(10):1436–7.
83. Leen AM, Rooney CM. Adenovirus as an emerging pathogen in immunocompromised patients. Br J Haematol 2005;128(2):135–44.
84. Howard DS, Phillips IG, Reece DE, et al. Adenovirus infections in hematopoietic stem cell transplant recipients. Clin Infect Dis 1999;29(6):1494–501.
85. Humar A, Kumar D, Mazzulli T, et al. A surveillance study of adenovirus infection in adult solid organ transplant recipients. Am J Transplant 2005;5(10):2555–9.
86. Hierholzer JC. Adenoviruses in the immunocompromised host. Clin Microbiol Rev 1992;5(3):262–74.
87. Komshian SV, Chandrasekar PH, Levine DP. Adenovirus pneumonia in healthy adults. Heart Lung 1987;16(2):146–50.
88. Hakim FA, Tleyjeh IM. Severe adenovirus pneumonia in immunocompetent adults: a case report and review of the literature. Eur J Clin Microbiol Infect Dis 2008;27(2):153–8.
89. Barker JH, Luby JP, Sean Dalley A, et al. Fatal type 3 adenoviral pneumonia in immunocompetent adult identical twins. Clin Infect Dis 2003;37(10):e142–6.
90. Case records of the Massachusetts General Hospital. Weekly clinicopathological exercises. Case 6-1979. N Engl J Med 1979;300(6):301–8.
91. Levin S, Dietrich J, Guillory J. Fatal nonbacterial pneumonia associated with Adenovirus type 4. Occurrence in an adult. JAMA 1967;201(12):975–7.
92. Dudding BA, Wagner SC, Zeller JA, et al. Fatal pneumonia associated with adenovirus type 7 in three military trainees. N Engl J Med 1972;286(24):1289–92.
93. Klinger JR, Sanchez MP, Curtin LA, et al. Multiple cases of life-threatening adenovirus pneumonia in a mental health care center. Am J Respir Crit Care Med 1998;157(2):645–9.
94. Landry ML, Greenwold J, Vikram HR. Herpes simplex type-2 meningitis: presentation and lack of standardized therapy. Am J Med 2009;122(7):688–91.
95. Echavarria M. Adenoviruses in immunocompromised hosts. Clin Microbiol Rev 2008;21(4):704–15.
96. Gray GC, McCarthy T, Lebeck MG, et al. Genotype prevalence and risk factors for severe clinical adenovirus infection, United States 2004-2006. Clin Infect Dis 2007;45(9):1120–31.
97. Leen AM, Bollard CM, Myers GD, et al. Adenoviral infections in hematopoietic stem cell transplantation. Biol Blood Marrow Transplant 2006;12(3):243–51.
98. Lindemans CA, Leen AM, Boelens JJ. How I treat adenovirus in hematopoietic stem cell transplant recipients. Blood 2010;116(25):5476–85.
99. Walls T, Shankar AG, Shingadia D. Adenovirus: an increasingly important pathogen in paediatric bone marrow transplant patients. Lancet Infect Dis 2003;3(2): 79–86.

100. Walls T, Hawrami K, Ushiro-Lumb I, et al. Adenovirus infection after pediatric bone marrow transplantation: is treatment always necessary? Clin Infect Dis 2005;40(9):1244–9.

101. Ison MG. Adenovirus infections in transplant recipients. Clin Infect Dis 2006; 43(3):331–9.

102. Ison MG, Green M. Adenovirus in solid organ transplant recipients. Am J Transplant 2009;9(Suppl 4):S161–5.

103. Koneru B, Atchison R, Jaffe R, et al. Serological studies of adenoviral hepatitis following pediatric liver transplantation. Transplant Proc 1990;22(4):1547–8.

104. McGrath D, Falagas ME, Freeman R, et al. Adenovirus infection in adult orthotopic liver transplant recipients: incidence and clinical significance. J Infect Dis 1998;177(2):459–62.

105. Seidemann K, Heim A, Pfister ED, et al. Monitoring of adenovirus infection in pediatric transplant recipients by quantitative PCR: report of six cases and review of the literature. Am J Transplant 2004;4(12):2102–8.

106. South MA, Dolen J, Beach DK, et al. Fatal adenovirus hepatic necrosis in severe combined immune deficiency. Pediatr Infect Dis 1982;1(6):416–9.

107. Khoo SH, Bailey AS, de Jong JC, et al. Adenovirus infections in human immunodeficiency virus-positive patients: clinical features and molecular epidemiology. J Infect Dis 1995;172(3):629–37.

108. Schnurr D, Bollen A, Crawford-Miksza L, et al. Adenovirus mixture isolated from the brain of an AIDS patient with encephalitis. J Med Virol 1995;47(2): 168–71.

109. Vigil KJ, Adachi JA, Chemaly RF. Viral pneumonias in immunocompromised adult hosts. J Intensive Care Med 2010;25(6):307–26.

110. Chemaly RF, Ghosh S, Bodey GP, et al. Respiratory viral infections in adults with hematologic malignancies and human stem cell transplantation recipients: a retrospective study at a major cancer center. Medicine 2006;85(5): 278–87.

111. August MJ, Warford AL. Evaluation of a commercial monoclonal antibody for detection of adenovirus antigen. J Clin Microbiol 1987;25(11):2233–5.

112. Shetty AK, Treynor E, Hill DW, et al. Comparison of conventional viral cultures with direct fluorescent antibody stains for diagnosis of community-acquired respiratory virus infections in hospitalized children. Pediatr Infect Dis J 2003;22(9): 789–94.

113. Fox JD. Nucleic acid amplification tests for detection of respiratory viruses. J Clin Virol 2007;40(Suppl 1):S15–23.

114. Heim A, Ebnet C, Harste G, et al. Rapid and quantitative detection of human adenovirus DNA by real-time PCR. J Med Virol 2003;70(2):228–39.

115. Lion T, Baumgartinger R, Watzinger F, et al. Molecular monitoring of adenovirus in peripheral blood after allogeneic bone marrow transplantation permits early diagnosis of disseminated disease. Blood 2003;102(3):1114–20.

116. Claas EC, Schilham MW, de Brouwer CS, et al. Internally controlled real-time PCR monitoring of adenovirus DNA load in serum or plasma of transplant recipients. J Clin Microbiol 2005;43(4):1738–44.

117. Suparno C, Milligan DW, Moss PA, et al. Adenovirus infections in stem cell transplant recipients: recent developments in understanding of pathogenesis, diagnosis and management. Leuk Lymphoma 2004;45(5):873–85.

118. Leruez-Ville M, Minard V, Lacaille F, et al. Real-time blood plasma polymerase chain reaction for management of disseminated adenovirus infection. Clin Infect Dis 2004;38(1):45–52.

119. Neofytos D, Ojha A, Mookerjee B, et al. Treatment of adenovirus disease in stem cell transplant recipients with cidofovir. Biol Blood Marrow Transplant 2007; 13(1):74–81.
120. Chakrabarti S, Mautner V, Osman H, et al. Adenovirus infections following allogeneic stem cell transplantation: incidence and outcome in relation to graft manipulation, immunosuppression, and immune recovery. Blood 2002;100(5): 1619–27.
121. Lenaerts L, De Clercq E, Naesens L. Clinical features and treatment of adenovirus infections. Rev Med Virol 2008;18(6):357–74.
122. Lenaerts L, Naesens L. Antiviral therapy for adenovirus infections. Antiviral Res 2006;71(2–3):172–80.
123. Toth K, Spencer JF, Dhar D, et al. Hexadecyloxypropyl-cidofovir, CMX001, prevents adenovirus-induced mortality in a permissive, immunosuppressed animal model. Proc Natl Acad Sci U S A 2008;105(20):7293–7.
124. Gavin PJ, Katz BZ. Intravenous ribavirin treatment for severe adenovirus disease in immunocompromised children. Pediatrics 2002;110(1 Pt 1):e9.
125. Bruno B, Gooley T, Hackman RC, et al. Adenovirus infection in hematopoietic stem cell transplantation: effect of ganciclovir and impact on survival. Biol Blood Marrow Transplant 2003;9(5):341–52.
126. Leen AM, Christin A, Khalil M, et al. Identification of hexon-specific CD4 and CD8 T-cell epitopes for vaccine and immunotherapy. J Virol 2008;82(1): 546–54.
127. Peters CJ, Khan AS. Hantavirus pulmonary syndrome: the new American hemorrhagic fever. Clin Infect Dis 2002;34(9):1224–31.
128. Ferres M, Vial P, Marco C, et al. Prospective evaluation of household contacts of persons with hantavirus cardiopulmonary syndrome in Chile. J Infect Dis 2007; 195(11):1563–71.
129. Wells RM, Sosa Estani S, Yadon ZE, et al. An unusual hantavirus outbreak in southern Argentina: person-to-person transmission? Hantavirus Pulmonary Syndrome Study Group for Patagonia. Emerg Infect Dis 1997;3(2):171–4.
130. Wells RM, Young J, Williams RJ, et al. Hantavirus transmission in the United States. Emerg Infect Dis 1997;3(3):361–5.
131. Khan AS, Khabbaz RF, Armstrong LR, et al. Hantavirus pulmonary syndrome: the first 100 US cases. J Infect Dis 1996;173(6):1297–303.
132. Hjelle B, Glass GE. Outbreak of hantavirus infection in the Four Corners region of the United States in the wake of the 1997-1998 El Nino-southern oscillation. J Infect Dis 2000;181(5):1569–73.
133. Young JC, Hansen GR, Graves TK, et al. The incubation period of hantavirus pulmonary syndrome. Am J Trop Med Hyg 2000;62(6):714–7.
134. Zavasky DM, Hjelle B, Peterson MC, et al. Acute infection with Sin Nombre hantavirus without pulmonary edema. Clin Infect Dis 1999;29(3):664–6.
135. Ketai LH, Williamson MR, Telepak RJ, et al. Hantavirus pulmonary syndrome: radiographic findings in 16 patients. Radiology 1994;191(3):665–8.
136. Moolenaar RL, Dalton C, Lipman HB, et al. Clinical features that differentiate hantavirus pulmonary syndrome from three other acute respiratory illnesses. Clin Infect Dis 1995;21(3):643–9.
137. Hallin GW, Simpson SQ, Crowell RE, et al. Cardiopulmonary manifestations of hantavirus pulmonary syndrome. Crit Care Med 1996;24(2):252–8.
138. Saggioro FP, Rossi MA, Duarte MI, et al. Hantavirus infection induces a typical myocarditis that may be responsible for myocardial depression and shock in hantavirus pulmonary syndrome. J Infect Dis 2007;195(10):1541–9.

139. Verity R, Prasad E, Grimsrud K, et al. Hantavirus pulmonary syndrome in northern Alberta, Canada: clinical and laboratory findings for 19 cases. Clin Infect Dis 2000;31(4):942–6.
140. Boroja M, Barrie JR, Raymond GS. Radiographic findings in 20 patients with Hantavirus pulmonary syndrome correlated with clinical outcome. AJR Am J Roentgenol 2002;178(1):159–63.
141. Nolte KB, Feddersen RM, Foucar K, et al. Hantavirus pulmonary syndrome in the United States: a pathological description of a disease caused by a new agent. Hum Pathol 1995;26(1):110–20.
142. Bharadwaj M, Nofchissey R, Goade D, et al. Humoral immune responses in the hantavirus cardiopulmonary syndrome. J Infect Dis 2000;182(1):43–8.
143. Terajima M, Hendershot JD 3rd, Kariwa H, et al. High levels of viremia in patients with the Hantavirus pulmonary syndrome. J Infect Dis 1999;180(6):2030–4.
144. Levy H, Simpson SQ. Hantavirus pulmonary syndrome. Am J Respir Crit Care Med 1994;149(6):1710–3.
145. Mertz GJ, Hjelle B, Crowley M, et al. Diagnosis and treatment of new world hantavirus infections. Curr Opin Infect Dis 2006;19(5):437–42.
146. Crowley MR, Katz RW, Kessler R, et al. Successful treatment of adults with severe Hantavirus pulmonary syndrome with extracorporeal membrane oxygenation. Crit Care Med 1998;26(2):409–14.
147. Mertz GJ, Miedzinski L, Goade D, et al. Placebo-controlled, double-blind trial of intravenous ribavirin for the treatment of hantavirus cardiopulmonary syndrome in North America. Clin Infect Dis 2004;39(9):1307–13.
148. Mills JN, Corneli A, Young JC, et al. Hantavirus pulmonary syndrome–United States: updated recommendations for risk reduction. Centers for Disease Control and Prevention. MMWR Recomm Rep 2002;51(RR-9):1–12.
149. Leen AM, Heslop HE. Cytotoxic T lymphocytes as immune-therapy in haematological practice. Br J Haematol 2008;143(2):169–79.

Influenza and Endemic Viral Pneumonia

Clare D. Ramsey, MD, MSc, FRCPC[a,b,c,*], Anand Kumar, MD, FRCPC[b]

KEYWORDS

- 2009 H1N1 • Viral pneumonitis • Viral pneumonia • Influenza
- Acute respiratory distress syndrome • Acute lung injury

KEY POINTS

- Viruses are an important cause of community-acquired pneumonia in both pediatric and adult populations.
- Disease surveillance systems are important in detecting outbreaks and particularly the emergence of novel viral pathogens capable of human transmission.
- Several common viral pathogens can lead to severe respiratory disease, including the most common virus, influenza A.
- Treatment of viral pneumonia is generally supportive; however, diagnostic testing to isolate the causative virus is important because some pathogens, such as influenza virus, have effective antiviral therapies.
- In the case of 2009 H1N1, early treatment with antiviral therapy appeared to be associated with improved outcomes.

EPIDEMIOLOGY OF VIRAL PNEUMONIA

Pneumonia is a common illness with estimates of approximately 450 million cases per year. According to the World Health Organization, lower respiratory tract infections account for approximately 7% of deaths per year worldwide.[1] Viruses are a common cause of community-acquired pneumonia, particularly among children. Among pediatric community-acquired pneumonia studies, where viral causes were specifically sought, the incidence of viral etiology of infection was 49%. The most common viruses isolated were respiratory syncytial virus (RSV) (11%), influenza virus (10%), parainfluenza virus (8%), and adenovirus (3%).[2] A Canadian study found that among adults

Disclosures: The authors have nothing to disclose.
[a] Section of Respiratory Medicine, Department of Medicine, University of Manitoba, RS 314, 810 Sherbrook Street, Winnipeg, Manitoba R3A 1R8, Canada; [b] Section of Critical Care, Department of Medicine, University of Manitoba, GC 425, 820 Sherbrook Street, Winnipeg, Manitoba R3T 2N2, Canada; [c] Department of Community Health Sciences, University of Manitoba, S113, 750 Bannatyne Avenue, Winnipeg, Manitoba R3E 0W3, Canada
* Corresponding author. RS 309, 810 Sherbrook Street, Winnipeg, Manitoba R3A 1R8, Canada.
E-mail address: cramsey@hsc.mb.ca

hospitalized with community-acquired pneumonia with an identifiable pathogen, 15% were viral and 20% bacterial, with 4% being mixed. The most common viral pathogens were influenza, human metapneumovirus, and RSV. Patients with viral infections were older, more likely to have cardiac disease, and in general more frail compared with adults with bacterial pneumonia. Furthermore, all cases of viral pneumonia occurred between October and May, whereas bacterial pathogens had no seasonal predilection. In this study, there were no differences in outcomes between viral or bacterial causes of pneumonia.[3] In a retrospective cohort analysis of adults admitted to an intensive care unit (ICU) with either severe community-acquired or health care–associated pneumonia, 115 of 198 patients had bronchoalveolar lavage and 159 of 198 had nasopharyngeal swabs for real-time polymerase chain reaction (RT-PCR). Of those with samples, 36.4% had a viral pathogen isolated and 35.9% had a bacterial pathogen isolated. Viral pathogens isolated in order of highest to lowest frequency were rhinovirus, parainfluenza virus, human metapneumovirus, influenza, and RSV. Again in this study, mortality was not different between bacterial and viral causes of pneumonia.[4]

This article focuses on viruses most commonly associated with severe community-acquired pneumonia, including those associated with recent epidemics.

INFLUENZA VIRUS

Influenza virus kills hundreds of thousands of people worldwide each year. In most cases, influenza infections are self-limited, mild illnesses lasting 4 to 5 days with predominantly upper airway symptoms. Among the most common severe complications and causes of death from influenza are viral pneumonia and/or secondary bacterial pneumonia.[5] In the absence of a pandemic, 11% to 19% of patients hospitalized with laboratory-confirmed influenza require treatment in the ICU.[6–10] Complications and death from influenza occur most commonly among the elderly, the very young, and those with chronic medical conditions. Chronic lung disease is the most common comorbidity associated with influenza infection, followed by neurologic disease, hemato-oncologic disease, and cardiac disease.[6] Risk factors for severe influenza complications are summarized in **Table 1**. A younger age of patients with critical illness is seen during pandemics, including the 2009 H1N1. In the historic 1918 pandemic, there was unexplained excess mortality in persons aged 20 to 40 years, with most deaths attributable to secondary bronchopneumonia, influenza-related lung disease, and associated cyanosis and cardiac collapse.[11] In the 1918 epidemic it was estimated that one-third of the world's population were infected with influenza, and the case-fatality rate was exceptionally high at greater than 2.5% in comparison with other pandemics. The number of deaths has been estimated to be at least 50 million.[12]

Pulmonary syndromes associated with the 1957 to 1958 influenza pandemic include an acute rapidly progressive pneumonia caused by the influenza virus alone, or concomitant viral and bacterial pneumonia.[13,14] The clinical course of patients with severe viral pneumonia was that of a rapid onset of severe progressive shortness of breath, tachypnea, cyanosis, and agitation caused by respiratory distress. A classic prodromal illness of high fever, chills, sore throat, aches, and dry nonproductive cough preceded the development of respiratory distress. Physical examination showed evidence of fever, respiratory distress, diffuse inspiratory crackles bilaterally, and occasional wheezes. Chest radiography (CXR) showed bilateral infiltrates similar to those in congestive heart failure (CHF) but without other clinical signs of volume overload. Although values of partial pressure of oxygen (Pao_2) are not provided, the low oxygen

Table 1
Prognostic indicators and risk factors for severe influenza complications

Risk Factor and Comorbidities	Comments
Age <5 y	Children <2 y and those with chronic cardiopulmonary disease at greatest risk
Age >65 y	Poor vaccine response, poor host response to influenza infection
Chronic cardiopulmonary diseases	COPD, asthma, congestive heart failure
Metabolic disease and chronic liver disease	Diabetes mellitus and cirrhosis increase the risk of influenza complications
Chronic neurologic illness	Neurocognitive and neuromuscular diseases associated with increased complications
Pregnancy	Particularly women in the third trimester
Obesity	BMI >35 kg/m^2 increased the risk of influenza complications on the 2009 outbreak
Hemoglobinopathy	Sickle-cell disease patients at increased risk
Immunosuppression	Glucocorticoids, chemotherapy, HIV, transplant recipients at increased risk
Children receiving salicylates	Increased risk of Reye syndrome
Aboriginal populations, poverty, poor access to health care services	Delayed treatment associated with increased risk of influenza complications
Secondary bacterial pneumonia	Bacterial pneumonia associated with longer ICU and hospital stays with more nosocomial complications and a greater mortality rate

Abbreviations: BMI, body mass index; COPD, chronic obstructive pulmonary disease; HIV, human immunodeficiency virus; ICU, intensive care unit.

From Opal S, Kumar A. Influenza. In: Vincent JL, Abraham E, Kochanek P, et al, editors. Textbook of critical care. 6th edition. Philadelphia: Elsevier Saunders; 2011; with permission.

saturations on high-level oxygen, radiographic characteristics, and lack of CHF would fit the description of acute respiratory distress syndrome (ARDS) secondary to viral pneumonia, as seen with the 2009 H1N1 pandemic.

Many believe that much of the excess mortality attributed to the 1918 influenza epidemic was related to secondary bacterial pneumonia with organisms such as *Staphylococcus aureus* and *Streptococcus pneumoniae*.[5,15] This opinion is supported by autopsy studies reporting severe bronchopneumonia with an ARDS-like illness, and cultured bacteria associated with pneumonic lesions; however, in some cases there was no evidence of bacterial pneumonia.[11,16,17] Good epidemiologic evidence supports the emergence of an antigenically novel influenza virus in 1918 with high virulence to which many younger people had never been exposed, which was likely a significant contributor to the high mortality rates in this younger age group.[12] In addition to the complication of severe respiratory failure, influenza infection has been associated with central nervous system, cardiac, skeletal, renal, and hepatic complications.[18]

INFLUENZA A 2009 H1N1

In the spring of 2009, an outbreak attributed to a new viral pathogen, swine-origin influenza A (2009 H1N1), led to a significant number of cases of severe hypoxemic respiratory failure attributable to viral pneumonia. The outbreak began in the Southwestern

United States and Mexico, with rapid spread throughout the rest of the United States, Canada, and then the rest of the world. This spread led the World Health Organization (WHO) to declare a phase-6 global pandemic alert on June 11, 2009.[19]

The number of patients requiring admission to an ICU for viral pneumonitis caused by 2009 H1N1 infection was much larger than rates due to seasonal influenza.[20] The increased incidence of critical illness, along with a high transmissibility rate and rapid increase in case numbers over a short period of time, created a significant stress on hospital resources in several countries, particularly in terms of ICU resources.[20,21] The need for invasive ventilatory support in some relatively underresourced nations in the Western hemisphere reportedly exceeded ICU capacity (Farmer C, personal communication, 2010).

Epidemiology and Risk Factors for Respiratory Failure Related to H1N1 2009

Since the onset of the pandemic in March of 2009, more than 214 countries and communities reported cases of pandemic 2009 H1N1 influenza, with more than 18,000 deaths.[22] In Australian provinces, approximately 5% of the population developed H1N1-related illness, 0.3% of infected patients were hospitalized, and 20% of hospitalized patients required ICU care, very similar to the proportions reported by the Public Health Agency of Canada.[23,24] During the pandemic in Argentina there were 1,390,566 cases of influenza-like illness and of those, 14,034 were admitted to hospital and 617 (4.4%) died as of January 2, 2010.[25] In the United Kingdom 13% of 2009 H1N1 patients, both adults and children, were admitted to either an ICU or high-dependency unit, with a mortality rate of 5%. Of those who died, 59% were previously healthy, and hospital mortality rate increased with increasing age.[26] Overall the case-fatality rate was low (<0.5%), and lower than generally reported for seasonal influenza, although there is much variability in estimates.[27–31]

The viral epidemic was initially suspected after an increasing number of young patients in Mexico were hospitalized with severe and, not infrequently, fatal pneumonia. In a reported series of the initial 2155 cases of severe pneumonia in Mexico, Chowell and colleagues[32] found that 87% of deaths and 71% of cases of severe pneumonia occurred in patients between ages of 5 and 59 years, which represented a significant shift in the age distribution of patients with severe disease or deaths from seasonal influenza. In Australia and New Zealand, 722 patients were admitted to an ICU within a 3-month period of time with confirmed 2009 H1N1. The mean number of admissions for viral pneumonitis within the same period in the prior 4 years was 57.[33]

Despite the young age of patients requiring ICU admission for respiratory failure, the highest death rate was among those older than 50 years.[34–36] However, because in comparison with seasonal influenza, 2009 H1N1 affected younger individuals, the number of years of life lost was substantial, estimated to be between 334,000 and 1973,000 years in the United States from May to December 2009.[37]

Among those requiring critical care in Canada, 67% were female with a mean age of 32 years. The majority of patients had at least 1 comorbidity, most commonly chronic lung disease (asthma, chronic obstructive pulmonary disease [COPD], bronchopulmonary dysplasia), obesity, hypertension, smoking, and diabetes. However, the majority did not have the kinds of major chronic organ failure typical of patients admitted to medical ICUs. The mean Acute Physiology and Chronic Health Evaluation II (APACHE II) score of ICU patients was 20, with major comorbidities present in 30%.[21] Similar patient demographics were noted in other countries, and many are known risk factors for influenza infection.[33,38,39] Indigenous persons from Australia and New Zealand, as well as Aboriginal Canadians (26%), were overrepresented among those who were critical ill.[21,33,40] Obesity, which interestingly has not been previously linked to complications of influenza, was a prominent risk factor for severe respiratory disease secondary to 2009 H1N1.[21,26,33,35,38,40–42] Pregnancy is well described as a risk factor for complications from seasonal influenza; however, the number of critically ill pregnant women with 2009 H1N1 pneumonitis was disproportionately large and led to excess mortality in this group.[42–45] In Australia and New Zealand, pregnant women had a relative risk of 13.2 of requiring ICU admission for their illness in comparison with nonpregnant women of childbearing age. Sixty-nine percent of women required mechanical ventilation and 11% died, all with viral pneumonitis and ARDS.[44] In California, 22% of pregnant women infected by 2009 H1N1 required ICU admission and 8% died, leading to an influenza-specific maternal mortality rate of 4.3 per 100,000 live births.[46]

Finally, factors associated with treatment were shown to correlate with severe disease. Canadian data showed that the interval from onset of symptoms to initiation of antiviral therapy or hospitalization was longer among patients with more severe disease (ICU admission or death),[24,40] and this was also shown to be true among hospitalized patients in the United States.[35,41] Observational studies of severe influenza H1N1 pneumonia suggest that early initiation of antiviral therapy is associated with improved outcomes.[47]

Clinical Presentation and Diagnosis

Although most cases of 2009 H1N1 were mild and self-limited, there were a significant number of cases with severe hypoxemic respiratory failure. Five clinical presentations with 2009 H1N1 were commonly noted: viral pneumonitis, exacerbations of asthma or COPD, exacerbations of other underlying disease (ie, CHF, chronic renal disease), secondary bacterial pneumonia, and croup/bronchiolitis in the pediatric population. The clinical presentation most frequently requiring ICU admission was that of viral pneumonitis, and most of these patients presented with rapidly progressive and refractory hypoxemia and bilateral alveolar infiltrates on CXR. Most of these patients fulfilled criteria for acute lung injury (ALI) or ARDS.[25,48]

Patients with viral pneumonitis and hypoxemic respiratory failure presented with symptoms of cough, dyspnea, and fever. These patients had rapidly progressive hypoxemia with high ventilatory demands, and in most case series greater than 70% to 80% of patients admitted to the ICU with this syndrome required mechanical ventilation.[21,35,41,49–51] Patients who presented with severe respiratory illness were hospitalized within a median of 2 to 6 days from onset of symptoms, and most requiring ICU admission did so within 24 hours of hospital admission.[21,25,39,41,49] In comparison with other causes of viral pneumonitis or seasonal influenza, an increased number of patients had gastrointestinal symptoms, typically diarrhea.[35,41,52–55]

The most common radiologic findings were bilateral patchy consolidation and/or ground-glass opacities, often worse in the lower lung zones (**Fig. 1**).[56] Among those requiring ICU admission and ventilation, at least 3 out of 4 lung quadrants on CXR were most commonly involved.[21,25,39,56] Computed tomography scans of the chest showed similar findings, with predominantly diffuse ground-glass infiltrates and consolidation.[56]

In Canada, ICU patients with 2009 H1N1 pneumonitis had a mean Pao_2/fraction of inspired oxygen (Fio_2) on admission of 147 mm Hg, and this remained on average lower than 200 among those remaining in the ICU at day 14. Seventy-three percent of patients had ALI at the onset of critical illness. Additional oxygenation and ventilatory support measures were not infrequently used, including high-frequency oscillatory ventilation (12%), nitric oxide (14%), neuromuscular blockade (30%), prone ventilation (5%), and extracorporeal membrane oxygenation (7%).[21] A similar degree

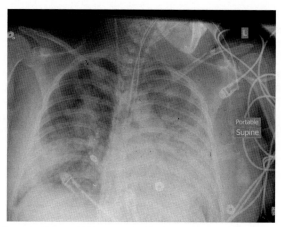

Fig. 1. Portable chest radiograph from a patient with H1N1 2009 viral pneumonitis and acute respiratory distress syndrome, showing diffuse bilateral airspace opacities.

of severe hypoxemia was noted in multiple case series from other countries.[25,38,49,57] Thoracic compliance was noted to be decreased in a subset of patients with 2009 H1N1–related hypoxemic respiratory failure, with a median of 22 mL/cm H_2O (interquartile range 21–34 mL/cm H_2O).[38] A significant number of patients developed at least 1 other organ dysfunction, and in some cases developed multisystem organ dysfunction.[21,38,39]

Duration of ventilation for 2009 H1N1 varied, with an average (median or mean reported) of 7 to 18 days.[21,38,51,52,58] The most common causes of death were severe ARDS with refractory hypoxemia and complications related to this, including infection, sepsis, or multisystem organ dysfunction. The most common infectious complication was secondary bacterial pneumonia, most frequently attributed to S aureus or S pneumoniae.[21,35,59]

Diagnosis of 2009 H1N1 2009 pneumonitis is made based on the compatible clinical syndrome as already described, and the detection of the H1N1 influenza virus by RT-PCR and/or viral culture. Viral cultures take up to 1 week for processing and thus RT-PCR, typically on nasopharyngeal swabs, is the preferred technique. During the 2009 H1N1 pandemic, it was noted that false-negative nasopharyngeal aspirates occurred in more than 10% of patients with viral pneumonitis. In severe cases of illness, tracheal aspirates or bronchoalveolar lavage specimens from intubated patients and repeated collection are recommended to increase the PCR diagnostic yield.[23,29]

Pathophysiology

Whether ARDS secondary to 2009 H1N1 is related to direct damage from the virus or to the host's immune response to the virus is unclear. Pandemic 2009 H1N1 virus can replicate in both the upper and the lower respiratory tract in comparison with seasonal influenza, which predominantly replicates in the upper respiratory tract.[60–62] In a retrospective study from Hong Kong, To and colleagues[63] examined the pattern of clinical disease, viral load, and immunologic profile between patients with varying severity of 2009 H1N1. Those who died or had ARDS had delayed clearance of viral load in their nasopharynx, had higher levels of proinflammatory cytokines and chemokines, and higher likelihood of viremia. There was significant correlation between the levels of interleukin (IL-6, IL-10, and IL-15) and disease severity. The association between high IL-6 and severe disease from influenza has been previously established.[64] Initial nasopharyngeal or endotracheal viral loads were similar among patients with differing disease severity; therefore, it would not appear to be viral load at the onset of infection that determines disease severity.[63]

Pulmonary Pathology

Most patients died of multisystem organ failure following admission for severe ARDS. On macroscopic examination, the lungs were noted to be heavy and diffusely edematous with areas of consolidation and hemorrhage.[65] Lung pathology typically showed diffuse alveolar damage (DAD), at times with associated areas of hemorrhage and necrotizing bronchiolitis (**Figs. 2** and **3**).

In a report from the Centers for Disease Control and Prevention (CDC) the most frequent histopathology in the airways of patients with 2009 H1N1 was inflammation and edema, with less frequent necrosis of the epithelium and hemorrhage. Lung tissue in all cases showed various stages of DAD, including edema, hyaline membranes, inflammation, and fibrosis. Seventeen patients had pulmonary thromboemboli. Immunohistochemistry showed viral antigens in airway epithelial cells, submucosal glands, and pneumocytes.[66] Viral antigen was also commonly seen in alveolar macrophages.[67] These studies show that H1N1 2009 virus has the ability to target both lower and upper respiratory tract infections, thus leading to DAD and clinical ARDS. Overall the pathologic findings were fairly similar to those published in autopsy studies from prior influenza epidemics in 1918 and 1957, including evidence of superimposed bacterial pneumonia.[13,14,68,69]

Management of ARDS Secondary to H1N1

Several studies examining risk factors for the development of ARDS related to 2009 H1N1 noted that time to treatment with antivirals was important: patients who received appropriate antiviral therapy with oseltamivir or zanamavir shortly after presentation for medical care had better outcomes.[41,46,48] Rapid initiation of antivirals when H1N1 infection is suspected is particularly important in those with risk factors for disease progression and those requiring hospitalization. Ideally, therapy should be started within 48 hours of symptom onset, but is also effective and recommended if

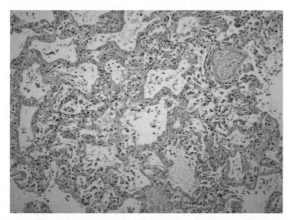

Fig. 2. Biopsy from a patient approximately 1 week into H1N1 2009 viral infection. This specimen demonstrates diffuse alveolar damage with hyaline membrane formation (hematoxylin-eosin, original magnification ×100). (*Courtesy of* Dr Julianne Klein, MD, FRCPC, University of Manitoba, Winnipeg, Canada.)

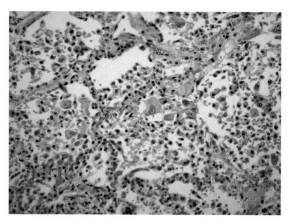

Fig. 3. Biopsy from patient with H1N1 2009 viral pneumonitis, demonstrating acute lung injury in the organizing phase. Type 2 pneumocyte hyperplasia and alveolar macrophages are prominent (hematoxylin-eosin, original magnification ×40). (*Courtesy of* Dr Julianne Klein, MD, FRCPC, University of Manitoba, Winnipeg, Canada.)

given later than this.[70] The recommended dose is 75 mg twice a day, although higher doses were given at some centers for critically ill and obese patients according to WHO recommendations.[71] Recent data suggest that 75 mg of oseltamivir administered twice per day via the orogastric route in critically ill patients consistently yields sufficient blood levels for near maximal (in vitro) suppression of viral replication.[72] Most patients also received broad-spectrum antimicrobial therapy, at least initially, while investigations were pending to determine the cause of respiratory failure. Current recommendations from the CDC state that antiviral treatment is recommended as early as possible in any patient with confirmed or suspected influenza who requires hospitalization, has severe, complicated, and progressive illness, or is at high risk for influenza complications (ie, <2 years and >65 years, immunocompromised, chronic disease, pregnant or postpartum, morbidly obese, Aboriginal, and residents of nursing homes or long-term care facilities). The current recommended therapy is either oseltamivir or inhaled zanamivir. However, in individuals with underlying respiratory disease, oseltamivir is recommended over zanamivir.[73] In critically ill patients with pneumonia, the viral RNA may be detected in lower airway secretions for several weeks after the initiation of oseltamivir. In patients with influenza pneumonia or evidence of clinical progression, an increased dose of the oseltamivir (150 mg twice daily in adults) and, more importantly, an increased duration of therapy for 10 days instead of 5 days, may be warranted.[29,74] Oseltamivir-resistant viruses have been isolated, but are not common. The resistance is via a His275Tyr mutation in viral neuraminidase, which confers high-level resistance to oseltamivir but not zanamivir. Most resistant isolates have been found in patients with prior oseltamivir exposure, and have been associated with mild self-limited disease. If oseltamivir resistance is suspected or confirmed, treatment should be with zanamivir.[29,75]

Most patients admitted to an ICU with 2009 H1N1 viral pneumonitis fulfilled the criteria for ALI or ARDS and required mechanical ventilation. Many patients initiated on noninvasive positive-pressure ventilation (NIPPV) failed this mode, and subsequently required intubation and invasive ventilation.[21,38] There are some reports of successful use of NIPPV, likely related to selection of less hypoxemic patients for this mode of treatment.[25] Concerns arose regarding transmission of H1N1 with NIPPV, as this mode of ventilation generates respiratory droplets and aerosols, which can reach a 0.5-m radius surrounding a patient receiving NIPPV.[76]

Most centers internationally ventilated 2009 H1N1 viral pneumonitis patients with low tidal ventilation (6 mL/kg of predicted body weight and plateau pressures <30 cm H_2O) whenever possible, as this is what has been recommended for ARDS based on results of the ARDSNet trial.[46,69,70,77–79] High levels of positive end-expiratory pressure (PEEP) were noted to be required to manage severe hypoxemia, with mean PEEP levels between 16 and 22 cm H_2O reported in some studies.[25,38,39,49] Other modes of ventilation were also used, including airway pressure release ventilation and high-frequency oscillation; however, there are insufficient data to conclusively state whether these modes had any impact on outcomes.[21,49] Similarly, recruitment maneuvers, prone positioning, and inhaled nitric oxide were used as salvage therapies for refractory hypoxemia, again with insufficient evidence to determine their effectiveness.[21,25,49,80]

Several studies have reported on the use of extracorporeal membrane oxygenation (ECMO) during the 2009 H1N1 pandemic. The largest of these series is from Australia, where 68 patients with severe ARDS (median Pao_2/Fio_2 of 58 and PEEP of 18 cm H_2O) were initiated on ECMO. Seventy-one percent survived their ICU admission and 21% died. By comparison, only 4 patients had been treated with ECMO for ARDS in the previous year in the same Australian centers.[58] Reports from other countries on the use of ECMO for ARDS related to H1N1 2009 pneumonia are much smaller, with mortality rates of between 56% and 67%.[81,82]

Avoidance of volume overload (and judicious diuresis) may also be associated with reduced duration of ventilation and length of stay in the ICU for most patients with ARDS.[83] This strategy was used and recommended in patients with ARDS related to 2009 H1N1.[84] Steroids were used in a variable number of patients across studies and for varying indications (sepsis, COPD or asthma exacerbation, stress-dose replacement therapy, or ARDS).[21,41,52] One study in Argentina examined the effect of treatment with corticosteroids, and found steroids to be safe and associated with improvement in lung injury score. However, there were only 13 patients and there was no real comparator group, as all patients received some degree of steroid therapy.[85] A study from the European Society of Intensive Care medicine H1N1 registry found that early use of corticosteroids in patients admitted to the ICU with H1N1 was associated with increased risk of superinfections, predominantly hospital-acquired pneumonia, with no mortality benefit.[86] Similarly, other studies found no mortality benefit or even harm with early steroid use.[87,88] At present there is insufficient evidence for routine use of steroids in 2009 H1N1 or other influenza-related ARDS. Some historical data and experience with recent influenza epidemics suggests the potential utility of convalescent serum in the management of severe influenza.[89,90] Although research on the issue is clearly required, the use of convalescent serum or immunoglobulin may become a useful treatment modality should future pandemic influenza A viruses be resistant to current antiviral agents.

ADENOVIRUS

Adenovirus is a common cause of mild upper respiratory illness in children; however, up to 20% of all children who are infected with adenovirus develop pneumonia.[91] Among adults, adenovirus accounts for 1% to 7% of respiratory infections, particularly among immunocompromised adults and those in closed or crowed settings.[91,92] Endemic cases occur throughout the year. In addition, epidemics have been reported among military recruits, long-term care facilities, and hospitals, with rapid spread of the virus. Adenovirus has also been shown to cause potentially fatal pneumonia, predominantly in immunocompromised hosts (especially transplant recipients).[93] Symptomatology is similar to that of other viral pneumonias, with fever, cough preceded by upper respiratory symptoms, and bilateral interstitial infiltrates on CXR. In cases of severe adenoviral pneumonia, case-fatality rates are high and may be above 50%.

Most cases of adenoviral pneumonia are due to serotypes 3, 7, 11, or 14. Transmission occurs via respiratory droplet secretions, tears, fecal-oral spread, or environmental surfaces. Infection-control measures are paramount in limiting disease spread.[93,94] The incubation period ranges from 2 to 14 days. Infections of the respiratory tract can also be associated with gastrointestinal symptoms (gastroenteritis or diarrhea). Detection of the virus is through PCR, serologic testing, or viral culture. PCR has the highest sensitivity and specificity, whereas viral culture can be insensitive and take up to 21 days.[91,95]

The treatment of adenovirus infections is supportive for mild disease; there are no approved antiviral drugs. Although often used in severe cases, ribavirin (a guanosine analogue) has not been shown to be effective in small clinical studies.[96] For immunocompromised patients and those with severe disease, cidofovir, a cytosine nucleotide analogue that inhibits DNA polymerase, has the greatest activity against the virus and is the preferred agent.[97] Several nonrandomized studies in hematopoietic stem cell transplant recipients have shown a favorable response to this agent.[98] Combination therapy with cidofovir and pooled intravenous immunoglobulin (IVIG) has been used, but data on the efficacy of this therapy are lacking.[98]

Severe Acute Respiratory Syndrome and Other Coronaviruses

The severe acute respiratory syndrome (SARS) coronavirus was first discovered in 2002/2003 when an epidemic originating in Southern China spread rapidly (in a limited number of cases) to the rest of Asia and then Europe, Canada, and the United States. SARS is a highly contagious virus, with high rates of spread identified in health care workers. The case-fatality rate during the epidemic was 9.6% and was strongly associated with increasing age (case-fatality rate of 43.3% in those older than 60 years).[99] SARS was noted to have multiple modes of transmission, including droplet and airborne spread as well as direct contact with contaminated surfaces.[100,101] In the nosocomial cases, contaminated surfaces included surfaces in the patient's own rooms.

The clinical presentation of SARS is one of a prolonged influenza-like prodrome of fever, cough, chills, myalgias, dyspnea, and headache. As the infection progresses the respiratory symptoms are more profound, and up to 20% of patients required ICU admission and mechanical ventilation after a median of 8 days from symptom onset.[102] The most common radiographic presentation was focal unilateral peripheral airspace disease, which progressed to multifocal unilateral or bilateral disease.[103,104]

Diagnosis is made based on clinical suspicion and contact with a known case, and is confirmed by either serologic testing or RT-PCR. RT-PCR for SARS has limited sensitivity and specificity, therefore repeated sampling is recommended.[105] As with influenza, tracheal aspirates may be helpful in intubated patients with severe pneumonia. Serologic testing is the most sensitive test but it takes several weeks for antibodies to develop, with a mean time to seroconversion of approximately 18 to 20 days.[106,107]

Treatment of SARS is supportive, with little evidence of any effective antivirals or other pharmacologic therapies.[108]

A novel coronavirus was discovered in September 2012, which has now been referred to as the Middle East respiratory syndrome (MERS) coronavirus. As of May 31, 2013, 50 cases have been confirmed with a death rate of 54%. Most cases have occurred within the Arab Peninsula and neighboring countries. Infection with the novel coronavirus has led to severe lower respiratory tract illness. There is a low rate of human-to-human transmission; however, concern has arisen that the virus may adapt to being more efficient at such transmission.[109]

Respiratory Syncytial Virus

RSV is an enveloped RNA virus in the paramyxovirus family, which is primarily associated with fall to winter epidemics of lower respiratory illness in infants and young children. Up to 70% of newborns are infected during their first winter. RSV infection in adults generally represents reinfection, and may be the etiologic agent in up to 2.4% of community-acquired lower respiratory tract infections.[110] Among the elderly, RSV infection is more common and may account for 10% of winter hospital admissions, with a case-fatality rate similar to that of influenza ($\sim$10%).[111] Risk factors for severe disease are advanced age, immunocompromised state, and chronic cardiopulmonary diseases, for which higher death rates have been reported.

RSV lower respiratory tract infection in adults presents as a wheezing illness in 90% of cases, along with crackles and a pneumonic infiltrate in 40%. However, the classic bronchiolitis picture seen in infants is rare in adult populations. Most adults present with nasal congestion, cough, and low-grade fever, which can be followed by dyspnea and wheezing. Often in adults the clinical features are difficult to distinguish from other respiratory viruses; however, myalgias and fever are less common, and wheezing and rhinorrhea more common, with RSV than with influenza infection.[112] CXR often demonstrates small focal infiltrates, but lobar infiltrates have been described.[92] Diagnosis is best made by RT-PCR of nasal aspirates and, if available, lower respiratory sample (bronchoalveolar lavage or deep tracheal suctioning) or viral cultures, which are less sensitive.

The aerosolized form of ribavirin is approved for treatment of RSV in children. Data from adult populations are limited. Ribavirin has been used in immunocompromised adults with upper and lower respiratory tract infections, either alone or in combination with IVIG (standard or RSV-IVIG).[113] Spread is via large droplets and fomites. Isolation and cohorting of infected patients is recommended.

HUMAN METAPNEUMOVIRUS

Human metapneumovirus (hMPV) is closely related to RSV, and primary infection often occurs in childhood; however, as with RSV, immunity is incomplete. In children the clinical manifestations are very similar to those of RSV. The incidence of symptomatic infection in adults is generally less than 5% in most studies.[114]

In a prospective study of hospitalized adults with cardiorespiratory illness during the winter season, hMPV was identified in 8.5% of the cohort. Of these patients, 13% and 12% required ICU admission and ventilatory support, respectively. The mortality rate overall was 7%. Coinfection with RSV, coronavirus, and influenza A was noted in up to 23%.[115] hMPV can result in pneumonia and respiratory failure, although this is less common than with influenza and RSV.[116] The clinical symptoms are indistinguishable from those of other respiratory viruses. Risk factors for severe disease are also similar to those for other viruses and include older age, immunocompromised state, and chronic cardiorespiratory disease. CXR reveals patchy infiltrates, predominantly in the lower lung zones. Identification of the virus optimally involves RT-PCR or direct immunofluorescence, as hMPV replicates very slowly and grows inefficiently using traditional viral culture methods.[114] The mainstay of treatment, as with most viral infections, is supportive. A few case reports and series have reported ribavirin to be a potentially effective treatment, although more studies are needed before this can be recommended.[117]

SUMMARY

Viruses are an important cause of community-acquired pneumonia in both pediatric and adult populations. Viral pneumonias tend to have a seasonal predilection and are often preceded by a prodromal illness. Disease surveillance systems are important in detecting outbreaks and particularly the emergence of novel viral pathogens capable of human transmission. Several common viral pathogens can lead to severe respiratory disease, including the most common virus, influenza A. Unfortunately, appropriate diagnostic testing is often not pursued or is unavailable, particularly in smaller community hospitals. Treatment of viral pneumonia is generally supportive; however, diagnostic testing to isolate the causative virus is important because some pathogens, such as influenza virus, have effective antiviral therapies. Specifically in the case of 2009 H1N1, early treatment with antiviral therapy appeared to be associated with improved outcomes.

ACKNOWLEDGMENTS

The authors would like to thank Dr Julianne Klein for providing pathology slides from patients with H1N1.

REFERENCES

1. The World Health Organization. The global burden of disease: 2004 update. Switzerland: Work Health Organization; 2008. Available at: http://www.who.int/healthinfo/global_burden_disease/GBD_report_2004update_full.pdf. Accessed May 27, 2013.
2. Ruuskanen O, Lahti E, Jennings LC, et al. Viral pneumonia. Lancet 2011; 377(9773):1264–75.
3. Johnstone J, Majumdar SR, Fox JD, et al. Viral infection in adults hospitalized with community-acquired pneumonia: prevalence, pathogens, and presentation. Chest 2008;134(6):1141–8.
4. Choi SH, Hong SB, Ko GB, et al. Viral infection in patients with severe pneumonia requiring intensive care unit admission. Am J Respir Crit Care Med 2012;186(4):325–32.
5. Khater F, Moorman JP. Complications of influenza. South Med J 2003;96(8): 740–3.
6. Coffin SE, Zaoutis TE, Rosenquist AB, et al. Incidence, complications, and risk factors for prolonged stay in children hospitalized with community-acquired influenza. Pediatrics 2007;119(4):740–8.
7. Moore DL, Vaudry W, Scheifele DW, et al. Surveillance for influenza admissions among children hospitalized in Canadian immunization monitoring program active centers, 2003-2004. Pediatrics 2006;118(3):e610–9.
8. Schrag SJ, Shay DK, Gershman K, et al. Multistate surveillance for laboratory-confirmed, influenza-associated hospitalizations in children: 2003-2004. Pediatr Infect Dis J 2006;25(5):395–400.
9. Burton C, Vaudry W, Moore D, et al. Children hospitalized with influenza during the 2006-2007 season: a report from the Canadian Immunization Monitoring Program, Active (IMPACT). Can Commun Dis Rep 2008;34(12):17–32.

10. Babcock HM, Merz LR, Fraser VJ. Is influenza an influenza-like illness? Clinical presentation of influenza in hospitalized patients. Infect Control Hosp Epidemiol 2006;27(3):266–70.

11. Morens DM, Taubenberger JK, Harvey HA, et al. The 1918 influenza pandemic: lessons for 2009 and the future. Crit Care Med 2010;38(Suppl 4):e10–20.

12. Taubenberger JK, Morens DM. 1918 Influenza: the mother of all pandemics. Emerg Infect Dis 2006;12(1):15–22.

13. Louria DB, Blumenfeld HL, Ellis JT, et al. Studies on influenza in the pandemic of 1957-1958. II. Pulmonary complications of influenza. J Clin Invest 1959; 38(1 Part 2):213–65.

14. Hers JF, Masurel N, Mulder J. Bacteriology and histopathology of the respiratory tract and lungs in fatal Asian influenza. Lancet 1958;2(7057):1141–3.

15. Brundage JF, Shanks GD. Deaths from bacterial pneumonia during 1918-19 influenza pandemic. Emerg Infect Dis 2008;14(8):1193–9.

16. Hirsch E, McKinney M. An epidemic of pneumococcus bronchopneumonia. J Infect Dis 1919;24:594–617.

17. French H. The clinical features of the influenza epidemic of 1918-19. In: Great Britain Ministry of Health. Reports on public health and medical subjects. Report on the pandemic of influenza, 1918-19. London: His Majesty's Stationery Office; 1920. p. 66–109.

18. Bhat N, Wright JG, Broder KR, et al. Influenza-associated deaths among children in the United States, 2003-2004. N Engl J Med 2005;353(24):2559–67.

19. World Health Organization. World now at the start of 2009 influenza pandemic. Statement to the press by WHO director. Geneva (Switzerland): 2009 Available at: http://www.who.int/mediacentre/news/statements/2009/h1n1_pandemic_phase6_20090611/en/index.html. Accessed May 27, 2013.

20. Kotsimbos T, Waterer G, Jenkins C, et al. Influenza A/H1N1_09: Australia and New Zealand's winter of discontent. Am J Respir Crit Care Med 2010;181(4): 300–6.

21. Kumar A, Zarychanski R, Pinto R, et al. Critically ill patients with 2009 influenza A(H1N1) infection in Canada. JAMA 2009;302(17):1872–9.

22. Norfolk SG, Hollingsworth CL, Wolfe CR, et al. Rescue therapy in adult and pediatric patients with pH1N1 influenza infection: a tertiary center intensive care unit experience from April to October 2009. Crit Care Med 2010;38(11):2103–7.

23. Fowler RA, Jouvet P, Christian M, et al. Critical illness due to influenza A 2009 H1N1. Critical Care Rounds [Internet]. 2009 August 2010; October 2009: [1–12 pp.]. Available at: http://www.medtau.org/pandemic/ccrounds.pdf. Accessed April 15, 2013.

24. Campbell A, Rodin R, Kropp R, et al. Risk of severe outcomes among patients admitted to hospital with pandemic (H1N1) influenza. CMAJ 2010;182(4): 349–55.

25. Estenssoro E, Rios FG, Apezteguia C, et al. Pandemic 2009 influenza A in Argentina: a study of 337 patients on mechanical ventilation. Am J Respir Crit Care Med 2010;182(1):41–8.

26. Nguyen-Van-Tam JS, Openshaw PJ, Hashim A, et al. Risk factors for hospitalisation and poor outcome with pandemic A/H1N1 influenza: United Kingdom first wave (May-September 2009). Thorax 2010;65(7):645–51.

27. Fraser C, Donnelly CA, Cauchemez S, et al. Pandemic potential of a strain of influenza A (H1N1): early findings. Science 2009;324(5934):1557–61.

28. Wilson N, Baker MG. The emerging influenza pandemic: estimating the case fatality ratio. Euro Surveill 2009;14(26).

29. Bautista E, Chotpitayasunondh T, Gao Z, et al. Clinical aspects of pandemic 2009 influenza A (H1N1) virus infection. N Engl J Med 2010;362(18):1708–19.

30. Presanis AM, De Angelis D, Hagy A, et al. The severity of pandemic H1N1 influenza in the United States, from April to July 2009: a Bayesian analysis. PLoS Med 2009;6(12):e1000207.

31. Hadler JL, Konty K, McVeigh KH, et al. Case fatality rates based on population estimates of influenza-like illness due to novel H1N1 influenza: New York City, May-June 2009. PLoS One 2010;5(7):e11677.

32. Chowell G, Bertozzi SM, Colchero MA, et al. Severe respiratory disease concurrent with the circulation of H1N1 influenza. N Engl J Med 2009;361(7):674–9.

33. Webb SA, Pettila V, Seppelt I, et al. Critical care services and 2009 H1N1 influenza in Australia and New Zealand. N Engl J Med 2009;361(20):1925–34.

34. Tuite AR, Greer AL, Whelan M, et al. Estimated epidemiologic parameters and morbidity associated with pandemic H1N1 influenza. CMAJ 2010;182(2):131–6.

35. Louie JK, Acosta M, Winter K, et al. Factors associated with death or hospitalization due to pandemic 2009 influenza A(H1N1) infection in California. JAMA 2009;302(17):1896–902.

36. Gomez J, Munayco C, Arrasco J, et al. Pandemic influenza in a southern hemisphere setting: the experience in Peru from May to September, 2009. Euro Surveill 2009;14(42). pii:19371.

37. Viboud C, Miller M, Olson D, et al. Preliminary estimates of mortality and Years of life lost associated with the 2009 A/H1N1 pandemic in the US and comparison with past influenza seasons. PLoS Curr 2010;2:RRN1153.

38. Miller RR 3rd, Markewitz BA, Rolfs RT, et al. Clinical findings and demographic factors associated with ICU admission in Utah due to novel 2009 influenza A(H1N1) infection. Chest 2010;137(4):752–8.

39. Perez-Padilla R, de la Rosa-Zamboni D, Ponce de Leon S, et al. Pneumonia and respiratory failure from swine-origin influenza A (H1N1) in Mexico. N Engl J Med 2009;361(7):680–9.

40. Zarychanski R, Stuart TL, Kumar A, et al. Correlates of severe disease in patients with 2009 pandemic influenza (H1N1) virus infection. CMAJ 2010; 182(3):257–64.

41. Jain S, Kamimoto L, Bramley AM, et al. Hospitalized patients with 2009 H1N1 influenza in the United States, April-June 2009. N Engl J Med 2009;361(20):1935–44.

42. Van Kerkhove MD, Vandemaele KA, Shinde V, et al. Risk factors for severe outcomes following 2009 influenza A (H1N1) infection: a global pooled analysis. PLoS Med 2011;8(7):e1001053.

43. Callaghan WM, Chu SY, Jamieson DJ. Deaths from seasonal influenza among pregnant women in the United States, 1998-2005. Obstet Gynecol 2010; 115(5):919–23.

44. Anzic Influenza Investigators. Critical illness due to 2009 A/H1N1 influenza in pregnant and post partum women: population based cohort study. BMJ 2010; 340:c1279.

45. Jamieson DJ, Honein MA, Rasmussen SA, et al. H1N1 2009 influenza virus infection during pregnancy in the USA. Lancet 2009;374(9688):451–8.

46. Louie JK, Acosta M, Jamieson DJ, et al. Severe 2009 H1N1 influenza in pregnant and postpartum women in California. N Engl J Med 2010;362(1):27–35.

47. Kumar A. Early versus late oseltamivir treatment in severely ill patients with 2009 pandemic influenza A (H1N1): speed is life. J Antimicrob Chemother 2011; 66(5):959–63.

48. Bernard GR, Artigas A, Brigham KL, et al. The American-European Consensus Conference on ARDS. Definitions, mechanisms, relevant outcomes, and clinical trial coordination. Am J Respir Crit Care Med 1994;149(3 Pt 1):818–24.
49. Siau C, Law J, Tee A, et al. Severe refractory hypoxaemia in H1N1 (2009) intensive care patients: initial experience in an Asian regional hospital. Singapore Med J 2010;51(6):490–5.
50. Centers for Disease Control and Prevention (CDC). Hospitalized patients with novel influenza A (H1N1) virus infection—California, April-May, 2009. MMWR Morb Mortal Wkly Rep 2009;58(19):536–41.
51. Lum ME, McMillan AJ, Brook CW, et al. Impact of pandemic (H1N1) 2009 influenza on critical care capacity in Victoria. Med J Aust 2009;191(9):502–6.
52. Champunot R, Tanjatham S, Kerdsin A, et al. Impact of pandemic influenza (H1N1) virus-associated community-acquired pneumonia among adults in a tertiary hospital in Thailand. Jpn J Infect Dis 2010;63(4):251–6.
53. Dawood FS, Jain S, Finelli L, et al. Emergence of a novel swine-origin influenza A (H1N1) virus in humans. N Engl J Med 2009;360(25):2605–15.
54. Human infection with new influenza A (H1N1) virus: clinical observations from Mexico and other affected countries, May 2009. Wkly Epidemiol Rec 2009; 84(21):185–9.
55. To KK, Wong SS, Li IW, et al. Concurrent comparison of epidemiology, clinical presentation and outcome between adult patients suffering from the pandemic influenza A (H1N1) 2009 virus and the seasonal influenza A virus infection. Postgrad Med J 2010;86(1019):515–21.
56. Agarwal PP, Cinti S, Kazerooni EA. Chest radiographic and CT findings in novel swine-origin influenza A (H1N1) virus (S-OIV) infection. Am J Roentgenol 2009; 193(6):1488–93.
57. Nin N, Soto L, Hurtado J, et al. Clinical characteristics and outcomes of patients with 2009 influenza A(H1N1) virus infection with respiratory failure requiring mechanical ventilation. J Crit Care 2011;26(2):186–92.
58. Davies A, Jones D, Bailey M, et al. Extracorporeal membrane oxygenation for 2009 influenza A(H1N1) acute respiratory distress syndrome. JAMA 2009; 302(17):1888–95.
59. Muscedere J, Ofner M, Kumar A, et al. The occurrence and impact of bacterial organisms complicating critical care illness associated with influenza A(H1N1) infection. Chest 2013;144(1):39–47.
60. Itoh Y, Shinya K, Kiso M, et al. In vitro and in vivo characterization of new swine-origin H1N1 influenza viruses. Nature 2009;460(7258):1021–5.
61. Munster VJ, de Wit E, van den Brand JM, et al. Pathogenesis and transmission of swine-origin 2009 A(H1N1) influenza virus in ferrets. Science 2009;325(5939): 481–3.
62. Maines TR, Jayaraman A, Belser JA, et al. Transmission and pathogenesis of swine-origin 2009 A(H1N1) influenza viruses in ferrets and mice. Science 2009;325(5939):484–7.
63. To KK, Hung IF, Li IW, et al. Delayed clearance of viral load and marked cytokine activation in severe cases of pandemic H1N1 2009 influenza virus infection. Clin Infect Dis 2010;50(6):850–9.
64. de Jong MD, Bach VC, Phan TQ, et al. Fatal avian influenza A (H5N1) in a child presenting with diarrhea followed by coma. N Engl J Med 2005;352(7): 686–91.
65. Mauad T, Hajjar LA, Callegari GD, et al. Lung pathology in fatal novel human influenza A (H1N1) infection. Am J Respir Crit Care Med 2010;181(1):72–9.

66. Shieh WJ, Blau DM, Denison AM, et al. 2009 pandemic influenza A (H1N1): pathology and pathogenesis of 100 fatal cases in the United States. Am J Pathol 2010;177(1):166–75.

67. Gill JR, Sheng ZM, Ely SF, et al. Pulmonary pathologic findings of fatal 2009 pandemic influenza A/H1N1 viral infections. Arch Pathol Lab Med 2010; 134(2):235–43.

68. Lindsay MI Jr, Herrmann EC Jr, Morrow GW, et al. Hong Kong influenza: clinical, microbiologic, and pathologic features in 127 cases. JAMA 1970;214(10): 1825–32.

69. Ng WF, To KF, Lam WW, et al. The comparative pathology of severe acute respiratory syndrome and avian influenza A subtype H5N1–a review. Hum Pathol 2006;37(4):381–90.

70. Dominguez-Cherit G, Lapinsky SE, Macias AE, et al. Critically ill patients with 2009 influenza A(H1N1) in Mexico. JAMA 2009;302(17):1880–7.

71. World Health Organization. Clinical management of human infection with pandemic (H1N1) 2009: revised guidance. 2009 [cited 2010 September 3]. Available at: http://www.who.int/csr/resources/publications/swineflu/clinical_management. Accessed June 10, 2013.

72. Ariano RE, Sitar DS, Zelenitsky SA, et al. Enteric absorption and pharmacokinetics of oseltamivir in critically ill patients with pandemic (H1N1) influenza. CMAJ 2010;182(4):357–63.

73. Centers for Disease Control and Prevention. Updated interim recommendations for the use of antiviral medication in the treatment and prevention of influenza for the 2009-2010 season. 2009. Available at: http://www.cdc.gov/h1n1flu/recommendations.htm. Accessed June 10, 2013.

74. World Health Organization. WHO guidelines for pharmacologic management of pandemic influenza A (H1N1) 2009 and other influenza viruses 2010 June 14, 2013. Available at: http://www.who.int/csr/resources/publications/swineflu/h1n1_guidelines_pharmaceutical_mngt.pdf. Accessed June 10, 2013.

75. Update on oseltamivir-resistant pandemic A (H1N1) 2009 influenza virus. Wkly Epidemiol Rec 2009;85:37–40.

76. Hui DS, Hall SD, Chan MT, et al. Noninvasive positive-pressure ventilation: an experimental model to assess air and particle dispersion. Chest 2006;130(3): 730–40.

77. Kaufman MA, Duke GJ, McGain F, et al. Life-threatening respiratory failure from H1N1 influenza 09 (human swine influenza). Med J Aust 2009;191(3):154–6.

78. Ventilation with lower tidal volumes as compared with traditional tidal volumes for acute lung injury and the acute respiratory distress syndrome. The Acute Respiratory Distress Syndrome Network. N Engl J Med 2000;342(18):1301–8.

79. Ramsey C, Kumar A. H1N1: viral pneumonia as a cause of acute respiratory distress syndrome. Curr Opin Crit Care 2011;17:64–71.

80. Funk DJ, Kumar A. Inhaled nitric oxide in patients with the acute respiratory distress syndrome secondary to the 2009 influenza A (H1N1) infection in Canada. Can J Anaesth 2013;60(2):212–3.

81. Roch A, Lepaul-Ercole R, Grisoli D, et al. Extracorporeal membrane oxygenation for severe influenza A (H1N1) acute respiratory distress syndrome: a prospective observational comparative study. Intensive Care Med 2010;36(11): 1899–905.

82. Freed DH, Henzler D, White CW, et al. Extracorporeal lung support for patients who had severe respiratory failure secondary to influenza A (H1N1) 2009 infection in Canada. Can J Anaesth 2010;57(3):240–7.

83. Wiedemann HP, Wheeler AP, Bernard GR. Comparison of two fluid-management strategies in acute lung injury. N Engl J Med 2006;354(24):2564–75.

84. Funk DJ, Siddiqui F, Wiebe K, et al. Practical lessons from the first outbreaks: clinical presentation, obstacles, and management strategies for severe pandemic (pH1N1) 2009 influenza pneumonitis. Crit Care Med 2010;38(Suppl 4):e30–7.

85. Quispe-Laime AM, Bracco JD, Barberio PA, et al. H1N1 influenza A virus-associated acute lung injury: response to combination oseltamivir and prolonged corticosteroid treatment. Intensive Care Med 2010;36(1):33–41.

86. Martin-Loeches I, Lisboa T, Rhodes A, et al. Use of early corticosteroid therapy on ICU admission in patients affected by severe pandemic (H1N1)v influenza A infection. Intensive Care Med 2011;37(2):272–83.

87. Diaz E, Martin-Loeches I, Canadell L, et al. Corticosteroid therapy in patients with primary viral pneumonia due to pandemic (H1N1) 2009 influenza. J Infect 2012;64(3):311–8.

88. Brun-Buisson C, Richard JC, Mercat A, et al. Early corticosteroids in severe influenza A/H1N1 pneumonia and acute respiratory distress syndrome. Am J Respir Crit Care Med 2011;183(9):1200–6.

89. Luke TC, Kilbane EM, Jackson JL, et al. Meta-analysis: convalescent blood products for Spanish influenza pneumonia: a future H5N1 treatment? Ann Intern Med 2006;145(8):599–609.

90. Zhou B, Zhong N, Guan Y. Treatment with convalescent plasma for influenza A (H5N1) infection. N Engl J Med 2007;357(14):1450–1.

91. Lynch JP 3rd, Fishbein M, Echavarria M. Adenovirus. Semin Respir Crit Care Med 2011;32(4):494–511.

92. Cesario TC. Viruses associated with pneumonia in adults. Clin Infect Dis 2012; 55(1):107–13.

93. Kojaoghlanian T, Flomenberg P, Horwitz MS. The impact of adenovirus infection on the immunocompromised host. Rev Med Virol 2003;13(3):155–71.

94. Russell KL, Broderick MP, Franklin SE, et al. Transmission dynamics and prospective environmental sampling of adenovirus in a military recruit setting. J Infect Dis 2006;194(7):877–85.

95. Terletskaia-Ladwig E, Leinmuller M, Schneider F, et al. Laboratory approaches to the diagnosis of adenovirus infection depending on clinical manifestations. Infection 2007;35(6):438–43.

96. Gavin PJ, Katz BZ. Intravenous ribavirin treatment for severe adenovirus disease in immunocompromised children. Pediatrics 2002;110(1 Pt 1):e9.

97. Ison MG. Adenovirus infections in transplant recipients. Clin Infect Dis 2006; 43(3):331–9.

98. Neofytos D, Ojha A, Mookerjee B, et al. Treatment of adenovirus disease in stem cell transplant recipients with cidofovir. Biol Blood Marrow Transplant 2007; 13(1):74–81.

99. Donnelly CA, Ghani AC, Leung GM, et al. Epidemiological determinants of spread of causal agent of severe acute respiratory syndrome in Hong Kong. Lancet 2003;361(9371):1761–6.

100. Poutanen SM, Low DE, Henry B, et al. Identification of severe acute respiratory syndrome in Canada. N Engl J Med 2003;348(20):1995–2005.

101. Booth TF, Kournikakis B, Bastien N, et al. Detection of airborne severe acute respiratory syndrome (SARS) coronavirus and environmental contamination in SARS outbreak units. J Infect Dis 2005;191(9):1472–7.

102. Christian MD, Poutanen SM, Loutfy MR, et al. Severe acute respiratory syndrome. Clin Infect Dis 2004;38(10):1420–7.

103. Bitar R, Weiser WJ, Avendano M, et al. Chest radiographic manifestations of severe acute respiratory syndrome in health care workers: the Toronto experience. Am J Roentgenol 2004;182(1):45–8.

104. Wong KT, Antonio GE, Hui DS, et al. Severe acute respiratory syndrome: radiographic appearances and pattern of progression in 138 patients. Radiology 2003;228(2):401–6.

105. Yam WC, Chan KH, Poon LL, et al. Evaluation of reverse transcription-PCR assays for rapid diagnosis of severe acute respiratory syndrome associated with a novel coronavirus. J Clin Microbiol 2003;41(10):4521–4.

106. Chen X, Zhou B, Li M, et al. Serology of severe acute respiratory syndrome: implications for surveillance and outcome. J Infect Dis 2004;189(7):1158–63.

107. Peiris JS, Chu CM, Cheng VC, et al. Clinical progression and viral load in a community outbreak of coronavirus-associated SARS pneumonia: a prospective study. Lancet 2003;361(9371):1767–72.

108. Stockman LJ, Bellamy R, Garner P. SARS: systematic review of treatment effects. PLoS Med 2006;3(9):e343.

109. MERS-CoV summary and literature update as of May 2013. Global Alert Response [Internet]. 2013 June 13, 2013 [cited 2013 May 31]. Available at: http://www.who.int/csr/disease/coronavirus_infections/update_20130531/en/index.html. Accessed June 13, 2013.

110. Dowell SF, Anderson LJ, Gary HE Jr, et al. Respiratory syncytial virus is an important cause of community-acquired lower respiratory infection among hospitalized adults. J Infect Dis 1996;174(3):456–62.

111. Falsey AR, Cunningham CK, Barker WH, et al. Respiratory syncytial virus and influenza A infections in the hospitalized elderly. J Infect Dis 1995;172(2):389–94.

112. Falsey AR. Respiratory syncytial virus infection in adults. Semin Respir Crit Care Med 2007;28(2):171–81.

113. Shah JN, Chemaly RF. Management of RSV infections in adult recipients of hematopoietic stem cell transplantation. Blood 2011;117(10):2755–63.

114. Falsey AR. Human metapneumovirus infection in adults. Pediatr Infect Dis J 2008;27(Suppl 10):S80–3.

115. Walsh EE, Peterson DR, Falsey AR. Human metapneumovirus infections in adults: another piece of the puzzle. Arch Intern Med 2008;168(22):2489–96.

116. Carrat F, Leruez-Ville M, Tonnellier M, et al. A virologic survey of patients admitted to a critical care unit for acute cardiorespiratory failure. Intensive Care Med 2006;32(1):156–9.

117. Shahda S, Carlos WG, Kiel PJ, et al. The human metapneumovirus: a case series and review of the literature. Transpl Infect Dis 2011;13(3):324–8.

Index

Note: Page numbers of article titles are in **boldface** type.

A

Abdominal catastrophes
    in ICU, **1017–1044**. *See also specific types, e.g.,* Abdominal compartment syndrome
        treatment of, 1032–1037
            antimicrobial, 1032–1034
            surgical, 1034–1037
Abdominal compartment syndrome, 1018–1021
    background of, 1018
    clinical presentation of, 1019–1020
    diagnosis of, 1020–1021
    epidemiology of, 1018–1019
    surgical management of, 1035
Abdominal organ transplant recipients
    life-threatening infections in, 960
ACCB. *See Acinetobacter baumannii* (ACCB)
Acidosis
    severe malaria and
        management of, 876
Acinetobacter baumannii (ACCB)
    resistant
        management of, 912–913
Acute acalculous cholecystitis, 1029–1031
    background of, 1029–1030
    diagnosis of, 1030–1031
    epidemiology of, 1030
Acute intestinal ischemia, 1021–1024
    background of, 1021–1022
    clinical presentation of, 1023–1024
    diagnosis of, 1023–1024
    epidemiology of, 1022–1023
Acute respiratory distress syndrome (ARDS)
    influenza A 2009 H1N1 and
        management of, 1075–1077
Adenoviral infections, 1052–1059, 1077–1078
    AIDS and, 1056–1057
    clinical manifestations of, 1053–1055
    congenital immune deficiency and, 1056
    diagnosis of, 1057–1058
    epidemiology of, 1053
    management of, 1058–1059
    microbiology of, 1052–1053
    solid-organ transplantation and, 1055–1056

Crit Care Clin 29 (2013) 1087–1103
http://dx.doi.org/10.1016/S0749-0704(13)00084-5
0749-0704/13/$ – see front matter © 2013 Elsevier Inc. All rights reserved.

criticalcare.theclinics.com

United States Postal Service

Statement of Ownership, Management, and Circulation
(All Periodicals Publications Except Requestor Publications)

1. Publication Title	2. Publication Number	3. Filing Date
Critical Care Clinics	0 0 0 - 7 0 8	9/14/13

4. Issue Frequency	5. Number of Issues Published Annually	6. Annual Subscription Price
Jan, Apr, Jul, Oct	4	$199.00

7. Complete Mailing Address of Known Office of Publication (Not printer) (Street, city, county, state, and ZIP+4®)

Elsevier Inc.
360 Park Avenue South
New York, NY 10010-1710

Contact Person
Stephen R. Bushing
Telephone (Include area code)
215-239-3688

8. Complete Mailing Address of Headquarters or General Business Office of Publisher (Not printer)

Elsevier Inc., 360 Park Avenue South, New York, NY 10010-1710

9. Full Names and Complete Mailing Addresses of Publisher, Editor, and Managing Editor (Do not leave blank)

Publisher (Name and complete mailing address)

Linda Belfus, Elsevier, Inc., 1600 John F. Kennedy Blvd. Suite 1800, Philadelphia, PA 19103-2899

Editor (Name and complete mailing address)

Patrick Manley, Elsevier, Inc., 1600 John F. Kennedy Blvd. Suite 1800, Philadelphia, PA 19103-2899

Managing Editor (Name and complete mailing address)

Adrianne Brigido, Elsevier, Inc., 1600 John F. Kennedy Blvd. Suite 1800, Philadelphia, PA 19103-2899

10. Owner (Do not leave blank. If the publication is owned by a corporation, give the name and address of the corporation immediately followed by the names and addresses of all stockholders owning or holding 1 percent or more of the total amount of stock. If not owned by a corporation, give the names and addresses of the individual owners. If owned by a partnership or other unincorporated firm, give its name and address as well as those of each individual owner. If the publication is published by a nonprofit organization, give its name and address.)

Full Name	Complete Mailing Address
Wholly owned subsidiary of	1600 John F. Kennedy Blvd., Ste. 1800
Reed/Elsevier, US holdings	Philadelphia, PA 19103-2899

11. Known Bondholders, Mortgagees, and Other Security Holders Owning or Holding 1 Percent or More of Total Amount of Bonds, Mortgages, or Other Securities. If none, check box ☐ None

Full Name	Complete Mailing Address
N/A	

12. Tax Status (For completion by nonprofit organizations authorized to mail at nonprofit rates) (Check one)
The purpose, function, and nonprofit status of this organization and the exempt status for federal income tax purposes:
☐ Has Not Changed During Preceding 12 Months
☐ Has Changed During Preceding 12 Months (Publisher must submit explanation of change with this statement)

13. Publication Title	14. Issue Date for Circulation Data Below
Critical Care Clinics	April 2013

15. Extent and Nature of Circulation		Average No. Copies Each Issue During Preceding 12 Months	No. Copies of Single Issue Published Nearest to Filing Date
a. Total Number of Copies (Net press run)		990	900
b. Paid Circulation (By Mail and Outside the Mail)	(1) Mailed Outside-County Paid Subscriptions Stated on PS Form 3541. (Include paid distribution above nominal rate, advertiser's proof copies, and exchange copies)	545	468
	(2) Mailed In-County Paid Subscriptions Stated on PS Form 3541 (Include paid distribution above nominal rate, advertiser's proof copies, and exchange copies)		
	(3) Paid Distribution Outside the Mails Including Sales Through Dealers and Carriers, Street Vendors, Counter Sales, and Other Paid Distribution Outside USPS®	189	156
	(4) Paid Distribution by Other Classes Mailed Through the USPS (e.g. First-Class Mail®)		
c. Total Paid Distribution (Sum of 15b (1), (2), (3), and (4))	▲	734	624
d. Free or Nominal Rate Distribution (By Mail and Outside the Mail)	(1) Free or Nominal Rate Outside-County Copies Included on PS Form 3541	68	62
	(2) Free or Nominal Rate In-County Copies Included on PS Form 3541		
	(3) Free or Nominal Rate Copies Mailed at Other Classes Through the USPS (e.g. First-Class Mail)		
	(4) Free or Nominal Rate Distribution Outside the Mail (Carriers or other means)	68	62
e. Total Free or Nominal Rate Distribution (Sum of 15d (1), (2), (3) and (4)	▲	68	62
f. Total Distribution (Sum of 15c and 15e)	▲	802	686
g. Copies not Distributed (See instructions to publishers #4 (page #3))	▲	188	214
h. Total (Sum of 15f and g)	▲	990	900
i. Percent Paid (15c divided by 15f times 100)		91.52%	90.96%

16. Publication of Statement of Ownership
☐ If the publication is a general publication, publication of this statement is required. Will be printed in the October 2013 issue of this publication. ☐ Publication not required

17. Signature and Title of Editor, Publisher, Business Manager, or Owner

Stephen R. Bushing – Inventory Distribution Coordinator
[signature]

Date: September 14, 2013

I certify that all information furnished on this form is true and complete. I understand that anyone who furnishes false or misleading information on this form or who omits material or information requested on the form may be subject to criminal sanctions (including fines and imprisonment) and/or civil sanctions (including civil penalties).

PS Form 3526, September 2007 (Page 1 of 3 (Instructions Page 3)) PSN 7530-01-000-9931 PRIVACY NOTICE: See our Privacy policy in www.usps.com

PS Form 3526, September 2007 (Page 2 of 3)

Moving?

Make sure your subscription moves with you!

To notify us of your new address, find your **Clinics Account Number** (located on your mailing label above your name), and contact customer service at:

Email: journalscustomerservice-usa@elsevier.com

800-654-2452 (subscribers in the U.S. & Canada)
314-447-8871 (subscribers outside of the U.S. & Canada)

Fax number: 314-447-8029

Elsevier Health Sciences Division
Subscription Customer Service
3251 Riverport Lane
Maryland Heights, MO 63043

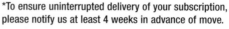
*To ensure uninterrupted delivery of your subscription, please notify us at least 4 weeks in advance of move.